W9-BXH-079

Reflections on Healing

RT
84.5
.R45
1997

Reflections on healing

KALAMAZOO VALLEY COMMUNITY COLLEGE
LIBRARY
KALAMAZOO, MICHIGAN 49003

GAYLORD M

RT
84.5
.R45
1997

Reflections on Healing

A Central Nursing Construct

Phyllis Beck Kritek, RN, PhD, FAAN
Editor

NLN Press   •   New York

Pub. No. 15-6511

KVCC KALAMAZOO VALLEY COMMUNITY COLLEGE LIBRARY

MAR 1 4 1997

Copyright © 1997
National League for Nursing
350 Hudson Street, New York, NY 10014

All rights reserved. No part of this book may be reproduced in print, or by pho-tostatic means, or in any other manner, without the express written permission of the publisher.

The views expressed in this publication represent the views of the authors and do not necessarily reflect the official views of the National League for Nursing.

Library of Congress Cataloging-in-Publication Data

Reflections on healing : a central nursing construct / Phyllis Beck
    Kritek, editor.
        p.   cm.
    Includes bibliographical references.
    ISBN 0-88737-651-1
    1. Nursing—Philosophy.   2. Healing.   3. Nursing—Psychological
aspects.   I. Kritek, Phyllis Beck, 1943—   .   II. Series: Pub.
(National League for Nursing) : no. 15-7254.
    [DNLM: 1. Nursing Care—psychology.   2. Mental Healing-
-psychology.   WY 100 R332   1997]
RT84.5.R45   1997
610.73'01—dc21
DNLM/DLC
for Library of Congress   96-50950
                                                                CIP

This book was set in Garamond by Publications Development Company of Texas. The editor and designer was Allan Graubard. The printer was Book Crafters. The cover was designed by Lauren Stevens.

Printed in the United States of America.

Dedication

The University of Texas Medical Branch (UTMB) School of Nursing at Galveston has a proud history. Founded in 1890, it is the oldest school of nursing west of the Mississippi and the first in the west to affiliate with a university, which it did in 1897. In 1923, it offered the first baccalaureate program, and in 1952, the first master's program in nursing in the state of Texas. It thus played a central role in the history of nursing in the west. It is located in Galveston, Texas, a barrier reef island off the coast which has its own colorful history of pirates, shipping, hurricanes, banking, fishing, oil rigs, and recreation. The history of each is inextricably intertwined, and nurses have been present as a dimension of both.

The nurses of UTMB are a legacy in their own right, with their own proud history. It has been one of healing. It is to these nurses, the nurses of UTMB of the past, present, and future, that this book is respectfully dedicated. May their tradition of healing grow and flourish.

Foreword

Healing. The word sounds so uncomplicated and comfortable, yet defining and understanding this concept is neither. Facilitating true healing is more difficult still, and recognizing it when we see it may be the most subtle work of all. These are the tasks which the faculty of the University of Texas School of Nursing at Galveston have taken on for themselves, with honesty, courage, and a sense of the breadth, depth, and beauty of their subject.

Like healing itself, this book is multidimensional, nonlinear and more than the sum of its parts. There are many views of healing represented in this collection of reflections. Yet there is also a theme, a unifying thread, which ties these diverse recollections together. That theme is wholeness, which is the meaning of the word *haelan,* from which the word heal derives. A focus on healing and wholeness is not new in nursing. What is new is the explicit claim that healing is what nursing is about. For while contemporary nursing claims Florence Nightingale as its founder, Nightingale's vision of the fullness of nursing as helping nature to heal has yet to come to fruition.

Healing has often remained a part of the hidden dimension of Western healthcare and nursing, living in the shadows of a disease-focused, high-tech, sick-cure system. If this approach actually worked, it would not be such a problem. But the fact remains that most of our modern illnesses are not acute but chronic, and they will not be cured but lived with for longer and longer periods of time. A true healthcare system, where people can receive adequate, nontoxic and noninvasive assistance in maintaining wellness and in healing for body, mind, and spirit, along with the most sophisticated, aggressive curing technologies in the world, has not yet been created. This fact has not escaped the attention of the healthcare-consuming American public, and they are saying no.

An average of 66 million Americans, roughly one-third of the population, are paying billions of dollars every year to access alternative and complementary treatment approaches, hoping to find healthcare that treats them as whole people in need of healing rather than broken parts requiring fixing. Yet even this emerging mega industry often falls into the trap of focusing on curing diseases instead of healing people. As insurance companies begin reimbursing for some of these complementary practices, they are increasingly prescribed in the same way as our traditional allopathic system prescribes—to cure disease, in three sessions or less.

Simply adding new tools of treatment to the same allopathic paradigm will not create a true healing healthcare system. Something else is required. A new vision, a new understanding of the meanings and methods of healing versus curing, and practitioners who are skilled in both are some of the basic elements needed for a transformed healthcare system. Or maybe there is already a vision which, rather than being created, needs to be remembered and treated as if it really matters.

The most contemporary sciences of our time are called, collectively, wholeness science or complexity science. These dynamic systems theories tell us that all living systems have two distinct drives or tendencies. One is toward wholeness, autonomy, self-actualization, and ultimately self-transcendence. The other tendency of all living systems is toward belonging, being a part of something larger, connecting, and interdependency. Arthur Koestler coined the term *holon* to describe this fact of simultaneous wholeness and partness. Each human being, as a living system, is a holon, a whole, integral entity, with its own pattern of organization of its parts (which are themselves holons), its own autonomy and unique identity striving toward actualization and transcendence, and, simultaneously, a part of the larger systems in which she or he is embedded, including relationships, family, and community systems and ultimately the entire physical world embedded in the universe.

These seemingly opposing forces must be in right relationship, must find harmony and balance with each other for the health of the system. If the tendency toward either wholeness or partness becomes too out of balance with the other, the system cannot survive. I would suggest that our current healthcare system is currently thrashing about trying to survive the imminent collapse which is a natural consequence of its almost exclusive dedication to partness at the expense of wholeness. Allopathy focuses almost exclusively on the person as a collection of isolated cells, tissues, and organs, separated from each other and from all other collections of parts including other persons, the surrounding community, environment, ecosystem, and cosmos. The institutions of allopathy are organized based on these parts, as are the specialists who admit patients to them. If one's focus remains only on the broken parts, one *cannot* be focused on healing, which by definition is about wholeness. And until there is a way of including healing in the focus of healthcare, there cannot be a true healing healthcare system.

These are not abstractions or philosophical musings, but the consequences of the way things are. It is simply the nature of things. For example, if the body cannot be cured of a disease, and the tendency toward wholeness, actualization, and transcendence remains, how and where will it manifest? What other dimensions of this person will continue to evolve and flower into more and more fullness? Every nurse has observed this process: We have each seen "incurable" patients transcend their pre-sickness realities into new ways of being and relating—to themselves, their disease, their significant others, their God. This is healing, and it is as natural as breathing. A focus on healing does not require us to create healing, but to see it, to feel it, to encourage it, to facilitate it, because healing, coming into right relationship at any level of the human experience and resulting in increased wholeness, decreased chaos and increased energy available for self-transcendence, is the most basic tendency of every living system. Becoming more holistic in our care is not a matter of inventing wholeness, but of recognizing it and acting as if it matters.

The faculty at the University of Texas School of Nursing at Galveston have taken on the great and bold adventure of seeing what is really true and acting as if it matters. Healing is not secondary, but primary, they are telling us. People are not collections of parts that need to be fixed, but whole bodymindspirits which are made for expansion of consciousness and self-transcendence. This is nature, I would add, the same nature that Nightingale instructs us to assist. This is the force of billions of years of evolution woven into every cell of our being. This is how things really are, and it matters very much.

"It is a tremendous challenge for nursing and a courageous leap for a group of nursing faculty in this time of healthcare transition with its emphasis on cost control and method of delivery to take a stand that healing is central to healthcare" writes Mary Fenton, dean of the school, and of course she is right. The American healthcare system stands poised in a moment of history between the no longer and the not yet. The system we have all grown up with has crumbled, yet the replacement for this system does not yet exist. While many turn their attention toward the tasks and almost frantic activities of survival during this tumultuous and frightening time, this faculty has taken a brave and daring step to actually propose a direction, if not a map, for moving into the "not yet." Like

Nightingale herself, they bring light, showing us the way, reminding us of what matters, leading us back to the future, back to our own professional roots as healers, and forward with a vision for a true healing healthcare system to carry us into the next century. Because a change in the part of a system always leads to a change in the whole, we can be certain that the commitment of this group of faculty to healing has already begun to impact on the larger system in which we teach and practice nursing.

JANET F. QUINN, PHD, RN, FAAN
Center for Human Caring
School of Nursing
University of Colorado Health Sciences Center

Acknowledgments

The work that makes a book like this happen is a complex process and involves substantial effort on the part of many. I would like to acknowledge those persons who helped make this book happen. The first and most obvious group are the authors themselves, many of whom risked sharing their personal stories to assist readers in learning to do the same. For all of the authors, their contributions were in themselves healing activities. For their gracious sharing and their patience with me as I cajoled, nagged, and encouraged them, I am grateful. Mary Donna Piazza provided all the graphic work for all of the chapters. She has the gift of giving her image-making the exact power and clarity we seek.

The administrative leaders of the school of nursing were supportive of this project from the outset. They have contributed to the book, but more importantly supported those who did. Hence, my thanks to Mary Fenton, dean, and Jeanette Hartshorn and Phyllis Waters, associate deans. I also want to thank the members of my department. As their chairperson, I sometimes was not as available as would have suited their needs. They were both forgiving and supportive and I am grateful for their understanding and their faith in me, a gift I have treasured. The support staff for the department, especially Yvette Viator, made a comparable contribution.

Perhaps no person did more to make this book happen than Chandra Ganesan, who also serves as the coordinator of our doctoral program development efforts. Chandra carried the lion's share of all organizing, typing, corresponding, and managing of the process of this book's development. She worked with the authors with grace and clarity, and chased down every imaginable detail. Chandra has the gift of blending professionalism with human warmth, and the touch of each is reflected in this book. She kept the project active when I fatigued. She also kept me honest and to the task. I owe her a gratitude that these words fail to capture. She was a gift to me.

Working with the process of publishing a book is always a series of negotiations. Allan Graubard, who worked with this book from its inception as an idea to its reality in your hands, was the ideal negotiator for me: he has the fine gift of knowing how hard to push, and conversely, when to back off and wait. I admire this in him; more importantly, I benefitted enormously from his sensitivity. He is also able to exercise a kind of wisdom coupled with realism that served me well repeatedly. I thank him for sharing his gifts. Nancy Marcus Land, who ushered us through the production phases, was professional, helpful, responsive, and fair minded. We were lucky to have her, and Chandra and I both valued her assistance.

During the preparation of this book, I was named the Florence Thelma Hall Distinguished Professor of Nursing. This was made possible through the generosity of Marie Hall, the daughter of Florence Thelma Hall. Her generosity and her vision have been valuable gifts to me, our school, and our university. These gifts have helped make this book possible, and I am grateful to her.

On a personal level, I want to acknowledge the two people in my life who continue to serve as my best teachers, supporters, advisers, and "kriteks," my two daughters Patricia Anne Kritek and Rebecca Marie Kritek. Their faith in me and their steady encouragement seem the hidden spring of life-giving water in my existence, and I can really never claim I have achieved anything without noting, with gratitude, their presence in my life. In their lives and in their characters I find reflected the wisdom of the healer.

PHYLLIS BECK KRITEK

Galveston, Texas
December 1996

Contents

Part Four: Healing in the Care of
Specific Patient Populations

Part Six: Healing as a Focus of Nursing Scholarship

Contributing Authors

Susan Scoville Baker, RN, CS, PhD
Associate Professor
School of Nursing
Texas A&M University
Laredo, Texas

Verolyn Barnes Bolander, RN, MS, CS
Associate Professor
The University of Texas School of
    Nursing at Galveston
Galveston, Texas

Kay Branum, RN, CCRN, PhD
Staff Nurse, Transplant Service
St. Luke's Episcopal Hospital
Houston, Texas

Karen A. Brykczynski, RN, RNCS,
    FNP, DNSc
Associate Professor
The University of Texas School of
    Nursing at Galveston
Galveston, Texas

Doris Campbell, RN, MSN, ANP
Assistant Professor
The University of Texas School of
    Nursing at Galveston
Galveston, Texas

Barbara Camune, RN, RNC, MSN,
    COGNP, CNM, DrPH(c)
Assistant Professor
The University of Texas School of
    Nursing at Galveston
Galveston, Texas

Barbara A. Carnes, RN, CS, PhD
Assistant Professor
The University of Texas School of
    Nursing at Galveston
Galveston, Texas

Rita S. Cascio, RN, PhD
Assistant Professor
The University of Texas School of
    Nursing at Galveston
Galveston, Texas

Audrey L. Chadwick, RN, MS
Assistant Professor
The University of Texas School of
    Nursing at Galveston
Galveston, Texas

Michele C. Clark, RN, PhD
Assistant Professor
The University of Texas School of
    Nursing at Galveston
Galveston, Texas

M. Jean Daubenmire, RN, MS
Associate Professor Emeritus
The Ohio State University College of
    Nursing
Consultant in Psychotheratic Practices
    including Guided Imagery &
    Therapeutic Touch
Columbus, Ohio

Geraldine Dorsey-Turner, RN, MS,
    PNA, CS
Faculty Associate
The University of Texas School of
    Nursing at Galveston
Galveston, Texas

Judith C. Drew, RN, PhD
Assistant Professor
The University of Texas School of
    Nursing at Galveston
Galveston, Texas

M. Christina R. Esperat, RN, PhD
Assistant Professor
The University of Texas School of
    Nursing at Galveston
Galveston, Texas

Mary V. Fenton, RN, DrPH
Dean and Professor
The University of Texas School of
    Nursing at Galveston
Galveston, Texas

Patricia Davis Gilmore, RN, MSN, JD
Assistant Professor
The University of Texas School of
    Nursing at Galveston
Galveston, Texas

Mary Anne Hanley, RN, MA
Consultant, School of Nursing
The University of Texas School of
    Nursing at Galveston
Austin, Texas

Rebecca A. Harbin, RN, BSN, CEN
BSN Student
The University of Texas School of
    Nursing at Galveston
Galveston, Texas

Jeanette Hartshorn, RN, PhD, FAAN
Professor and Associate Dean for
    Academic Administration
The University of Texas School of
    Nursing at Galveston
Galveston, Texas

Alice Hill, RN, PhD
Associate Professor
The University of Texas School of
    Nursing at Galveston
Galveston, Texas

Jean Bell Ivey, RN, MSN, CPNP, DSN
Assistant Professor
The University of Texas School of
    Nursing at Galveston
Galveston, Texas

Helen K. Kee, RN, PhD
Assistant Professor
Director, Graduate Program in
    Nursing Administration
The University of Texas School of
    Nursing at Galveston
Galveston, Texas

Priscilla W. Koester, RN, RNCS, PhD
Assistant Professor
The University of Texas School of
    Nursing at Galveston
Galveston, Texas

Phyllis Beck Kritek, RN, PhD, FAAN
Professor and Chair, Mental Health
    Management
Florence Thelma Hall Distinguished
    Professor
Director, Doctoral Program
The University of Texas School of
    Nursing at Galveston
Galveston, Texas

B. J. Landis, RN, CFNP, PhD
Assistant Professor
The University of Texas School of
    Nursing at Galveston
Galveston, Texas

Roberta K. Lee, RN, DrPH, FAAN
Professor
The University of Texas School of
    Nursing at Galveston
Galveston, Texas

Phylicia H. Lewis, RN, MS, MSN,
    ARNP
Family Practice ARNP
The University of Texas School of
    Nursing at Galveston
Galveston, Texas

Barbara G. Mason, RN, RNC, EdD
Associate Professor (Retired)
The University of Texas School of
    Nursing at Galveston
Galveston, Texas

Elnora P. Mendias, RN, CSFNP, PhD
Assistant Professor
The University of Texas School of
    Nursing at Galveston
Galveston, Texas

Donna L. Morris, RN, CNM, DrPH
Associate Professor
The University of Texas School of
    Nursing at Galveston
Galveston, Texas

Corinne M. Oppermann, RN, MSN
Assistant Professor of Nursing, and
    Assistant Dean for Student Affairs
The University of Texas School of
    Nursing at Galveston
Galveston, Texas

Virginia Rahr, RN, MSN, EdD
Associate Professor
The University of Texas School of
    Nursing at Galveston
Galveston, Texas

Harriett L. Riggs, RN, CPNP, PhD
Associate Professor (Retired)
The University of Texas School of
    Nursing at Galveston
Galveston, Texas

Patricia Romick, RN, MS, RNCS
Assistant Professor
The University of Texas School of
    Nursing at Galveston
Galveston, Texas

Doris J. Rosenow, RN, CCRN, PhD
Associate Professor
Department of Nursing and Health
    Sciences
Texas A&M—Corpus Christi University
Corpus Christi, Texas

Linda R. Rounds, RN, FNP, PhD
Associate Professor
The University of Texas School of
    Nursing at Galveston
Galveston, Texas

M. Kay Sandor, RN, PhD
Assistant Professor
The University of Texas School of
    Nursing at Galveston
Galveston, Texas

Peggy L. Standard, RN, MSN, MA, LPC,
    LMFT
Assistant Professor
The University of Texas School of
    Nursing at Galveston
Galveston, Texas

Poldi Tschirch, RN, CS, PhD
Assistant Professor and Director of
    Undergraduate Programs
The University of Texas School of
    Nursing at Galveston
Galveston, Texas

Ruth Tucker, RN, RNC, PhD
Associate Professor
The University of Texas School of
    Nursing at Galveston
Galveston, Texas

Phyllis J. Waters, RN, MS
Assistant Professor and Associate
    Dean for Practice
The University of Texas School of
    Nursing at Galveston
Galveston, Texas

Introduction

PHYLLIS BECK KRITEK, RN, PHD, FAAN

On February 28, 1994, the faculty of the University of Texas Medical Branch (UTMB) at Galveston School of Nursing formally adopted the central construct of "healing" as the organizing principle of their doctoral program in nursing. This decision followed several months of study, discussion, open forums, and reflection. Faculty sought a doctoral program emphasis congruent with the traditions, values, and beliefs of their school and reflective of the interest, expertise, scholarship, and clinical competencies of their faculty. The decision emerged more as a naming than as a choosing process, more an outcome of effectively engaging in self-description than in re-invention.

The formal action focused on a doctoral program white paper that is occasionally referenced in the book you now hold. This white paper, which is redrafted and presented as the first paper in this book, served as a springboard to a much richer, more diverse collection of reflections, observations, studies, stories, and poetry which reflect an array of approaches to this central construct of healing. That collection became this book.

All of the authors have some direct affiliation with UTMB; most are currently active faculty members. Each contributor identified a perspective on healing they wished to share with a larger audience. The variance was then, and continues to be, striking. It is clearly a robust construct. It is also a demonstration of the richness a faculty can bring to an important dimension of professional nursing.

ATTENDING TO HEALING

The decision to share the ideas in this book is an aspect of a larger decision, one about attending to healing as central to nursing. Several of the unintended changes in healthcare delivery patterns that characterize the U.S. systems of care intensify the urgency of that larger decision. As a discipline, nursing has always elected to invest in healing as both a process and an outcome. It has been less deliberate in its clarity and coherence in articulating that commitment. As a result, while we give a good deal of lip service to the centrality of healing, we find ourselves daily called upon to make decisions and take actions that ignore this centrality. More compelling issues capture our attention: length of stay, cost containment, efficiencies of delivery, payment protocols and methodologies, technologies of choice, administrative details, provider mix, product lines, and quality improvement initiatives. Because healing is not in actuality given centrality, these compelling concerns are too often conceptualized and acted upon with little or no attention given to the overriding construct of healing.

For many nurses, and many healthcare providers, this situation has become quite disturbing. It is even more disturbing for patients, their families and friends, and a society that finds healthcare a burgeoning industry with decreasing interest in the human dimension of that care. There is no doubt that the lessons from corporate America being learned in healthcare agencies today are both valuable and necessary. That the human dimension should become so painfully overshadowed by these corporate concerns, however, serves no one well. Healing brings us back, perhaps abruptly, to a more precise, and hopefully prescient, focus on the human dimension. We have need for further reflection on this construct.

We, as a faculty, learned that such reflection changed many things for us. In time, we made the decision to give healing centrality in our undergraduate program of study, in our masters' programs, in our faculty practice initiatives, and in our community service. While healing began as an articulation of our focus of scholarship, it became apparent to us that it had the potential to serve as a unifying principle for all our endeavors. We recognized that this robust construct guided us on a path that was full of discovery, but also full of satisfaction and improved clarity. We recognize that we are beginners on that path, but it is a path full of meaningful challenges and opportunities for hope.

REFLECTING ON HEALING

This book is neither comprehensive nor exhaustive; it is rather what the title states: a collection of reflections. Because it attends to the human dimension of healthcare, an attempt has been made to reflect the rich variety of images and forms such reflections can take: essays, philosophical analyses, poetry, scientific papers, parables—the array of voices one can discover in reflecting.

This book is thus titled *Reflections on Healing* with intent. It springs from my sense of the era in which it has emerged, an era characterized by an awareness of the limits of scientific knowing but not yet certain of the array of ways of knowing available to us, and likely to serve us well as humans. It is also largely crafted in the voice of women, and bears the stamp of that particular worldview. This voice, still tuning up in the larger culture, is often more reflective than dogmatic, more exploratory than certain. It is my conviction that such efforts at reflection take us further than any final answer implying a closed door. It thus may serve to provide an impetus to better questions to ask as well as to roadmaps to better answers to those questions.

Both among themselves and within the larger culture, nurses tend to be viewed as doers, people who take action. It is rare for us to present ourselves, or be perceived as reflective. This has served no one well. The intimacy and power of the practice of nursing is best conducted from the spirit of a reflective mind, and we would all benefit from a collective effort to lay claim to this reflective mind. It is in the act of reflection that the stuff of dialogs and discovery emerge, and for that reason, the book not only provides reflection but encourages it in the reader.

THE USES OF THIS BOOK

It is my hope, and that of its many contributors, that this book of reflections will serve as an impetus to all nurses to ponder more deliberately on the nature of healing in our discipline, and its centrality. It may indeed be viewed as an antidote to the dehumanizing trajectory followed by much of the current healthcare dialog. It is also our hope that those beginning their careers in nursing, our students, will have access to this book as a way of shaping their philosophy of nursing. While many textbooks will tell them of the science and tasks of nursing, this book should provide impetus to reflect on the most human dimensions of the discipline, and the attending power in doing so. It is also our hope that this book will encourage others to join this dialog, and that many additional books on professional nursing's role in healing will emerge.

The book is structured so that any of the six parts can be read separately, in any preferred order, and that each contribution can be read independent of the total structure. It is also assumed, however, that each component adds a further insight into the concept of healing, and that the strength of the book lies in the richness of its diversity. No one view is intended to prevail, and each voice adds some new perspective to the whole. In that sense, the book is best imaged as a tapestry, with each contribution serving as a thread of reflection. It is our hope that you will get to know all the threads in an effort to know the tapestry.

A FINAL THOUGHT

It is a truism in the study of human behavior that we tend to become that which we focus upon with intention and consistency. One of the unplanned outcomes of preparing these manuscripts, for all the authors, is a heightened awareness of their own personal involvement in the concept of healing, their passions and commitments, and their convictions about the centrality of healing to their practice of nursing. It has thus become, in some sense, a process of healing, of finding a greater wholeness as a professional nurse. We have learned that reflecting on healing is indeed itself a healing process.

Finally, we hope that your journey through our reflections will not only stimulate, enlighten, and enliven you, but also serve as a healing force in your life.

PART ONE

REFLECTIONS ON HEALING: A CENTRAL NURSING CONSTRUCT

PHYLLIS BECK KRITEK, RN, PHD, FAAN

In reflecting on a concept, I always wish to start with as wide a lens as possible to take in the broad scope. There is an alternative which is taking one dimension, then another, and teasing the meaning of each apart, attempting to link them together as one would a puzzle. The latter approach is often used in our culture as the first step in discovery, since the analytic mode predominates both in our scholarship and perhaps even in our daily living. We are a pragmatic culture, and focus in on a single dimension more often than on the whole. This may explain why everything we create seems to eventually reveal itself as having an harmful impact on some dimension of our lives.

Holistic thinking, which has a more synthetic quality to it, is often dismissed as too overwhelming, abstract, or diffuse. As a result, the wholeness of healing, one which the authors of this book attempt to describe, stands in sharp contrast to the common patterns we manifest as too often constricted or limited in scope and depth. It was with this realization in mind that I conceived of the present book. I have attempted to practice what I preach, to manifest what I believe, and to honor the synthetic approach, especially because it is so rarely used that the resultant imbalance in our literature is discomforting. Hence, you will find here and hopefully benefit by a rich variety of reflections on the essence of healing.

None of these reflections purports to be a final, total, or correct answer. While the authors share substantive commitment to the ideas they present, they also present unique perspectives that, again, will hopefully enrich the reader. An additional trait of our culture, deeply biased toward a competitive, argumentative, and even warlike approach to ideas, views differing ideas as an invitation to a contest. Only one idea can be true, and we must

1

engage in argument and competition until one idea is declared true. I think quite differently about this, and start from the assumption that no one has the complete truth, this being a reality of the human condition, but each person has some vision or perspective that can be of value to others. It is in this bringing together of diverse ideas that the impetus to create new relationships emerges, and a careful reading of the history of science will document this readily. Nonetheless, so attached are we to the competitive image of scholarship that we still search for a "winner" who then claims the honor of presenting the "best, therefore truest," answer to our questions. Even the best of today's answers, however, imperfect because of our being human and humanly imperfect, become the force behind the emerging of tomorrow's good questions.

It is in the interaction of many good ideas, none of them final or best, that the creative dimension of reflection reveals itself. It is in this sense that *Reflections on Healing* has been prepared as a book that can create new dialog. In our individual and collective search for truth, a careful and generous contribution of ideas assists us immensely.

Part One provides an opportunity to explore the essential nature of healing through a variety of lenses. The word *essential,* in both the dictionary and thesaurus, is associated with terms such as *inherent, basic, necessary, primary,* and amusingly, *quintessential.* These terms speak to the fundamental nature or core of a concept. Hence, the authors provide a perspective on the inherent and necessary nature of healing.

Part One also opens with a revised edition of the white paper that publicly started us on the path that we, as a nursing faculty, have chosen as a central theme in the University of Texas Medical Branch at Galveston doctoral program, and subsequently, as the core concept for all programs and activities. I wrote this paper to clarify how healing itself related to current and emerging nursing practice, and to initiate a dialog at the institutional level. Hence, a primary focus here is on contexting *healing* for a community of scholars committed and acclimated to traditional allopathic medicine and leery of emerging approaches to healthcare and alternative or complementary therapies. Although this latter viewpoint actually can provide a much richer picture of the potential for discovery embedded in the construct of healing, even within the biases and beliefs of traditional Western medicine and healthcare systems, as this white paper demonstrated, the promise of scholarship on healing processes in nursing could reveal rich potential for knowledge generation.

The paper describes the historic limits we have placed on our understanding of healing, the multidimensional character of the concept, and the increasing readiness we have shown to abandon healing practices in favor of the more readily rewarded and admired technologies that characterize our healthcare today. In this paper, too, healing is explored through a taxonomy of the expanding number of planes of meaning inherent in the concept. Exemplars of these planes of meaning or axes of the taxonomy are described and contexted in current health practices.

Mary Fenton's paper moves beyond this description and relates healing to the concept of humanistic caring. Her premise is that cost-effective and high quality care can best be attained through incorporation of humanistic caring as an essential dimension of healing. Viewing such caring as both a process and an outcome, she posits that healing is the end result of a humanistic approach to healthcare and that, when such is missing, healing does not occur.

Reviewing thirty years of previous research that utilized Fenton's tool for measuring humanistic care, she notes that we indeed have the capability to operationalize and measure this construct, and therefore are able to create an expanding body of literature that demonstrates the intrinsic relationship between humanistic caring and healing processes and outcomes. Her concluding premise is that in today's healthcare climate, because we can measure humanistic caring, we can also demonstrate its impact on outcomes, identifying length of stay as a potential means for measurement. As dean of the School of Nursing, Mary's passion for the concept of humanistic caring is indeed one of several reasons why this concept has energized so many of us toward engagement in this path of discovery.

Alice Hill provides a compelling and creative glimpse of healing from yet another perspective. In telling the story, the narrator not only describes action and outcomes, but also provides an image of meaning. As Beck (1996) notes, a narrative outlook uses story to provide understanding through the narrator's point of view, presenting a positional mental frame of reference. A narrative outlook, he notes, has "certain consistent features." He describes these features as the story belonging to the narrator and one that generates a struggle among story characters which manifests as "contrasting ideologies" (p. 11). The story Alice tells does this very well, and is powerful in providing a description of her own healing process from an ugly encounter with racism as a young college student.

While never naming the dimensions of healing that she views as essential to healing, Alice Hill nonetheless provides a compelling image of such healing, a story of the self-determination, integrity, and courage that the need for healing draws forth from a human. She demonstrates the nature of a healing relationship in her interactions with her mother, reveals the time component essential to healing, manifests the self-compassion needed to move through the process of healing, and with an understated revelation of inner strength presents to the reader the discoveries and outcomes of a deliberate healing process.

Poldi Tschirch, who approaches essence from its basis or roots, guides us through an analysis of Florence Nightingale's vision of nursing and healing. She begins with Nightingale's observation that the nurse is the central provider in assuring that the healing process is enabled, and notes the timelessness of this perspective. Nightingale consistently presents the patient as the focus of healthcare, and nature as the primary agent of healing. She sees the nurse as removing the obstacles to healing and creating an optimal environment for enabling this natural process. She actually describes illness as the physical manifestation of the patient's healing process.

Poldi explores both the internal and external environments that Nightingale attends to, the fact that nurses are a "healing presence" for the patient, and nursing's commitment to the whole person, in effect, to wholeness as an outcome of healing. Nurses are advised to use every power at their disposal to create the conditions for healing to occur. Nightingale's vision, contexted in today's healthcare system, could profitably be reexplored as a guide to the healing potentials that nurses assume responsibility for and, perhaps more sobering, the healing activities we have abandoned. This particular window on the essence of healing reminds us that we started out at a place that we may now be struggling to rediscover.

Exploring the essence of a concept inevitably involves an explanation of philosophies of nursing, and the theoretical constructs, conceptual frameworks, and theories that we use as guides. Phyllis Waters and Jean Daubenmire exemplify this activity especially well. They describe and explain a conceptual model for what they call therapeutic capacity, a competency in nurses that answers their opening questions: How do nurses facilitate healing and are there ways to help nurses to expand their therapeutic capabilities? They posit that the nurse brings unique capabilities to the healing environment which evoke the endogenous process of healing in the patient. They observe that the lack of such a conceptual model limits the nurse's understanding and delays the development of practices that create a healing environment and engage the patient's consciousness in the healing process.

Building on Martha Rogers and Margaret Newman, in their model they identify three central dimensions of therapeutic capacity: clinical intervention, caring dynamics and transpersonal efficacy, the latter described as a conscious process of centering, intentionality, connecting and repatterning. They define transpersonal efficacy as the ability to create a shared corridor of consciousness that facilitates the patient's endogenous process. Its impact, they posit, is exponential in nature. They conclude by observing that the goal of healing is human evolution in consciousness, creating harmony. This conceptual framework serves as a wonderful exemplar of the types of theoretical tools that we have need of to begin to develop a body of knowledge focused on healing. It also ably demonstrates what a given philosophical outlook might devise as an innovative expression of the essence of healing.

Mary Anne Hanley provides yet another genre as an opportunity for expressing an essence of healing: the parable. The dictionary describes *parable* as a fable or a short story with a moral dimension; a tale that is allegorical or symbolic in nature, demonstrating a principle through the telling of a story. In Hanley's short story, she describes a dramatic human event, a serious injury suffered by a friend's child, and places healing in the context of nursing practice at the concrete and practical level. She also introduces the book's first exploration of what are called in our country "alternative therapies": therapeutic touch, reflexology, guided imagery, visualization, and meditation. Her story actually serves to demonstrate that another term used for these therapies, "complementary," can be readily demonstrated in a situation where traditional medicine is excellent at dealing with some dimensions of severe trauma effectively and substantively complemented by the addition of other modalities.

As a result, one of the lessons or morals of this story emerges clearly: it is in the best interest of the patient to have as many facilitating therapies as the situation evokes, and that includes both traditional and emerging therapies. Emerging is perhaps a misnomer, since some cultures use one or more of these approaches and have done so for centuries. Others have been used without consciousness or a clear conception of the actions taken. Hanley demonstrates the interactive effect of these approaches.

She concludes with the simple statement "the healing continues," and in doing so highlights another essential character of healing: it does not have a beginning, a middle, and an end but is characteristically an ongoing process continuously revealing new facets of ourselves and our efforts at right relationship with ourselves and with the world in which we live. This too is a moral with powerful implications for healthcare providers who harbor the arrogant assumption that they can determine and complete a healing process. The parable provides a unique kind of catalyst to our reflections on a construct because it activates our moral imagination and calls forth from us new insights that are uniquely contexted in our personal worldview.

One way of highlighting the essence of a concept is to note the dimensions neglected, ignored, or denied expression. The next two papers provide such an opportunity. In the first, B. J. Landis explores the spiritual dimensions of healing. While nursing has always laid claim to a commitment to spiritual aspects of care, we have tended to give such care relatively little focus, tending to circumvent it rather than to confront it, and giving it lip service or accepting it as a covert force in nursing. Yet, if we posit that healing involves wholeness, then attention to a dimension of the human that is critically important to many, perhaps most people, is essential and necessary.

Landis begins by noting that we need to develop numerous models for understanding exactly how the nurse incorporates a patient's spirituality in the enablement of healing. She posits that spirituality in humans has four characteristics: it synthesizes, it enables and motivates, it evokes transcending oneself to bond with other humans, and it acknowledges the supernatural as a dimension of the human person. It is the expression of the human spirit. She advises that it is essential to address this dimension of the human if we are to change our focus from physical cure to healing, acknowledging that all facets of humanness are essential to the wholeness sought through healing. She observes that we frequently speak of the mind/body split, and in doing so indicate that we have elected to omit the human spirit in our discussion.

Defining healing as an "active process of mobilizing one's inner resources toward achieving balance and wholeness," she explores the importance of attending to spirituality since it is one of a patient's most powerful inner resources. She presents her own spirituality, which is Christian, but acknowledges that there are many others, and that nurses who wish to be efficacious in enabling healing will profit from an awareness of these many others.

Discussing energy based theories of health, including Eastern approaches of Ayurveda and Chinese systems, Landis also points to nursing's therapeutic touch modality, and identifies the relationship these systems have with the spiritual dimension of care, noting that each assumes this dimension as a central feature of the approach described. In doing so, she raises our consciousness about views concerning the essential nature of healing that differ substantively from Western traditions and indeed start from a very different place, one that assumes spirituality to be a central or core aspect of the healing process.

Judy Drew highlights another dimension of healing that is more often notable through neglect than through consciousness or attention: the ethnocultural context of healing. One imbalance that emerges from an overemphasis on analytic scholarship is decontexting. Judy draws us back into context, and in a scholarly fashion demonstrates the essential nature of the context of healing and the scope of its influence. She posits that from the viewpoint of the patient, the ethnocultural context is central, and the nurse who fails to grasp this creates conflicts that not only fail to enable healing but actually interfere with healing outcomes.

According to Judy Drew, the patient is the only one who can define healing, and this starts when the patient defines an illness and determines an action to be taken. The patient controls in what way an illness is recognized, interpreted, understood and managed, and this process is shaped by the ethnocultural context of each person. Hence, illness and healing as realities are highly subjective and dependent on the beliefs and values of a given culture: these are social experiences. If the things we do as healthcare providers to enable healing are highly congruent with a given culture's beliefs, there is little conflict; if not congruent, the conflict, unfortunately characterized by mistrust and suspicion, can become the primary phenomenon we find ourselves addressing.

In the main, she notes, we seek healthcare that is culturally congruent with our own, but for some people this is not possible and for many there are no options but the prevailing traditional systems. The dominant biomedical perspective is often impervious to change and can feed or exacerbate the patient's conflict when cultural incongruity enters the mix. Judy's analysis highlights the ease with which a nurse, seeking to enable healing, can ignore this central characteristic of the healing process and actually impede healing. Both Judy Drew and B. J. Landis help us reflect on the irrationality of attempting to assist patients in their search for wholeness while ignoring or neglecting some essential trait of healing and its importance to the patient.

I wrote the last paper in Part One to catalyze a more robust discussion of nursing ethics, which too often seems mired in a constrictive perspective bounded by the assumptions of traditional or allopathic approaches to illness. Most often, it explores the impact of our fascination with technology as not merely the most interesting and compelling dimension of healthcare, but sometimes as the only dimension. Our current moral debates, it seems, are driven by technological expansion, very constructive in its potential for good but largely developed with a serious time lag in understanding the moral dilemmas of what we create.

It has always seemed to me that this dilemma was best exemplified by Albert Einstein, whose discoveries were essential to the development of an atomic bomb. He concurrently was an ardent passivist, an articulate opponent of the German holocaust, himself a Jew who helped many members of the Jewish community in Europe escape by contributing his own personal funds, and a man who recommended to Harry Truman use of the atomic bomb in World War II. It was his conviction that the Germans were nearing readiness for the use of an atomic bomb and it was wiser for us to develop it first and to use it first (Einstein, 1954). This strange dilemma of creating the future and then discovering its moral implications seems a trait of humans, and one which we would be wise to explore.

In this final paper, I explore the multidimensional complexity of healing and the wholeness of the patient as an intrinsic assumption of our understanding of healing. Taking the patient at diverse levels of analysis, we include the community, which can include the world community. If this global community is indeed a whole that, like the individual, can experience fragmentation and disharmony, then the choices we make either enhance or diminish, even at the global level, the balance we seek through healing.

In conducting a careful analysis of the traditions of healthcare in the United States and the most recent expression of these, the corporatization of healthcare, an awareness of the centrality of moral choice becomes apparent. To have acted without awareness of harms does not make the harms less harmful. In this country, the focus on what I call *in extremis* care, attention to the extremes of illness, dysfunction, and trauma, creates a certain environment where healing is either discounted, misconceived, or confused with the interruption of symptoms. Hence, the moral act or "good" of enabling the healing process can be effectively dismissed and dismantled.

I explore the metaphors of choice we use to describe our healthcare, predominantly those equating time with money and disease with an evil to be conquered. Since policy follows metaphor, we craft a system of care that essentially deletes healing activities. They are not easily contained in time intervals and are irrelevant if one is actually waging a war on disease. In this atmosphere, the ethical choices follow the metaphors, and success and failure are measured in this fashion. If we intend to develop a body of knowledge exploring healing, then the moral dimension of these processes, not only at the personal level but also at the system, national and global level, warrant early focused attention. It is my conviction that since nursing is the central healthcare provider in processes of healing, it is nursing's task to take on, particularly at the system and policy levels, a delineation of the moral issues that surround facilitation of healing and to disseminate this information proactively. I note that for the feminist ethicist, this inevitably involves risk and can incur censure, and that it is these realities we might wisely first confront.

Part One manifests substantial diversity. It also points to some common themes: the implications of the wholeness sought as the outcome of healing processes, the current and historical centrality of the nurse in this process, healing as a call to expand and refine modalities and dimensions of healthcare currently under-emphasized or misunderstood, the complexity and transformative potential of healing, and the presence of pitfalls or habitual omissions we might be wise to attend to at the outset. These themes point to some essential characteristics of healing; they also serve to highlight some of the sources of variance that influence healing. They do not in any way exhaust the meaning of *healing,* but serve well to catalyze reflection on the essence of healing, to start the dialog.

REFERENCES

Beck, R. R. (1996). *Nonviolent story: Narrative conflict resolution in the gospel of Mark.* Maryknoll, New York: Orbis Books.
Einstein, A. (1982). *Ideas and opinions.* New York: Crown Publishers.

CHAPTER 1

Healing: A Central Nursing Construct-Reflections on Meaning

PHYLLIS BECK KRITEK, RN, PHD, FAAN

Healing is a term that evokes a sense of familiarity, both in healthcare providers and in all persons struggling with a perceived need or desire for ourselves or those we care about or care for. We experience in a personal and compelling way the need for healing, and find ourselves drawn to answers to a recurrent question evoked by our life experiences: Can I heal from this? The range of potential meanings we give to healing can thus be extensive and diverse. Within healthcare communities, the term also has a deep and rich history, and thus a range of meanings. Each discipline tends to explain this history on its own terms, with its own meanings and cultural expectations. This at once expands the meaning in one respect, and, if it is viewed as an exhaustive description, can also confine that meaning.

Healing is the gerund of the word heal, the latter an Old English word meaning whole. This provides the foundation for meanings emergent from English-speaking cultures, and is then dependent on the scope and depth of meaning given to the idea of wholeness. The nature of a gerund is equally significant, a term derived from a verb but used as a noun. To heal is the activity of becoming whole, and healing is thus a process that becomes an object, an activity that becomes a knowable entity in its own right.

History, traditions, beliefs, cultural mores, and current societal context all influence the meaning any person or group assigns to the idea of healing. This provides depth, richness, specificity, and focus. It also builds into a pursuit of wholeness the potential confinement of any given limited understanding of wholeness. The intellectual limit is itself a deterrent; the impact the limitation has on the well-being of humans is a bit more troublesome. It also creates the anomalous situation where a sought-after wholeness is conceptualized and pursued in a manner that implicitly or explicitly denies or ignores dimensions of the human condition that are essential to achieving that wholeness.

These fundamental insights unveil an array of challenges that frame the study and integration of healing processes. There is a subtle but enduring catch-22 in explorations of healing that wisely evokes curiosity in the scholar and the scientist as well as the human in search of the good life. What had at first seemed simple and straightforward can become complex and confusing with the healing process deterred, interrupted, delayed, or aborted. Healing is a good deal more than it seems.

Margaret brings her son to the local community hospital emergency room from the local high school soccer field in a small town in Indiana. She is anxious, even agitated, and the hospital emergency room staff walk her through an admission process that confuses her further, and makes her wonder if her son's injury is about money and profit, structures and policies, or about her sixteen-year-old and his future. A series of negotiations ensue to determine who can care for her son, what providers are appropriate. The concerns are around organizational structures and institutional policies. The provider who can best meet her son's needs never emerges as a consideration. She senses this.

The physician who meets with her son in the noisy little cubicle they have been assigned orders an X-ray of his leg, and advises her, upon analyzing it, that he will need a confirmation from an orthopedic specialist tomorrow, but for now he will cast the leg. The fractures are such that he feels a long-term immobility followed by an interrupted soccer career is the future for her son. He tells her this as the son listens. She looks at her son's face and becomes more anxious, watching the fear escalate in his eyes, a signal no one but her seems to notice. She wonders if the doctor knows what he is saying to this young man, and its impact.

The casting process is completed, directions are given for a return to a designated physician the next day, crutches are provided, and a nurse meets with Margaret and her son to discuss the immediate needs he will be experiencing, primarily focused on pain management and increased immobility. This is a small town, and Margaret and the nurse know one another from the high school activities for parents that they attend together. They achieve an easy and spontaneous rapport, but as she listens to the nurse, Margaret becomes even more anxious. The nurse assures both Margaret and her son that she thinks the fracture can be managed, that the physician they will see tomorrow is excellent, that bone fractures tend to mend quickly and successfully in young people, and that the pain and swelling will subside readily.

Margaret looks at her son, whose face is now showing even greater strain and pain, and knows he is thinking only of the soccer career that may have just ended, the loss of comraderie and membership in a club he wants to stay in, the loss of public identity and local respect, and perhaps, the loss of the scholarship that was his only viable ticket to college. Her pain for him and herself is escalating as she listens to the assurances about pain management and limb elevation. No one seems to understand that everything they are saying and doing is irrelevant to both her and her son, and that his dreams of soccer successes are dying in the little cubicle, along with a part of her soul and her son's soul. They are however, polite and grateful, and leave with two prescriptions for drugs, a new set of crutches, a phone number and address of an orthopedic surgeon, and a broken dream no one ever seemed able to imagine.

As this story illustrates, healing for Margaret's son is to a high degree framed within the boundaries of the providers' worldviews, and Margaret is essentially invited to share in and embrace that worldview. She seems uncertain if she should even introduce the broader dimensions of healing, the months of immobility and their strain on her family relationships, the loss of income from her son's job, the depression she fears her son is facing, the loss of a family dream, the denial of a child's future. A fractured bone, the best possible conditions for attending to that bone, its role in the skeletal system, its integration with muscle and body fluids, its impact on nerve endings, and ultimately, its healing process takes focus.

There is some modest acknowledgment of the emotion attendant to pain management, the fear of potential unhealed bone, the need to understand the nature of the fracture intellectually, and the social context of immobility. There is also a willingness to provide even more specialized attention to these issues from an expert. The wholeness seems intent on the bone, however, not the child. Whole universes of reality are denied or ignored, and Margaret and her son are left to drive home from the emergency room with a grocery list of issues and healing that never became an identified dimension of their disrupted sense of wholeness.

HEALING AS NURSING CONSTRUCT

All healthcare providers in some fashion attend to the ultimate goal of healing, and view their work, if not themselves, as healers. In the United States, this basic assumption is often lost in the swirl of activities and interventions, policies and procedures, but the underlying goal remains as an assumption guiding the activities. Nursing has a particular affinity for this goal because of its historic commitment to an holistic approach to patients and their health concerns. Nurses embrace the idea of healing readily, and think of themselves as persons engaged in healing the whole person, the family, and indeed, even the communities where they serve. Nurses assume that their actions, as professionals, aim to facilitate wholeness in others through an interaction based on a mutuality of purpose, acknowledging, as they do so, the multi-dimensional nature of humans with a variety of health related experiences. They acknowledge the human desire for a state of achieved, restored, maintained or reclaimed wholeness, view this as a human good, and believe that assisting others toward this goal is a human good.

Wholeness can be conceptualized both as an objective abstraction and as subjective perception. It can thus be further understood, in any concrete situation, as some admixture of these complementary conceptualizations. As an objective abstraction, the concept, applied to humans, points to an ideal rather than a reality, since no human is actually whole. In this sense, it is a goal or a destination embedded in the evolutionary process of human development. Its scope and depth are bounded only by the specific person who is defining the nature of wholeness.

Specific individuals can also subjectively define for themselves the level of wholeness they seek or desire. This too is bounded by their personal definition of the nature of wholeness, and may or may not coincide with the definitions of those from whom they seek help. Because of the multidimensional nature of human wholeness, both parties may experience dissonances where their definitions of wholeness are either more confining and limited or more robust and complex than those presented to them.

Nurses are educated to attend to both subjective and objective meanings of healing and wholeness, and engage in interactions with others where both meanings guide nursing responses. The ambitiousness of this intention is only superficially acknowledged, and the skills and knowledge necessary to excel in such an effort are not yet delineated. Good will, finely tuned intuitive skills, years of experience and learning from one's errors have been more conducive to such mastery than the guidance provided by a comprehensive educational program that enables needed competencies. The goal, laudable in itself, is also not furthered as a comprehensive dimension of nursing education or practice, nor is it a definable element in the overall healthcare provided in the United States. Recognizing the disturbing nature of this reality has given impetus to the need to better understand the nature of healing processes in the practice of professional nursing.

As is perhaps apparent, the pursuit of wholeness through healing is not uniquely a dimension of the domain of nursing, but how nurses participate in this process is unique. Better understanding the processes of healing in nursing is of value to nurses and those for whom they care. In addition, a more comprehensive understanding of healing processes in nursing should enhance an overall understanding of healing and be of value to others, both those attempting to assist in healing and those seeking such assistance. Because nursing has consistently embraced an holistic understanding of persons seeking healthcare, this exploration of nursing's role in healing processes gives promise of addressing a multidimensional understanding of those who seek to heal themselves and others.

HEALING IN HISTORICAL CONTEXT

Healing, or human wholeness, can only be understood within a given historical context; it changes and evolves over time. It acquires its meaning from diverse eras and cultures, social systems that support and reinforce selected beliefs and behaviors. As a result, any effort to systematically investigate healing phenomena of nursing begins with the acknowledgment of and benefit from this diversity. While building on this past, such investigations also provide the opportunity to explore alternatives that will further the evolutionary development of our collective understanding of the meaning of healing. In this sense, context is both constraint and opportunity.

Constraints warrant scrutiny. Historians and sociologists have amply documented the systematic suppression of nursing perspectives and the systematic oppression of nurses as scholars and healthcare providers. In this light, nursing scholars are called upon to investigate not only the aspects of healing practices unique to nursing, but also those dimensions of nursing that have been suppressed, and the oppressed group behaviors in nurses that delimit healing practices.

Suppression and oppression as historical realities in nursing have often led to marked distortions about nurses as healers and nursing as healing, distortions that in some cases are manifested and sustained by nurses themselves if not actively imposed on them. Understanding healing practices in nursing inherently requires an honest appraisal of these facts. This has a particular impact on the effort to develop a scholarship of healing processes and practices in nursing.

For several centuries now, the United States, as both a participant and purveyor of a Western worldview, has embraced a paradigm of knowledge generation shaped by Cartesian assumptions about reality. As practiced, these assumptions emphasize detached observation—examining, measuring, and estimating an external reality—vis à vis a knower somehow separate from the known. This "received view" has proven robust in a variety of investigatory activities, but has increasingly revealed its limits, particularly in current perceptions of human wholeness.

Thus, while nursing has participated in the activities of, and benefits from, this view of science, nursing's commitment to holistic interpersonal healthcare goes well beyond the artificial boundaries accepted by adherents to Cartesianism. Nurses have variously found themselves either coopted into this constricted worldview, ineffectively rebellious toward it, or withdrawn from it in a state of uncertainty or hopelessness. As a result, the full scope of the nurses' role in the healing interaction with patients has been neither well-identified nor studied. In addition, the active discounting of alternative worldviews has prohibited nurses from assuring the systematic evolutionary development of the central construct of healing as it is given meaning, day to day, by nurses and their patients. Margaret and her son directly experienced the consequences of that state of affairs.

An honest confrontation with these historical and current realities heightens awareness of the need to address such deficiencies in existing nursing knowledge and to generate the knowledge base needed to assure practicing nurses active, informed, and competent involvement in their role in healing processes. The nurse approaches the patient from a perspective of personal humanity, acknowledging that same humanity in the patient. No healing encounter can accurately be described as one between a detached observer and an object. To do so is to strip the patient and the nurse of their individual subjective expressions of humanity, destroy or disrupt the mutuality of intent between the nurse and the patient, all prohibitory of healing encounters. Hence, this constricted view of knowledge generation, while able to provide some useful components leading to an understanding of healing, is unable to capture the dimensions and nuances of the whole.

Beyond the Boundaries of the Prevailing Paradigm

As an investigative approach, detached observation was first and best devised to explore physical or material phenomena. By isolating a physical object and differentiating it from all other like objects, the knower discovered its unique properties and potentials. The periodic chart of chemical elements is a useful exemplar here. Relating various objects within a given domain also became possible—as exemplified in the development of an array of chemical compounds. Detached observation, however, did not provide a useful template for relating these objects to those outside the domain, including non-physical phenomena from differing domains sharing a common context. It also did not reveal the relationship of the object to the knower.

This reductionistic, analytic approach to understanding physical phenomena gave us vast reservoirs of new information, but did so by separations, divisions, discriminations and subsequent controlled relating processes. As a result, and as the fragmentation of knowables into separate units proceeded, the capacity of any knower to perceive holistically diminished. In addition, the acknowledgment of any phenomenon as real which could not or would not subject itself to this mode of scrutiny became suspect. The emphasis on observables as the preferred focus also gradually came to define the only accepted focus, the only possible perception of reality.

Scientists hoped then to find causal relationships among objects as reflected in desired outcomes. In time, they began to work toward predicting outcomes, and exerting the needed controls to assure such outcomes. Increasingly, the real became a sterile compendium of mechanistic and materialistic givens that scientists tinkered with in the hope of teasing out new possibilities for prediction and control.

This historical development of knowledge generation shapes our current understanding of healing and wholeness. Due to our gradual fragmentation of the dimensions of humanness, healing activities are currently focused on establishing, achieving, or regaining a sense of cohesion among various "parts" or "facets" of a human person. For most of us, we experience this as a desire for personal integrity, and we assume it is a reasonable goal. We humans are complex creatures with a capacity for self-awareness, and thus possessing a related capacity to sense to some degree both a diversity of facets and varying levels of integration among these facets. If some facets are denied reality, or if pathways to a meaningful integration of any facets are denied reality, our capacity to discover wholeness and healing suffers. Because each of us has the capacity to deter our own wholeness through denial of selected human facets, we can also create situations where, as healthcare providers, we assist persons in sustaining such deterrents.

A pragmatic set of questions confront the contemporary student of healing as a result. What are the facets or dimensions of the human condition? What are the relationships among these dimensions? What forces lead to coherence among these dimensions? What deters such cohesion? How do we attend to these deterrents and forces of coherence?

Prevailing paradigms tend to focus intensively on a preferred set of givens. To determine the adequacy of a paradigm, one must ask, then identify "what is missing." If there are vested interests in retaining a current paradigm, this question can prove disturbing, even threatening, to those who embrace the paradigm. Yet, if selected realities are denied existence, the paradigm is inadequate to meet the challenge of the serious scholar.

The paradigm which now prevails in the United States embraces such a set of preferred givens, and implicitly denies the reality of others, particularly the obverses of these givens—leading to imbalance, the denial of important influential factors, and the distortion of knowledge generation activities. Hence, the serious student of healing, seeking to study the nature of wholeness, must constructively explore these distortions and reveal them in order to meet the rigors of the task of discovery.

Revealing such obverses, however, is only a partial response to the intellectual challenge that confronts the scholar. One must then conciliate these obverses in some fashion, so that pathways to healing can be ascertained, described, and pursued. Hence, moving beyond the prevailing paradigms involves both the clear delineation of constructs systematically denied reality followed by the even more daunting task of finding ways to conciliate these constructs with their more readily acknowledged obverses. In this regard, the task of exploring healing opens wide vistas of scholarship, much of it unchartered territory or territory proclaimed as non-existent or irrelevant.

Professional nursing is fortunate, however, in that it has both traditionally and operationally sustained convictions about these realities despite their denial. An expert nurse would have noticed the struggle Margaret and her son were experiencing, would have asked them each what this event meant, would have explored the implications of an event that could change their lives despite its seemingly uncomplicated nature and predicted physical outcomes. Professional nurses have experienced directly the patient's search for cohesion among all facets of self during a health event. They have also learned of the kind of cohesion that is possible.

Much of this is largely a function of working closely, in deep personal contact and mutuality, with humans who seek healing despite deterrents placed in their way, even by those of prevailing paradigms. Thus the capacity to discover is available, and requires only the systematic, rigorous, and disciplined pursuit of clarity and comprehension. This discovery, shared, gives promise of making a substantial contribution not only to nursing knowledge but more provocatively, to the overall wellness of all humans. Hence, the systematic investigation of healing processes opens the window to discovery of new realities and relationships, accommodating both the "known" dimensions of the prevailing paradigm and the emergent dimensions of hitherto unexplored realities.

Balance here must prevail as well. Scholars of healing need to attend to both analysis and synthesis. Current models of knowing are invaluable tools, but are best augmented by alternative models of knowing such as aesthetic knowing, hermeneutics, ethical knowing, and deconstructionism. Because healing is an integrative process, the interactive and inter-relational dimensions of human reality need to be acknowledged and explored with an intent to understand the process of creating constructive connections and effective mutualities, both among humans and within the human. In such explorations, the capacity to conciliate seemingly opposite forces becomes a focus of interest. Coming full circle, acknowledgment of the import and impact of context becomes an explicit dimension of study.

These approaches essentially posit that, beyond the abstract analysis of the detached observer, there is a substrate of reality where shared existence offers explanations beyond those achieved through separations and detachments. In this sense, the nurse scholar studies the implicit and explicit fact that nurses interact with patients from a common ground of being, where the nurse is disposed to encounter the "other," the patient, not as a depersonalized object but as an expression of a shared existence, a shared human condition. While such personal experience is incontrovertible, its impact on the process of healing is poorly understood and in some cases actually denied reality. To continue to deny this reality is to actively elect to prohibit healing, since such a denial communicates to the patient the very fragmentation and disunity that is the antithesis of the wholeness sought in the healing processes.

Historically, nurses have sustained their awareness of and respect for this dimension of healing through intuitive encounters with patients that seemed to "fall outside" the boundaries of accepted healthcare practices. Such encounters have often been turning points in the process of healing, and reveal a relational synergy between nurse and

patient. Both nurses and patients have valued these encounters, and recognized their significance both in themselves, and as a dimension of the
process of healing. Exploring such encounters formally and systematically in an effort to unveil their inherent power and potential for facilitating the healing process is now a necessity. In this sense, the formal
validation of realities too often viewed as murky or unreal can become
more readily apparent, and thus available to the practicing nurse who
elects to respond to the patient's search for healing experiences and
opportunities.

CONCEPTUAL DIMENSIONS OF A FORMAL AND
SYSTEMATIC INVESTIGATION OF HEALING

The practicing nurse approaches the patient assuming that some desire
for "wholeness" is present and can be discovered through interaction
with the patient. This assumption frames the nurse's commitment to
holistic care, a "gestalt-like" process of human interaction and mutuality.
The actual organization of nursing knowledge and process of nursing decision making, however, is focused on a variety of dimensions that are
ways of knowing what it means to be human. These dimensions are recognized as interactive and interdependent in nature. The ability to isolate
and the desirability of isolating one or another for purposes of discrimination and clarification is also recognized. Such discriminatory activity is
constructive in itself, but is recognized as occurring within and in interaction with the whole. This tension of part and whole is acknowledged as
difficult and demanding, but more congruent with reality than an illusional overemphasis on one or the other perspective.

Having accepted the utility of differentiating these dimensions for
closer scrutiny, one can then identify several dimensions of human
health that are appropriate to the study of healing in nursing. These dimensions can actually be conceptualized as a taxonomy of sorts, or a matrix of interacting dimensions of variance among humans seeking
healing, including dimensions that focus on humans from the following
perspectives: physical beings, emotional beings, intellectual beings, social beings, moral beings, and spiritual beings. Hence, one might study
tissue integrity in wound healing (a primarily physical focus) or the ethical dilemmas of end-of-life decisions which honor a human's desire for
wholeness (a primarily moral focus), by way of example. This taxonomy
of dimensions provides one intellectual device for the systematic study

of nursing phenomena as expressions of the process of healing. It is, however, only one of several potential "axes" of study, axes referring here to a "main line or direction, motion, growth, or extension" or "one of the reference lines of a coordinate system" (Webster's New Collegiate, 1981).

Additional axes can be identified that can provide alternate approaches to nursing phenomena related to healing processes. For example, a second axis might focus on the units of analysis the nurse uses in conceptualization and decision making. Professional nurses acknowledge a range of units of analysis, each focused on greater levels of complexity and scope, through cellular physical healing to bodily organs, physical systems, holistic individual human functioning, families, groups, and communities, including a global community in search of healing processes. The formal investigation of nursing phenomena is further organized with the use of this axis of units of analysis. By way of example, one could study the implications of healing processes as a response to violence. Doing so using the unit of analysis of organ system after trauma differs substantively from doing so using the unit of analysis of urban communities with a high incidence of hand gun injuries or homicides. Both fall within the domain of nursing, but each differs substantively due to the unit of analysis selected by the nurse scholar.

A third conceptual axis also emerges from professional nursing's metaparadigm, which identifies four essential elements in any theoretical conceptualization of nursing: the nurse, the patient, the context, and health itself. Here healing involves the nurse and the patient interacting within a given context in response to a health experience in which the nurse works in a pattern of mutuality with the patient, facilitating healing in response to a patient's elicitation of nursing involvement and expertise. These four fundamental elements are always present in the healing encounter in nursing, but manifest in a rich variety of patterns which can be the focus of formal investigations. Exemplars could include such diverse studies as health teaching interventions for early breast and prostate cancer detection in rural communities, or quality case management parameters of home infusion programs of care, or health policy implications of changing school nurse prescriptive authority legislation. The diversity is substantive, yet each explores a particular meaning of the healing encounter between the nurse and the patient. Such studies would expand, amplify, and enrich the theoretical understanding of nursing thus far evolved, and benefit patients seeking healing encounters.

Current nursing information systems compile and classify data using additional axes of interest to the student of healing in nursing. These include taxonomies of nursing assessment parameters, nursing diagnoses, nursing interventions and nursing outcomes. Each of these indicate additional axes where investigations of the involved phenomena as expressions of some dimension of the healing process can be profitably scrutinized. In addition to these data systems which are unique to nursing, the analogous systems of other health disciplines and the emerging data systems on innovative and alternative healthcare approaches may yield foci of study or indicate a need for formal investigation of the interface of interaction with phenomena within the domain of nursing.

Some axes of the study of healing processes in nursing will be less characteristically involved with the investigation of one or more dimensions of these various taxonomic systems of classification of phenomena and more directly focused on the lived experiences involved in the healing processes. In these axes, the nature of phenomena are explored for enhanced comprehension and the potential identification of additional dimensions of importance to professional nurses and their patients. These investigations point to issues such as unidentified sources of variance, the parameters of quality care provision, and the uses of intuitive knowing. Dimensions of healing that elude simplistic quantification or are distorted by such efforts might reasonably be pursued within axes of emphasis such as these.

Analysis of the actual meaning of "wholeness" as an expression of health evokes another such axis as defined above. One dictionary definition of health describes "wholeness" as a "flourishing condition," signifying wholeness as integral or integrity *within* and *among* dimensions. More commonly in current health practices, "wholeness" presents as a manifestation of levels of wellness or illness.

Nurses acknowledge the subjective and individual interpretation of the meaning of wellness and illness, flourishing condition, and death for each patient, thus allowing the patient primacy in defining and pursuing wellness. Indeed, patients may define their interest in wellness or wholeness within boundaries significantly more constrictive than those of the healthcare system. The nurse serves as a respondent, and facilitates healing within the boundaries of this patient definition. Where the patient may lack awareness of the constrictive nature of such personal boundaries, the nurse may further serve as a health educator, seeking to unveil the implications of limiting boundaries not known by the patient or exploring with the patient the nature of individual deterrents to more generous boundaries of wellness.

Wholeness or integrity in this sense is not an arbitrary abstraction but a concrete human perception. It is not determined by the absence of presence of disease or the severity or terminal nature of disease. It is more accurately conceptualized as the range, scope and depth of the patient's responses to a health event, or a series of health events. It focuses on the lived experience, the meaning given such an experience, and the outcomes that emerge. The profound nature of the search for human wholeness and healing is explored. Understanding these processes gives substance to the concept of healing, expands and enriches the meanings nurses and others might give to patient experiences, and may thus change the ways care is provided.

In this axis of healing processes, the patient is the central focus and the lived experience of the health event is a more transient and changing process in which the nurse plays a role. The patient seeks the assistance of the nurse in this process because of the unique expertise of the nurse. The nurse facilitates the healing sought by the patient. Using this conceptualization, the healing process extends across a broad spectrum of health experiences, ranging from the pursuit of high level wellness to the desire to die with dignity and meaning.

This approach to healing acknowledges that the patient can and will take a "position" on a spectrum of relatively "objectively" determined criteria for "human health" and will seek wholeness from that position on the spectrum. The nurse responds to the patient in the light of that position, and various positions call forth alternative responses by the nurse. The assumption of "wholeness achieved" is not the focus of healing, but the pursuit of wholeness within the human limits of a given health event or experience. Human limits manifest themselves not only in the human condition manifested by the patient, and the meanings assigned that condition by the patient, but also within a diversity of health and context factors. Thus healing within professional nursing acknowledges the human condition not so much as something to be denied, transcended or controlled, but something to be honored and addressed constructively in active mutuality with the patient. Such an approach reflects sensitivity to the more subjective and relative nature of the meaning of healing as it expresses itself in the lives of real humans.

A second axis that approaches healing from a more phenomenological perspective involves explorations about the sources of healing. Diverse scholars of healing, beginning in the West with Hippocrates, consistently give attention to the fact that healing arises from within the person seeking healing. All humans are in some sense the primary source of their own healing, innately seeking wholeness and integrity as persons. This pursuit of wholeness is, however, also shaped by the distortions, misconceptions and self limitations that characterize the human condition. Humans thus concurrently experience themselves deterring their own healing, yet seeking this healing. One such expression of this seeking of healing is to solicit help from others, among them nurses.

Nurses, by actively seeking their own wholeness, enrich their capacity to assist others in their efforts at wholeness. In addition, environments and communities that further healing can be created to assist this inner source of healing and wholeness, both in patients and in nurses. Thus, investigations of self healing, healing of the healers, and creation of healing environments and communities become another significant dimension of inquiry in a program of study that investigates the nature of healing processes in nursing.

These various approaches to healing provide nurse scholars with organizing frameworks of study and enable practicing nurses to refine their focus on the nature of healing practices in which they participate. The approaches might best be understood as axes or planes of meaning which interact. Each axes becomes a plane of decision making and action that clarifies nursing activities focused on healing. In time, a rich array of insights about and awarenesses of the processes of healing in nursing can emerge. These should have a substantive impact on the quality of health-care patients receive from professional nurses.

THE NURSE AS A HEALER

Traditional conceptualizations of healing in the United States have tended to reflect the systematic biases of the culture, shaped by a dominant paradigm, and thus have introduced systematic biases into research on this topic. The United States has given primacy to the physical dimensions of health and healing, and focused primarily on disease or illness states. Thus healing has often been equated with the curing of a physical disease or dysfunction.

While this indeed can be one potential expression of the process of healing, to view it as the only one restricts both the scope and depth of the concept, and places unnecessary and undesirable restrictions on the definition of healing. It also assumes that healing is achieved when selected indicators of a given physical disease or dysfunction are no longer apparent to the healthcare provider. It is a definition that is determined by the provider, and denies to a high degree any role of the patient in the process of healing, or reduces the role to one of passive compliance with healthcare provider prescriptions, advice and admonitions. It implicitly denies the self agency of the patient in the healing process.

This concept of healing is not congruent with the central tenets of nursing practice and the professional nurse's understanding of the human condition. Professional nursing assumes the self agency of the patient, and posits that the patient is the central force in the healing process, the nurse one who assists and responds. Thus healing is a process within the patient's lived experience, and nurses are healthcare providers with expertise to facilitate this process.

This conceptual approach to healing contrasts with the more constrictive and control focused definitions of healing that often determine healthcare practices in the United States. For many nurses, the impact of this culture-bound definition has served to place artificial boundaries on their practice or led to an actual lack of awareness of the role of the nurse in the healing process of the patient. Further, the prevailing conceptual approach can create environments where the nurse is continuously subjected to distorted or unrecognized judgments of the nurse's intention, motivation, or intervention, evoking self doubt and uncertainty in the nurse. Thus, investigations of the denial or denigration of substantive nursing realities become a potential focus of study.

In addition, the formal investigation of healing from this more robust nursing perspective has been largely neglected due to this confusion. An honest effort to address this area of neglect gives promise of expanding nursing's body of knowledge about this central but poorly understood process. It seems ironic that the ultimate aim of the healthcare encounter should be the most shadowy dimension of our nursing activities, but we have the option to address this deficiency.

As becomes readily apparent, both the conceptual delineation of this alternate view of healing, and the formal investigation of nursing phenomena from this perspective would serve to substantively alter current practices and outcomes. To the degree that nurses perceive themselves as healers, or persons engaged in a practice of healing, the absence of knowledge about healing becomes a serious deterrent to quality care. In addition, the multidimensional nature of healing is neglected, and patients are afforded healthcare that confines them within the limits of an increasingly indefensible understanding of wholeness.

HEALING AND THE FUTURE OF HEALTHCARE

For most practicing nurses, the current healthcare delivery climate in the United States is undergoing the most intense and rapid changes of their careers. Students entering this climate no doubt wonder at the responses of the established professional nurse. It is in many ways a vulnerable time for nurses, where the convictions they have historically embraced can be given short shrift more easily, since many were not clearly articulated or documented in the past. The nurse caring for Margaret and her son may indeed simply have been swept up in the norms of her environment, losing touch with the values and beliefs that have guided her in the past.

The changes visiting practicing nurses are also experiencing a change in scope as we collectively evolve toward a global community. This evolution itself creates new vistas and is reflected in innovations such as telecommunications, global economies, and shared technologies. AIDS is a useful exemplar of the nature of a disease that can only be understood if viewed as a global phenomenon. This global perspective comes slowly to persons accustomed to predictable boundaries in their worldview, which may have only extended to the local or national level. Healthcare providers today are called upon to understand and respond to potential and real ecological and human disasters such as the Chernobyl incident or the sequelae of the Gulf War. The World Health Organization, in the Alma Alta Declaration of 1978 embraced a goal of global primary care provision for all people, reiterated and clarified in Riga in 1988 with the initiation of the campaign for "Health for all by the year 2000." This initiative constitutes a clear and clearly proactive agenda for all people around the planet who are invested in the processes of healing. How is our understanding of healing shaped by a given culture? What do persons in contexts quite different from our own know about healing that we have failed to learn? What do we have to share? We have only begun to tease apart the difficult implications of these questions.

At the national level, the on-going process of rapid change in healthcare delivery patterns and structures continues unabated, unveiling both improvements and devastating problems, with a range of mixed reports in between these extremes. It is rare for any of these changes to attend even modestly to the lived experience of the patient and the patient's healing encounters with the nurse. The United States is the only "developed" country that has not declared healthcare as a right. At a time when other nations are vigorously pursuing the WHO initiative, the United States was reframing its societal role from one of service to a self-definition as an "industry," a fact made even more ironic given the futurists assurance that the industrial age is waning. This emphasis on the industrial model, while congruent with the United States' attachment to a mechanistic approach to human wholeness, intensifies our emphasis on healthcare as expensive technologies and "profitable" hyperspecialization and chemical treatment.

The patient as a vulnerable yet self-determining moral agent, as the central focus of healthcare, has suffered in this transition, and indeed groups of such patients became a strong force in the impetus to health-care reform. The current debate on reforms tends to focus on fear as a primary motive, and threatens the patient with even greater limits on self agency and sensitivity to individuality. The awareness of the potential impact of proposed reforms on the efforts of any human to evoke healing, and the capacity of others to facilitate this process seems remote, if not totally denied. To create a clear and competent voice that acknowledges the realities that characterize and enhance human healing seems imperative if this debate and its outcomes are to avoid furthering the dehumanizing practices and moral bankruptcy of the healthcare delivery systems of this country. The implicit invitation to cynical solutions is incompatible with the history and traditions of professional nursing in this country, and thus requires astute and careful reflection, deliberation, and action. These add dimensions to the preparation of nurse scholars at this time in this country.

The historic suppression and oppression of nursing's viewpoint stands as a challenge to all nurses facing the healthcare futures that characterize our times. As healthcare reform progresses, the nurse as healer becomes an increasingly compelling concern. It will take both courage and creativity for nursing to address this concern. Perhaps the most startling insight we may discover is this: reforms that assure patient wholeness and healing may actually be reforms that improve access, decrease cost, improve funding practices, assure quality, and honor the right of all humans to equity in healthcare. We seem unable to imagine this possibility, caught as we are in the propensity for zero sum game thinking. Imagining a healing future despite the confusions of the times becomes a sizable challenge, but one that calls forth the best in all of us. It is a challenge worthy of a discipline committed to the work of healing.

CHAPTER 2

Healing: The Outcome of Humanistic Care

MARY V. FENTON, RN, DRPH

Healing, in the context of this collection of writings, has been described as "the interactive process that emerges when patients within a specified health context seek the expertise of the professional nurse to facilitate progression toward a desired 'wholeness'" (Kritek, 1994). This definition includes some of the esoteric words that academia, the healthcare profession, and nursing school accreditation bodies would expect and require if a school of nursing faculty announced that they had chosen the concept of healing as a basis for developing nursing scholarship and research, educational programs, and clinical practice models. Although this definition would meet such established criteria, it is more important to know how the concept is translated into healthcare for people, families, and communities. It is also important to determine how you would know when healing occurs and how you would measure its effect. The relationship between healing and humanistic care is a natural one and has been defined and studied intensively over the last thirty years. This chapter will synthesize much of this work in an attempt to conceptualize and legitimize the past and future humanistic basis of nursing practice's contributions to healing.

Exploring the concept of healing as an outcome provides a forum to explore and institute humanistic care as a legitimate and appropriate approach to the delivery of healthcare in any setting. It is much more difficult to quantify the aspects of humanistic care and its effect on healing than the number and length of visits to a healthcare provider. This aspect of care has largely been ignored in the healthcare reform debate. However, humanistic interventions are quantifiable, and instruments have been developed, studied, and published in the literature.

In this chapter I focus on humanistic care to promote healing in a context of cost-effective, high quality healthcare. Using healing as both a process and an outcome, more humane and ethical decisions can be made concerning what type of healthcare is necessary, the best method of delivery, and the measurement of outcomes.

HEALING AND HEALTHCARE

The term *healing* is familiar, but to some it would have meaning only at the physiological level. Those persons who focus on the more psychosocial and cultural end of the spectrum might conjure up a vision of a religious healer or shaman praying over an ill person. Some would argue that healing can only be defined as a process; others would say it is also an outcome. The term *healing* is not well understood in our high-tech society. Yet it is a concept that greatly affects our lives and the lives of those we care about.

Healthcare is in a state of transition, not only in relationship to cost and method of delivery but also in terms of what is expected of consumers and healthcare providers. The old paradigm of healthcare that consisted of cost-unaware, technologically driven, institutionally based, specialized care governed by the professions and focused on the individual patient and provider in a competitive model is giving way. The new paradigm is focused on cost-accountable, humanistic, community-based, managed primary care with team providers in a partnership model. However, whether the new paradigm will truly be operationalized into our healthcare systems is still questionable. The government, the healthcare industry, academia, and healthcare providers are all concerned with the outcomes of healthcare. However, the profit motive of the large managed care corporations has resulted in a focus on cutting costs by limiting access to specialists or by utilizing certain types of delivery systems or intervention therapies rather than on patients' needs.

Nursing's attempts to demonstrate that the environment, the nature of the care, and the interaction between patient and provider may have a profound impact on the outcome of the care are often ignored in the race to the bottom line. Instead, more emphasis is being placed on how many patients can be seen by one provider in one hour or how many hospital RNs can be replaced with less trained workers without endangering patients. Much of the cost of our health system is wasted because it does not consider the whole patient, his or her life and environment, or his or her past and future. Many patients who seek healthcare are not only seeking a diagnosis or a prescription, but are also seeking to heal their lives physically, mentally, emotionally, culturally, spiritually, and socially.

Diagnosis and treatment of an infection with an antibiotic does not always answer the question as to why this person's immune system was susceptible at this time and place to this infectious agent. As a society, we have limited ways that people can seek help for pain and suffering unless there is a demonstrable physical cause. People often turn to a healthcare system that is ill-prepared to provide the solace or remedy they seek. People seek help for symptoms that they may describe as physical as a way to gain access to the healthcare system though their real problems may have emotional, spiritual, or social underlying or related causes (Roberts, 1994). Then they are confused—as is their care provider—when they cannot be diagnosed or treated successfully. Or the symptoms may be relieved only to return because only the symptoms were treated, leaving the underlying causes unidentified.

THE EFFECT OF HUMANISTIC HEALTHCARE ON HEALING

Most healthcare literature supports the notion that delivery of humanistic healthcare is a highly desirable goal. However, it is a complex concept that has not always been well defined or developed through systematic research endeavors. The literature ranges from descriptions of how to make healthcare environments more humanistic by architectural design to multiple studies of medical students and residents to determine if they lose their humanistic orientation through their medical education process. Much of the literature is anecdotal and based upon opinions about what health professionals should do in order to provide more humanistic care.

Nursing's efforts to provide humanistic environments and care that promotes healing in all dimensions of patients' lives spans the century. But only in the last half of the century have attempts been made to quantify the outcome and effect of a humanistic-focused nursing approach to healthcare. The end result of a humanistic approach to healthcare is healing. Evidence exists that healing has occurred in the most unlikely of cases and situations when the patient's will to live has promoted and sustained the healing process. A humanistic approach by caregivers increases the likelihood that such healing will occur. The focus of nursing is, thus, to facilitate healing.

The word *humanistic* is found throughout all definitions and theories of nursing. Martha Rogers, the well-known nursing theorist, explicitly defined nursing as a humanistic science with concern for mankind as central to the process of nursing (Rogers, 1970). Other nursing theorists including Orem (1971) and Roy (1974) view the nurse as a humanistic clinician. In 1980, the American Nurses Association made the statement that "nurses are guided by a humanistic philosophy having caring coupled with understanding and purpose as its central feature" (American Nurses Association, p. 18). Humanistic care in nursing is most often exemplified by Patterson and Zderad's interactive humanistic nursing theory. They define nursing as "peak experiences related to health and suffering in which the participants in the nursing situation are and become in accordance with their human potential" (Patterson & Zderad, 1976, p. 7). Although the word *humanistic* is highly identified with their writings about nursing, the theory is somewhat limited by its focus on the experience of the nurse and the patient primarily at the moment of interaction (Meleis, 1991).

Although nursing defines itself as a highly expressive, supportive, and humanistic process, it is not always evident that practicing nurses consistently incorporate these values into their roles. Jourard's (1971) classic studies describe the bedside manner of nurses who work in hospitals as stereotyped behavior used to satisfy the nurses' needs and reduce their anxiety. Lorber (1975), in an investigation of the behavior of surgical patients and the reactions of physicians and nurses to that behavior, found that patients who complained and interrupted well-established routines were termed "problem patients" and were subject to earlier discharge, neglect, and referral to a psychiatrist.

Further incongruence is described in nurse-patient interaction studies done in the 1960s and 1970s in which nurse-patient interaction was studied in relation to psychological and physiological measures of the success of coping with illness or surgery (Pride, 1968; Schmitt & Wooldridge, 1973; Skipper & Leonard, 1968). Some of the commonalities in the experimental humanistic approaches were transmission of accurate information about the hospital experience, exploration of the meaning of illness and hospitalization to the patient, and facilitation of the expression and acceptance of patients' feelings, fears, and anxieties (Lindeman & Van Aernam, 1971; Thornton & Leonard, 1964). The control groups usually received one of the following approaches: routine hospital care with no contact with the researcher, a friendly yet task-oriented approach with little interpersonal interaction, or information about the hospital experience without opportunity for the patient to express feelings or reactions to it (Dumas & Leonard, 1963; Elms & Leonard, 1966). The assumption in these studies was that routine care did not include the personalized variables found in the experimental approach (Diers, Schmitt, McBride, & Davis, 1972; Tryon & Leonard, 1966). Therefore, although nursing has described itself as humanistic, these nurse-patient interaction studies and their results indicated that the researchers did not believe a humanistic approach routinely occurred in hospital settings.

The most important finding of these studies is that the humanistic patient-centered approach did contribute to positive outcomes both physiologically and psychologically. Much of this body of knowledge was summarized in a meta analysis of 34 controlled studies (Mumford, Schlesinger, & Glass, 1982) that demonstrated that on the average, surgical or coronary patients who are provided information and emotional support to help them master their illness do better than patients who received routine care. Use of hospital days post-surgery or post-heart attack as outcome indicators showed that psychological intervention reduced hospitalization by at least two days as compared to the control groups. Humane and considerate care is not only valuable in promoting better outcomes but is shown to be cost effective. Use of days hospitalized post-surgery does not guarantee that healing as defined as wholeness has occurred in its entirety, but it is an outcome measure that in today's cost-centered healthcare environment has high legitimacy and will attract the attention of even the most rigid cost-cutting bureaucrat, administrator, or care provider.

THEORY VERSUS PRACTICE: MEASURING HUMANISTIC BEHAVIORS

Although the term *humanistic care* appears to be central to nursing's definitions, theories, and paradigms, there is no universal definition of humanistic healthcare. One of the clearest definitions was put forth by the sociologist Jan Howard in her book *Humanizing Health Care* (Howard & Strauss, 1975). After an exhaustive review of the literature, she defines humanistic healthcare as, "care that enhances the dignity and autonomy of patients and health professionals alike" (Howard, David, Pope, & Ruzek, 1977, p. 12). She further proposes eight theoretical components as requirements for the delivery of humanistic healthcare: irreplaceability, holistic selves, freedom of action, status equality, shared decision making and responsibility, empathy, positive affect, and inherent worth (Howard, 1975).

Irreplaceability occurs when staff believe that all humans are unique and irreplaceable and have a right to respond differently to illness. The component *holistic selves* implies that all dimensions and roles of a patient's life are relevant to health and disease and that culture and religious beliefs play a large part in response to illness. In *freedom of action,* the amount of individual freedom of choice reflects the degree to which humanism or dehumanism exists. In *status equality,* healthcare providers treat patients as equals if the interaction is considered to be humanizing. The component *shared decision making and responsibility* reflects the idea that all patients, regardless of education or knowledge, have the right to participate as much as possible in decisions about their care. *Empathy,* in a humanistic context, implies that healthcare providers see the world from the vantage point of their patients so that they can understand the patients' needs and respond appropriately to them as individuals. *Positive affect* implies that affect in humanizing relationship tends to be positive and that dehumanizing interactions involve surpluses of negative and neutral emotions. *Inherent worth* implies that all human beings are objects of value to themselves if not to others, and that persons should not have to prove their worth to receive adequate healthcare (Howard, 1975).

Based on Howard's theoretical model of dimensions pertinent to the domain of humanistic care, Fenton (1987) developed and tested a scale to measure the degree of humanistic healthcare in hospital settings as perceived by nursing personnel. This was done in an attempt to demonstrate that the theoretical construct of humanistic care could be operationalized and understood at the nurse-patient level. The interactions demonstrated in the earlier nurse-patient interaction studies as psychological interventions correlated highly with the definitions of Howard's dimensions of humanistic care and the actions that compose the Scale of Humanistic Behaviors. Rigorous application of reliability and validity indexes yielded a final scale of 70 items measuring four dimensions: shared decision making and responsibility, holistic selves, status equality, and empathy.

The Scale of Humanistic Nursing Behaviors has been used in a variety of research studies. For example, Groden (1988) compared humanistic nursing care in hospital and hospice settings; Zalon (1988) compared nurses' empathy for patient's pain as a function of the degree of humanistic care in the nursing environment; Aillon (1989) studied the relationship among organization climate variables, nurse characteristics, and humanistic caring behaviors; Webb (1989) determined that the scale could be adapted for cultural differences in perceptions of humanistic care; O'Connor (1989) and Tice (1990) correlated patient satisfaction and years of experience of professional nurses with humanistic behaviors; Donoghue (1990) compared perceptions of humanistic behaviors in nursing and nurses' experience; and Feringa (1992) used the scale to assess humanistic behaviors within the context of nursing in Botswana.

The results of these studies confirmed the reliability and validity of the Scale of Humanistic Nursing Behaviors; demonstrated that the scale could be adapted to other cultures; and showed that humanistic behaviors by nurses are most highly correlated with area of practice, type of unit and collegial environments. The development and use of this instrument demonstrates that the concept of humanistic care can be operationalized in nursing in healthcare settings and that nurses exhibit behaviors that reflect humanistic behaviors. The commonalities of the concepts that describe humanistic healthcare throughout the literature are remarkable. The definitions may vary slightly, but the concepts and constructs that support the definitions are strikingly similar.

HUMANISTIC CARE VERSUS CARING

More recently, humanistic care in nursing has been related to the concept of *caring*. The terms caring and humanistic care are often used interchangeably in definitions and theories of nursing; however a universal definition of caring has not been accepted. Nursing literature of the past ten years has defined caring as a central unifying theme of nursing (Benner & Wrubel, 1989; Leininger, 1984, 1986; Watson, 1985). This focus on the concept of caring represents an evolution of the development of the expressive, supportive, empathic, and compassionate interpersonal process that is central to the definition of nursing as a humanistic process. Part of the development of this unified caring perspective consisted of conducting a critical analysis of caring concepts, factors, and activities. The concepts were analyzed and reduced in number without losing their original meaning and divided into two categories, humanistic concepts and scientific concepts (Watson, 1985).

According to Watson (1985), humanistic concepts focus on human experiences and expressions of feelings and concern through such concepts as faith, trust, growth, empathy, compassion, hope and self-actualization. Scientific concepts focus on the scientific and empirical factors of nursing action which can be expressed through such concepts as helping, supporting, protecting, decision making, health promotion and maintenance, clinical judgments regarding technological monitoring, environmental restructuring, and maintaining human integrity. The humanistic concepts were translated into five unique nursing qualities that Watson asserts represent the basic essences in professional nursing caring relationships: actualization; instillment of faith and hope; concern and love for another; experiencing-with and being there; and interpersonal valuing and involvement. The scientific concepts were also translated into entities which reflect independent nursing actions integral to health and illness care: nursing therapeutics; restructuring of environments; health promotion and maintenance; caring nurse-patient/client relationships; maintaining human wholeness and integrity; technological management and monitoring.

These humanistic nursing qualities and scientific nursing actions are then used to form the structure for a professional nursing caring paradigm. The commonalities in the description of humanistic care and caring are quite evident and may overlap and be so complementary that it is impossible to separate one concept from the other. It may be that the combining of the two terms into humanistic caring may be the more encompassing of the concepts and behaviors that compose the two concepts.

However, most patients and their families would not know that such a humanistic model or nursing caring paradigm existed or that it was the basis for the manner in which their nurse interacted with them. They would be more focused on whether their immediate physical needs were met, whether they felt comfortable and reassured that their nurse was capable and confident of identifying and addressing their needs. Their actual experience of a nurse using such a paradigm would be one of not having to worry about what was going to happen next, of being relieved of much of the stress of coping with illness and being in a strange environment where most of their normal everyday activities are either highly controlled or denied. Patients of such nurses describe them as wonderful and caring, but they would seldom say, "my nurse used a professional nursing caring paradigm in taking care of me."

Kyle (1995) found a distinct incongruence between patients' and nurses' perceptions of caring in her review of the literature regarding research on caring. Nurses identified expressive behaviors more frequently as care indicators than patients. Patients identified instrumental or technical competencies as care indicators more often than nurses. One explanation that has been offered is that expressive humanistic nursing behaviors are more obvious when absent than when present (McKenna, 1993). Other authors have suggested that patients may not be receptive to expressive caring behaviors until physical needs are met and that as patients gain confidence in nurses performing tangible interventions, the more expressive activity becomes more important (Brown, 1986; Komorita, Doehring, & Hirchert, 1991; Mayer, 1987). In other words, the theoretical basis of providing a humanistic and caring nursing environment has yet to become part of the average patient's understanding of what to expect from professional nursing care. In order to do this, our care must be operationalized in a way that people can see it, measure it, and understand it. Our terms must be defined in language that is understandable to all. If humanistic care is to continue to be thought of as the central core of nursing, a critical focus must be continued development of valid and reliable instruments and research methods to measure its presence and its outcomes upon patient care.

SUMMARY

There is ample evidence that humanistic care can be defined and measured and that it contributes to healing as a process and an outcome. The question is how to integrate the operationalization of humanistic care into healthcare delivery systems which fail to realize that facilitating healing will improve their bottom-line cost. This question can only be answered by research which includes the development of reliable and valid tools to measure the outcomes of humanistic care and its effect on healing. It is a tremendous challenge for nursing and a courageous leap for a group of nursing faculty in this time of healthcare transition with its emphasis on cost control and method of delivery to take a stand that healing is central to healthcare.

REFERENCES

Aillon, B. (1989). *The relationship among organizational climate variables, selected nurse characteristics and nurse caring behavior.* Unpublished manuscript, Russell Sage College, Troy, NY.

American Nurses Association. (1980). *Nursing: A social policy statement.* Kansas City, MO: American Nurses' Association.

Benner, P., & Wrubel, J. (1989). *The primacy of caring.* Menlo Park, CA: Addison-Wesley.

Brown, L. (1986). The experience of care: Patient perspectives. *Topics of Clinical Nursing, 8*(2), 56–62.

Diers, D., Schmitt, R. L., McBride, M., & Davis, B. L. (1972). The effect of nursing interaction on patients in pain. *Nursing Research, 21,* 419–428.

Donoghue, J. (1990). *Humanistic care and nurses' experiences.* Unpublished master's thesis, La Trobe University, Abbotsford, Melbourne, Victoria, Australia.

Dumas, R. G., & Leonard, R. C. (1963). The effect of nursing on the incidence of post-operative vomiting. *Nursing Research, 12,* 12–25.

Elms, R., & Leonard, R. (1966). Effects of nursing approaches during admission. *Nursing Research, 15,* 39-47.

Fenton, M. V. (1987). Development of the Scale of Humanistic Nursing Behaviors. *Nursing Research, 36*(2), 82-87

Feringa, M. M. (1992). *Perceptions of humanistic behavior in nursing.* Unpublished master's thesis, Deborah Retief Memorial Hospital, School of Nursing, Mochudi, Botswana.

Groden, M. (1988). *Humanistic nursing care in the hospital and hospice setting.* Unpublished master's thesis, University of Connecticut.

Howard, J. (1975). Humanization and dehumanization of health care. In J. Howard & A. Strauss (Eds.), *Humanizing health care.* New York: Wiley.

Howard, J., David, F., Pope, C., & Ruzek, S. (1977). Humanizing health care: The implications of technology, centralization and self-care. *Medical Care, 5 Supplement, 15,* 11-26.

Howard, J., & Strauss, A. (Eds.). (1975). *Humanizing health care.* New York: Wiley.

Jourard, S. (1971). *The transparent self.* New York: Van Nostrand.

Komorita, N. I., Doehring, K. M., & Hirchert, P. W. (1991). Perceptions of caring by nurse educators. *Journal of Nursing Education, 30*(1), 23-29.

Kritek, P. (1994). *Healing, a central nursing construct.* Unpublished doctoral program White Paper, The University of Texas Medical Branch School of Nursing, Galveston, Texas.

Kyle, T. V. (1995). The concept of caring: A review of the literature. *Journal of Advanced Nursing, 21,* 506-514.

Leininger, M. M. (1986). Care facilitation and resistance factors in the culture of nursing. *Topics in Clinical Nursing, 8*(2), 1-11.

Leininger, M. M. (1984). Care: The essence of nursing and health care. In M. M. Leininger (Ed.), *Care: The essence of nursing and health care.* Thorofare, NJ: Slack.

Lindeman, C., & Van Aernam, B. (1971). Nursing intervention with the surgical patient: Effects of structured and unstructured pre-operative teaching. *Nursing Research, 20,* 319-331.

Lorber, J. (1975). Good patients and problem patients: Conformity and deviance in general hospital. *Journal of Health and Social Behavior, 16,* 213-225.

Mayer, D. K. (1987). Oncology nurses' versus cancer patients' perceptions of effective caring behaviors: A replication study. *Oncology Nursing Forum, 14*(3), 48-52.

McKenna, G. (1993). Caring is the essence of nursing practice. *British Journal of Nursing, 2*(1), 72-76.

Meleis, A. I. (1991). *Theoretical nursing: Development and progress* (2nd ed.). Philadelphia: J. B. Lippincott.

Mumford, E., Schlesinger, H. J., & Glass, G. V. (1982). The effects of psychological intervention on recovery from surgery and heart attacks: An analysis of the literature. *American Journal of Public Health, 72*(2), 141-146.

O'Connor, P. (1989). *Service in nursing: Correlates of patient satisfaction.* Unpublished doctoral dissertation, Case Western Reserve University, Cleveland, Ohio.

Orem, D. (1971). *Nursing concepts of practice.* New York: McGraw-Hill.

Patterson, J., & Zderad, L. (1976). *Humanistic Nursing.* New York: Wiley Biomedical Publications.

Pride, L. F. (1968). An adrenal stress index as a criterion measure for nursing. *Nursing Research, 17,* 292-303.

Roberts, S. J. (1994). Somatization in primary care. *Nurse Practitioner, 19*(5), 47, 50-56.

Rogers, M. (1970). *An introduction to the theoretical basis of nursing.* Philadelphia: F. A. Davis.

Roy, C. (1974). The Roy adaptation model. In H. Riehl & C. Roy (Eds.), *Conceptual models for nursing practice.* New York: Appleton-Century-Crofts.

Schmitt, F. E., & Wooldridge, R. J. (1973). Psychological preparation of surgical patients. *Nursing Research, 22,* 108-116.

Skipper, J., & Leonard, R. (1968). Children, stress and hospitalization: A field experiment. *Journal of Health and Social Behavior, 9,* 275-287.

Thornton, T. N., & Leonard, R. C. (1964). Experimental comparison of effectiveness and efficiency of three nursing approaches. *Nursing Research, 13,* 122-125.

Tice, M. E. (1990). *A study of the relationship between humanistic nursing care and years of experience of professional nurses.* Unpublished master's thesis, University of Akron, Akron, Ohio.

Tryon, P., & Leonard, R. (1966). A clinical test of patient-centered nursing. *Journal of Health and Human Behavior, 7,* 183-192.

Watson, J. (1985). *Nursing: Human science and human care.* Norwalk, CT: Appleton-Century-Crofts.

Webb, D. M. (1989). *Examining Bahraini, Indian, and Philipino nurses' perceptions of the degree of humanistic health care provision.* Unpublished master's thesis, University of Texas Graduate School of Biomedical Sciences at Galveston, Galveston, Texas.

Zalon, M. L. (1988). *Nurses empathy for patients' experience of pain as a function of the degree of humanism in the nursing environment, the patient's age and length of time since surgery.* Unpublished doctoral dissertation, New York University, New York, NY.

CHAPTER 3

A Paradigm Shift: A Code for Life and the Right to Heal

ALICE HILL, RN, PHD

She had seen the sun rise over the breakfast table many mornings. She knew exactly where each ray of sun would strike and the reflections precipitated by its presence. Little did she know that this day would change her life forever. This day would cause her to question the very essence of her being, her upbringing, and all that life had meant to her over the years. She was eighteen years old with all the charm and grace of any woman. It was the beginning of her sophomore year in college, her goals were clear and she knew without a doubt that they would become a reality. She would be a nurse, a Registered Nurse.

Born in the Bible Belt, she was fully indoctrinated with the religious beliefs of the Baptists. She understood right from wrong, or at least she thought she did until that day. There was a "code for life" that she had learned from her parents during the past eighteen years, and she lived this code without question: (1) do right by *ALL* people; (2) look for good in mankind; (3) don't assume the worst in any situation; (4) don't walk away just because you are losing; (5) finish what you start; (6) give people a second chance; and (7) know that your strengths come from within.

Today, a day that had started just like any other day, with the beautiful sunrise, the smell of the fresh country air, and an unparalleled serenity—this would be the day that would challenge her "code of life"; a day that would cause her to question the very foundation on which her life had evolved.

As she boarded the bus to go to her first class, she engaged in idle chatter with her friends. They talked about three things that were significant only to eighteen, nineteen, and twenty-year olds—men, fashion, and men. Without a doubt they had all the answers. As they giggled and went into class, they became serious for the next fifty minutes.

As she left her friends to walk across campus for her next class, she thought to herself, "One more semester here, then I will be ready to start my nursing courses. Won't that be wonderful? Me, a nurse, working in pediatrics with sick kids." She had it all figured out, she would see this kid in a room one morning and go in and . . . what's this? Those guys don't look too friendly, she thought to herself, "I'll just turn and go the other way to avoid a confrontation . . . Oh, no I think they are following me." Then she heard one say, "You n_____, what are you doing on OUR campus? Don't you know that it's people like you low life n_____ that make society what it is today?"

For the first time in her life she was truly afraid, afraid for her life, afraid that she would die. Just then one of the young men approached her, his hair combed to one side, small freckles over his face, ears protruding, and probably weighing no more than 130 pounds. She wanted to run but her feet would not move, she was frozen in place. Never before had she been so afraid. What could she do? The young man moved within what seemed like inches of her face, and said, "We want you and your friends off this campus, now!" Then in an instant he spat on her face—and walked away.

Frightened and in tears she ran to where she had left her friends, but they had gone to another class. She looked for someone who could, or would help—teachers, administrators, campus security—probably not. She was indeed an unwelcome "guest" by all standards. But she knew she had to try. She had to find out if there was someone in authority that would condemn that type of action. She went to what was known as Student Services. She made her complaint, but knew by the complacent attitudes that nothing would be done.

She left campus that day without attending her other two scheduled classes. When she got home her mother, who was also her friend, was there, ready to listen to her nonstop chatter about her day. But this time it was different.

She wanted her mother to explain to her why she had been taught to look for good in people, and why she had to do right by people? Why was she led to believe that if you did right, right would come back to you? She told her mother that there was no way she was going back to that University, and there was nothing that she or her father could do that would change the way she felt.

Her mother was totally confused. She knew something was dreadfully wrong, but could not imagine what had brought on such horrible reactions in her daughter, a daughter who was the eternal optimist. Her mother said, "I can't help you unless you tell me what happened. If your father and I did something so horrible, let us know before you completely crucify us."

"Mama," she said, "how can you stand there and tell me that I can't give up, how can you tell me to finish what I start? How can you do that to me? You can't possibly know what I had to face today. You and daddy have fed me these lines for years, and like a fool I believed them, well not any more!"

"Honey," her mother said, "If you don't tell me what is bothering you, I will never be able to help you try and sort through all of this. Calm down and tell me what's really eating at you."

"Today, mama, I was called a n_____. Of course, I have heard the word used before, and I've heard it used on television. But I have never been confronted with the word—to my face. Mama, they spat on me. They spat in my face. Now mama, you can't expect me to go back there. You can't expect me to look for good in those people. You can't expect me to stand up to this kind of abuse. I know you mama, and you wouldn't, you couldn't want me to have to contend with this and try to learn at the same time."

Her mama listened, her heart breaking as her daughter talked. Her eyes filled with tears, and she told her daughter, "It's not what I think that's important, it's what you think." She told her mama, "Well I know what I feel, and by the Grace of God, I will withdraw from that University at first light tomorrow morning."

Her mama said, "That choice is yours, and even though your father and I want more than anything for you to finish your dream, I would never want you to do anything that would jeopardize your health and well being. But if you will listen to me for just one moment, I have a short story I would like to tell you, one that I have not told any of my daughters. When your father and I decided to purchase this property, the very place where you are standing today, a man, whose home is three miles up the road, did everything in his power to block the sale. Although we couldn't prove it, he had our cattle killed, and one night one of our crops was mysteriously destroyed. Your father and I could have easily backed down, and probably should have, considering that your oldest sister was just a baby. But your father and I decided to see it through. We told my father, and oddly enough he had some friends in high places that stepped in to help resolve the problem. You see, honey, we could have given up, we could have believed that all people were bad, and we could have allowed the other people to win, but we said no. This is what we wanted, there was no good reason why we couldn't have it, and we decided to stick it out, no matter what the cost."

"But, mama," she said, "I am not you or daddy, I will not take that from anyone." "So then," her mother said, "what you are telling me is that you are going to allow someone to destroy your dreams. You are going to let someone dictate how you will spend the rest of your life. You are going to lie down, and allow someone to take away from you the one thing that is truly yours?" The pain she felt was too great, and all she could hear was her mother's voice spouting what she felt was useless wisdom for today's society.

As she left the room, her mother uttered these last words, "Look inside yourself; look to your inner strength." She thought to herself again, "I've heard and believed in those words all my life. And today all these words are meaningless. My code for life has been shattered, for good."

The next morning as she left for school, she told her mother that she had made a decision—a decision that made no sense to her right then, but in time she hoped it would. Although her mother was eager to know what her daughter had decided, she did not push, she just said, "Have the best day of your life."

That evening, she went home and told her mother that she had decided to stay in school. Not because she believed in her parents' code for life, but because she wanted to "show them all." She told her mother, "Don't expect me to believe that there is good in everyone; that if I do right, right will come my way; and that I should give people a second chance." She did not believe that worked for her anymore. Her mother never said a word; she just turned her head and smiled. Somehow she knew her daughter would be all right.

More than twenty-five years have passed since that incident, and she rarely speaks of that day any more. The day that changed her life forever. Although she vowed to change her "code for life," time helped her to resolve the conflicts and heal the pain she felt that day. She now knows that: (1) there is good in "most" people; (2) there comes a time when you should quit, but not without a good fight; (3) you do right, because it is right; (4) some people deserve a second and maybe even a third chance; (5) it is important, but not necessary, to finish what you start; (6) you should give yourself the right to make mistakes; (7) one's true strengths come from within; and (8) following any traumatic situation you must give yourself time to heal. It is your right.

In memory of the friends whose lives were cut short, and to my parents for trying to make it all make sense.

CHAPTER 4

Nightingale on Healing

POLDI TSCHIRCH, PHD, RN, CS

No single individual has had a more profound influence on the modern profession of nursing than its acknowledged founder Florence Nightingale (1820–1910). She gained international reknown and enormous prestige from her work as superintendent of nurses at the English General Military Hospitals during the Crimean War (1854–1856). She was one of the most effective and influential advocates for social reform in the 19th century. Her School of Nursing at St. Thomas' Hospital in London, which opened in 1860, served as a model for nursing education. Her conceptual model and moral vision of nursing shaped the profession during its formative years in the latter half of the 19th century.

Nightingale's model, in its interpretation of the nurse's role in relation to healing, offers fundamental and unchanging truths about the unique contribution of nurses to patient care. The concept of healing plays a central role in her definitions of health, illness, and nursing. She places the nurse at the center of the healing endeavor. She was the first to clearly articulate the nurse's role as healing presence, as the caregiver *principally* responsible for creating a healing environment. She advocated the use of the tools of science *as they further the healing mission.* She placed the patient at the center of the nurse's concern, with all observations and attention focused on the responses and needs of the patient as a person. While the context and content of nursing practice have changed dramatically, this vision of the nurse's role is timeless. This paper will examine the place of healing within Nightingale's conceptions of health and illness, the role of the nurse in creating a healing environment, and will critically evaluate the implications of her 19th-century model for nurses in the 21st century.

CONCEPTIONS ON HEALTH AND HEALING

Nightingale's text *Notes on Nursing* (1898) was a critical contribution to nursing reform and nursing education. This widely read and influential work presented her definition of nursing, her understanding of the concepts of sickness and health, and the relationship of the laws of hygiene and sanitation to the promotion of health. Although not a textbook of nursing (it did not describe methods of nursing practice), it established a philosophy for trained nursing with the patient as the focus of the nurse's work.

Nightingale conceptualizes illness as the physical manifestation of the body's healing processes:

> *Shall we begin by taking it as a general principle—that all disease, at some period or other of its course, is a more or less reparative process, not necessarily accompanied with suffering: an effort of nature to remedy a process of poisoning or of decay, which has taken place weeks, months, sometimes years beforehand, unnoticed, the termination of the disease being then, while the antecedent process was going on, determined? (Nightingale, 1898, p. 7)*

The symptoms of disease represent the body's effort to restore health, efforts that can be impaired by insufficient attention to creating the proper conditions for healing to occur:

> *The symptoms or the sufferings generally considered to be inevitable and incident to the disease are very often not symptoms of the disease at all, but of something quite different—of the want of fresh air, or of light, or of warmth, or of quiet, or of cleanliness, or of punctuality and care in the administration of diet, of each or of all of these. The reparative process which Nature has instituted and which we call disease, has been hindered by some want of knowledge or attention, in one or in all of these things, and pain, suffering, or interruption of the whole process sets in. (Nightingale, 1898, p. 8)*

Her conception of wellness identifies a health continuum:

> *The same laws of health or of nursing, for they are in reality the same, obtain among the well as among the sick. The breaking of them produces only a less violent consequence among the former than among the latter—and this sometimes, not always. (Nightingale, 1898, p. 9)*

Illness occurs when the body's normal processes are overwhelmed by environmental stressors or deprivations. Wellness is the state resulting from proper attention to the elements of or necessary conditions for health: fresh air, sufficient light, warmth, quiet, cleanliness and proper diet. Her careful, detailed observations of patterns of illness and experience with the filthy conditions of 19th-century hospitals provided a strong basis for her views.

Nightingale's definitions of health and illness are further refined in the paper *Sick Nursing and Health Nursing,* (1894), which was read at the International Congress of Charities, Correction and Philanthropy held in Chicago in 1893:

> *What is sickness? Sickness or disease is nature's way of getting rid of the effects of conditions which have interfered with health. It is nature's attempt to cure. . . . What is health? Health is not only to be well, but to be able to use well every power we have. (p. 444)*

In this paper, Nightingale articulates a powerful definition of health. It is not simply the absence of disease, but a state of full realization of the powers of body, mind, and spirit.

Nightingale's conceptions of health and illness were shaped by long-held beliefs within the scientific community about the functions of the body and the relationship between the environment, behavior, and illness. The body was seen as a system in which all local phenomena affected the wellbeing of the whole organism, which depended on maintaining equilibrium between bodily resources and the demands placed on them (Smith-Rosenberg & Rosenberg, 1973). The economic model of the nervous system, widely espoused in the 19th century, represents this conceptual framework. The body was believed to have a finite store of energy and overstimulation could lead to depletion of nervous force, debility, and illness (Sicherman, 1978). This view is evident in Nightingale's description of the central concern of nursing. "[Nursing] ought to signify the proper use of fresh air, light, warmth, cleanliness, quiet, and the proper selection and administration of diet—all at the least expense of vital power to the patient" (Nightingale, 1898, p. 8).

Nightingale was committed to a holistic view of the body/mind/environment interaction. Illness arose when the body's natural healing powers were overwhelmed by violations of the principles of sanitation and hygiene in unhealthy environments. This understanding was a critical element in her formulation of the nurse's role.

CREATING A HEALING ENVIRONMENT

Nightingale's definition of nursing flows from her conceptions of health and illness:

> *What is nursing? Both kinds of nursing [sick nursing and health nursing] are to put us in the best possible conditions for nature to restore or to preserve health—to prevent or to cure disease or injury."* (Nightingale, 1894, p. 446)

She places nurses at the center of the healing endeavor. She had little faith in therapeutic interventions as such. Their efficacy arose from the extent to which they foster the body's healing processes:

> *It is often thought that medicine is the curative process. It is no such thing; medicine is the surgery of functions, as surgery proper is that of limbs and organs. Neither can do anything but remove obstructions; neither can cure; nature alone cures. (Nightingale, 1898, p. 133)*

She defines distinct and different roles for nursing and medicine. In her schema, the physician is responsible for identification of causes of disruption in normal bodily functions, determination of the effects on body systems and removal of these "obstructions" to the body's healing processes. The nurse creates the environment in which healing takes place, through careful attention to the condition of the patient's environment, both external and internal, and detailed and constant observation of responses to environmental influences. Her actions and her caring presence focus on promoting natural healing processes.

The External Environment

The word "atmosphere" appears frequently in Nightingale's writings, and is of concern to her on several levels—the health of the larger environment, the patient's immediate physical environment, and the body's inner environment. A "pure atmosphere" is an important consideration in selecting the site for hospitals. The occurrence and spread of infectious diseases like cholera, dysentery, tuberculosis, and smallpox were directly attributable to the accumulation of filth, crowded living conditions, and water contamination characteristic of life in many crowded 19th-century cities. The same conditions prevailed in most hospitals before the reform movement in which Nightingale, and the trained nurse, played such a key role in the second half of the 19th century. The striking success of her work and that of the Army Sanitary Commission in reducing death rates from 42% to 2% through proper sanitation measures and improving hygiene and diet in the military hospitals in the Crimea (1854–1856) provided clear evidence of the impact of environment on disease incidence (Kalisch & Kalisch, 1986). Much of her reform career was devoted to advocacy for public hygiene principles in the hospital, workhouse, and home environment.

Nightingale's emphasis on the importance of environmental influences in sustaining the body's natural healing powers is reflected in the detailed attention given to every aspect of the patient's environment:

The very first canon of nursing, the first and the last thing upon which a nurse's attention must be fixed, the first essential to a patient, without which all the rest you can do for him is as nothing, with which I had almost said you may leave all the rest alone, is this: To keep the air he breathes as pure as the external air, without chilling him. (Nightingale, 1898, p. 12)

She offered detailed instructions on how to air the patient's room without sacrificing necessary warmth. Her suggestions for the pavilion design, positioning and size of windows, spacing of beds in relation to windows, space in cubic feet allotted to each patient in *Notes on Hospitals* (1863) reflects the critical importance of adequate ventilation and light in creating a healthful environment. These instructions on providing space, light, and air recur constantly in her work on army hospital reform, rural hygiene, district nursing of the poor, and the structure for workhouse infirmaries.

She devoted a section in *Notes on Nursing* (1898) to "Health of Houses," detailing the hazards of untrapped drain pipes, dirty carpets, unswept chimneys, old papered walls, and the oblong sink, which she considered an "abomination." "That great surface of stone, which is always left wet, is always exhaling into the air" (p. 26). She viewed society as a whole, rich and poor, as ignorant of the laws of hygiene:

I have met just as strong a stream of sewer air coming up the back staircase of a grand London house from the sink, as I have ever met at Scutari; and I have seen the rooms in that house all ventilated by the open doors, and the passages all unventilated by the closed windows, in order that as much of the sewer air as possible might be conducted into and retained in the bedrooms. It is wonderful. (Nightingale, 1898, p. 26)

Attention to cleanliness and care of bedding were essential to the healing environment. The effluvia emitted by the diseased body poisoned the atmosphere and interfered with the healing process. It was essential that the nurse give meticulous attention to the "healing space" surrounding the body:

> . . . *if she allows her sick to remain unwashed, or their clothing to remain on them after being saturated with perspiration or other excretion, she is interfering injuriously with the natural processes of health just as effectually as if she were to give the patient a dose of slow poison by the mouth.*
>
> *The amount of relief and comfort experienced by sick after the skin has been carefully washed and dried, is one of the commonest observations made at a sick bed. But it must not be forgotten that the comfort and relief so obtained are not all. They are, in fact, nothing more than a sign that the vital powers have been relieved by removing something that was oppressing them. (Nightingale, 1898, p. 93)*

The Inner Environment

Another important nursing role was to support the patient's healing potential by attempting to recreate the natural balance within the body. Nightingale's views in this area clearly reflect her holistic view of health and illness, in which one threatened system jeopardizes the whole organism. The nurse must protect the patient from noxious stimuli that drain vital energy, thus impairing the body's natural healing powers. She makes a very clear linkage between the health of mind and body. Stimuli that create anxiety or emotional distress sap vital healing energy, thus, her very specific strictures about anticipating needs and maintaining watch over the patient's schedule, mail and visitors:

> *Apprehension, uncertainty, waiting, expectation, fear of surprise, do a patient more harm than any exertion. Remember, he is face to face with his enemy all the time, internally wrestling with him, having long imaginary conversations with him. Rid him of his adversary quickly, is a first rule with the sick. (Nightingale, 1898, p. 38)*

She was also concerned about the effect of noise on the patient's well-being. She viewed it as essential that the nurse create a calm and quiet environment, conducive to rest and healing. Her instructions were again very specific: distinguishing "necessary" from "unnecessary" (and more harmful) noise, how to awaken a patient, the way to walk and speak in the patient's presence. "A nurse who rustles (I am speaking of nurses professional and unprofessional) is the horror of a patient, though perhaps he does not know why" (Nightingale, 1898, p. 47).

She was very sensitive to the impact of the physical environment on the patient's state of mind:

> *To any but an old nurse, or an old patient, the degree would be quite inconceivable to which the nerves of the sick suffer from seeing the same walls, the same ceiling, the same surroundings during a long confinement to one or two rooms. . . The nervous frame really suffers as much from this as the digestive organs from long monotony of diet, as e.g., the soldier from his twenty-one years "boiled beef."* (Nightingale, 1898, p. 58)

She felt that whenever possible the nurse should avoid confining the patient to one room. She scoffed at contemporaries who refused to place flowers or plants in the sick-room because of their misplaced views about the unhealthiness of growing things in the sick room. She suggested (1969) that variety in the shape, color and hue of the objects in the patient's room are "actual means of recovery" (Nightingale, 1898, p. 59).

Diet was another important aspect of strengthening the patient's inner environment. She was very critical of the lack of attention to diet paid by most caregivers. "Every careful observer of the sick will agree in this that thousands of patients are annually starved in the midst of plenty, from want of attention to the ways which alone make it possible for them to take food" (Nightingale, 1898, p. 63). She recommended careful consideration of the patient's needs and habits to determine when, how much and what type of nourishment should be offered. She offered specific advice about how to prepare and serve eggs, vegetables, beef tea, and arrowroot; how to keep milk fresh and the follies of serving gelatin. The focus was on close observation of the patient's needs and responses to diet treatment.

Using the Tools of Science for Healing

Nightingale viewed nursing as proper work for women, based on women's caring nature and Christian duty. She did not consider a womanly caring nature sufficient to provide effective care of the sick, however. She viewed scientific training and development of method and discipline essential to nursing work:

Nursing the sick is an art, and an art requiring an organized, practical and scientific training, for nursing is the skilled servant of medicine, surgery and hygiene . . . Training is to teach the nurse how God makes health and how He makes disease. Training is to teach a nurse to know her business, that is, to observe exactly in such stupendous issues as life and death, health and disease . . . Training is to teach the nurse how to handle the agencies within our control which restore health and life, in strict, intelligent obedience to the physician's or surgeon's power and knowledge; how to keep the health mechanism prescribed to her in gear. (Nightingale, 1894, p. 446)

Training in the principles of hygiene and sanitation, care of the patient and the home or ward were essentials. Most important was training in skills of observation:

The most important practical lesson that can be given to nurses is to teach them what to observe—how to observe—what symptoms indicate improvement—what are the reverse—which are of importance—which are of none—which are the evidence of neglect—and of what kind of neglect. (Nightingale, 1898, p. 105)

Her own prescriptions for patient care were based on her meticulous observations and recording of data of all kinds relating to the health of patients. The importance of careful observation of patient responses, habits and needs is integrated throughout *Notes on Nursing.* In every section, she identifies the type of observations that must be made in regard to diet, rest, warmth, mood; she lectures the reader on false conclusions that can be drawn by the careless observer or nurse who poorly understands the laws of hygiene. Science was a tool to be used in observing the manifestations of disease, which represented the body's healing efforts, and understanding how to sustain these healing energies. One of her most important contributions to nursing reform was in building a bridge between the womanly art of caring and the tools of science.

THE NURSE AS A HEALING PRESENCE

Nightingale sought to establish nursing as a legitimate field of endeavor for women outside the home, within a 19th-century culture and ideology of womanhood which perceived woman as physically and intellectually more fragile than men; more spiritual and moral (Smith-Rosenberg & Rosenberg, 1973). Women possessed moral authority within the home, which was their proper sphere. The physical and moral dangers of public life, including the filthy, disorderly and dangerous world of the 19th-century hospital, were not for them. Nightingale's personal history is a fascinating study in the struggles of one woman to break free of the constraints of this ideology and carve a meaningful role in public life. One element in her success in creating her own reform career and in legitimizing trained nursing as an acceptable endeavor was her linkage of 19th-century beliefs about women's caring nature and caring as a proper role for women with scientific training.

Like other women social reformers in the 19th century, she sought to expand the boundaries of the "home," which was women's proper sphere, to include the larger society in relation to issues that concerned the health and welfare of women, children, and families. The presence of trained nurses in hospitals would bring not only scientific understanding about principles of hygiene, sanitation, and disease management, but also an uplifting moral atmosphere.

Consistent with her holistic view of health and illness, the patient's moral state influenced and was influenced by disease. In her report to the governors of the Harley Street Nursing Home (Verney, 1970), where she served as superintendent from 1853–1854, before her appointment as superintendent of nurses in the Crimea, she described both the medical and moral progress of her patients. She reviewed the status of the patient population:

Of those now in the house:

3 cases are waiting for death. . .

To these the house has been an incalculable benefit—miracles of Medical Science, they have benefited still more morally

3 cases are being rapidly cured of obstinate skin disease
1 of self-mismanagement
2 are greatly benefiting
7 are either trifling, hysterical or incurable cases
───
16

It is therefore concluded that

> I. *Of the Patients admitted during the last six months*
> *4/12 have derived the greatest benefit*
> *3/12 neither good nor harm*
> *5/12 have manifestly deteriorated morally and medically.*
> *(pp. 14-15)*

Her representation of the patient's moral condition in this report reflects her holistic view of health and illness. Every dimension of the individual's nature—physical, emotional, spiritual, and moral—is engaged in the healing process. Her conception of nursing built upon women's caring nature and the nurse as a "Christian soldier" in the battle against disease, taking action against the ignorance, dirt and disorder that lead to disease and moral decay.

The nurse herself was an instrument of healing, not only through her actions, but through her person and presence. Her voice, her step, her movements, even the rustle of her skirts have an impact on the patient's well-being. Her recommendations for nursing education reflect the need for sound moral character and moral training for the good nurse:

> *Discipline is the essence of moral training. The best lady trainer of probationer nurses I know says, "It is education, instruction, training—all that, in fact, goes to the full development of our faculties, moral, physical, and spiritual." (Nightingale, 1894, p. 447)*

Her model for the nurse training school, with its strict rules for the appearance, conduct and regulation of the student's behavior both on the wards and in the nurses' residence reflect her convictions about the importance of the nurse's moral character in promoting public acceptance of the field as respectable work for women and in exercising a positive influence on the patient's physical, emotional, and moral well-being.

Nightingale in the 21st Century

No individual has had greater impact on the trajectory of nursing's development as a healing practice and an intellectual discipline than Florence Nightingale. Her legacy to contemporary nurses is a subject of ongoing debate within the communities of nursing and feminist scholars. Some see her as a visionary thinker and reformer, others as a product of the Victorian age, whose vision for nursing is limited by the gender, class, and racial biases of her time. Historian Susan Reverby argues that the continuing struggle of contemporary nurses for professional self-determination is an outgrowth of the failure of nursing's ideology of duty to empower nurses to achieve this goal. Joann Ashley's groundbreaking work *Hospitals, Paternalism and the Role of the Nurse* (1976) documented the systematic oppression of the profession by male-dominated hierarchies in hospitals and the medical profession, an oppression perpetuated by nursing leaders who failed to effectively challenge male authority. It can be argued that Nightingale, as the principal architect of nursing's ideology, limited her vision for nursing by accepting and working within 19th century social conventions, with the results Ashley and Reverby describe.

Given the influence of the 19th-century social context on Nightingale's work, can her vision still provide meaning and direction for nursing as the 21st century approaches? The answer is unquestionably, yes. Changing perspectives on her struggles with 19th century sexual politics may affect our understanding of her contributions as a leader. However, her profound and original insights on the nature of health and illness, on the process of healing and the place of nursing within that process are not bound by time or social context.

Nightingale's conception of the nurse as healing presence and creator of a healing environment has great relevance for the profession today. Some of her specific concerns in relation to the patient's environment in the hospital and home were based in the problems of the 19th-century world she inhabited, and have been resolved by the relative success of the public health reform movement she supported, at least in modern industrialized nations. Proper sanitation, pest control, sewage treatment, and clean water have resulted in dramatic reductions in many infectious diseases, a result she demonstrated effectively in the military hospitals of the Crimea. Nations lacking the resources to adequately provide these services continue to struggle with patterns of illness much like those of Nightingale's era.

Nightingale's specific concerns with sinks, carpets, and petticoats was contextual; the relevance of her central concern for the patient's environment and its impact on healing emerges. The cleanliness of the hospital environment is still essential to the patient's well being. Her patients were at risk for dysentery and typhoid, ours for methicillin-resistant staphylococcus aureus. It would be an interesting challenge to re-write some of the chapters in *Notes on Nursing:* "Noise," "Variety," "Taking Food," "What Food," for the 1990s. Sources of noise and methods of administering nutrients have changed. The existence of interaction between patient and environment has not.

Nightingale's concern that the nurse use the tools of science to support the healing process is one that contemporary nurses would do well to revisit. Her intent was to enhance the nurse's ability to support "nature's healing powers" through use of scientific knowledge. The revolution in science and technology over the last century has created a climate in which the ultimate goal of the healing endeavor seems to become lost. The tools of science are often used to "engineer" the healing process, rather than to nurture it. The tools, rather than the body's healing potential, are seen as the true source of healing and technology dominates the interactions between patients and caregivers. Promotion of sleep and rest, comfort, concern for proper nutrition, traditional concerns of nursing and essential elements in supporting healing, too often receive far less attention than round-the-clock interventions and monitoring activities.

Contemporary nurse theorists and clinicians challenge this paradigm, in a sense "re-discovering" or refocusing and expanding upon Nightingale's conceptions. Energy is a central concept in the work of theorists Martha Rogers and Myra Levine, echoing Nightingale's focus on the patient's "vital powers." The holistic nursing movement emphasizes interventions that support the "inner" environment's healing potential. Relaxation exercises, guided imagery, biofeedback, and therapeutic touch are predicated on the mind/body interaction that Nightingale recognized in her observations about the influence of anxiety and the patient's emotional state on healing. In her work on clinical knowledge development, theorist Patricia Benner (1984) defines "the helping role" as one of the domains of nursing practice. Two competencies she has described as essential elements of that domain are "The Healing Relationship: Creating a Climate for and Establishing a Commitment to Healing" and "Presencing: Being with a Patient." Nightingale saw the nurse herself as an agent of healing, with her tone of voice, expression, movements, appearance influencing the patient's well-being. The current interest in presence as a tool for healing acknowledges the relevance of her thinking.

Nightingale's conception of the nurse's healing role represents the core of nursing's unique contribution to patient care. The nurse *is* a healing presence. The nurse is the caregiver *principally* responsible for creating a healing environment. It is the nurse's responsibility to use the tools of science *as they further the healing mission*. The patient is the center of the nurse's concern and the nurse's observations focus on the person, responses and needs of that individual. Her articulation of this conception of the nurse was visionary and of timeless importance. The context and content of nursing practice has changed dramatically over the past 150 years, but our role is still as she envisioned it. We sustain the patient's potential for healing, with the tools of science and our healing hands.

REFERENCES

Ashley, J. (1976). *Hospitals, paternalism and the role of the nurse.* New York: Teachers College Press.

Benner, P. (1984). *From novice to expert: Excellence and power in clinical nursing practice.* Menlo Park: Addison-Wesley.

Kalisch, P. A., & Kalisch, B. J. (1986). *The advance of American nursing.* Boston: Little, Brown and Co.

Nightingale, F. (1863). *Notes on hospitals* (3rd ed.). London: Longman, Green.

Nightingale, F. (1898). *Notes on Nursing: What it is and what it is not.* New York: Appleton & Co. (Original work published 1860).

Nightingale, F. (1894). Sick nursing and health nursing. In J. S. Billings & H. M. Hurd, (Eds.), *Hospitals, dispensaries and nursing.* Baltimore: The Johns Hopkins Press.

Reverby, S. (1987). *Ordered to care: The dilemma of American nursing, 1850-1945.* Cambridge: Cambridge University Press.

Sicherman, B. (1978). The uses of a diagnosis: Doctors, patients and neurasthenia. In J. W. Leavitt & R. L. Numbers (Eds.), *Sickness and health in America,* pp. 25-38. Madison: The University of Wisconsin Press.

Smith-Rosenberg, C., & Rosenberg, R. (1973). The female animal: Medical and biological views of woman and her role in nineteenth century America. *The Journal of American History, 60,* 332-335.

Verney, H. (Ed.). (1970). *Florence Nightingale at Harley Street: Her reports to the governors of her nursing home, 1853-1854.* London: J. M. Dent & Sons, Ltd.

CHAPTER 5

Therapeutic Capacity: The Critical Variance in Nursing Practice

PHYLLIS J. WATERS, MS, RN

M. JEAN DAUBENMIRE, MSN, RN

Experienced nurses, educators, patients, and their families recognize that there are observable differences in how nurses practice. In the hospital, one frequently hears nurses characterize another's practice. "She's a great nurse; I'd be glad to have her take care of my mother"; "The nurses on that unit will take good care of you," or alternately, "I wouldn't want a member of my family put on that unit." What makes the difference? Is it clinical judgment, technical competence, caring? Or is it all of these factors and more? While all nurses are assumed to have some basic competencies, there are nurses who appear to have a capacity to effect observable therapeutic outcomes and healing experiences. What constitutes the critical variance in practice among nurses that leads to observable differences in patient experiences and outcomes? How do nurses facilitate healing? Are there ways of helping nurses to expand their therapeutic capabilities?

In our search for answers to these questions, we have coined the term "therapeutic capacity" as a way of referencing nursing practice that produces healing outcomes—"the unique capabilities that the nurse brings to the healing environment to evoke the endogenous healing process." The healthcare paradigm within which one practices influences the therapeutic capacity of nurses and the healing experiences of patients. We have developed a conceptual framework to describe therapeutic capacity. Though early in its development, we hope this conceptual framework describing therapeutic capacity, the process involved, its development,

The authors wish to acknowledge the significant contributions of Sharon Stout Shaffer.

and its impact on patient outcomes will be useful in creating new models of practice to facilitate healing.

HEALTHCARE PARADIGM INFLUENCES

The healthcare paradigm within which nurses practice has a determining influence on their professional thinking and behavior. The dominant paradigm that creates the context for contemporary nursing defines health as the positive pole on a continuum with illness as the negative pole, assuming varying states between these two points.

This health vs. illness dichotomy sets the stage for the patient being perceived as less than whole or in need of repair, the nurse and other providers being perceived as the "fixers." Most healthcare structures, processes, and outcomes reflect this perspective. In this dichotomous paradigm, nurses have primarily focused on the presenting problems of the patient as they relate to the diagnosed disease process and treatment plans. Therefore, nursing education emphasizes identifying problems and delineating the nurse's role in problem resolution. As a result, many nurses perceive their role as "doing battle" with the disease process on behalf of the patient. Their armament is their ability to assess, intervene, and effectively reverse the patient's disease or symptoms. The goal is to "fix" the patient's problems—the patient remains passive, healthcare providers active. Even the term "healthcare provider" implies the patient receives health from an outside source or provider.

Nurse–patient interactions are focused on getting the problem solved, not necessarily responding to the patient's needs as he or she perceives them. As a result, patients may experience nursing practice as highly instrumented, contrived, and in some instances, interpersonally indifferent. This type of interaction does not engage the patient. Since the patient is the one who possesses what is necessary to heal, this lack of engagement does not serve to facilitate or support the healing process. Some provider interactions are so stressful to patients that they actually interfere with healing.

As a profession, nursing has espoused caring for the "whole person," with "whole" encompassing physical, mental, emotional, and spiritual aspects. However, it is difficult for nurses to relate to patients as "whole" while practicing in a paradigm that views health as the absence of disease. With wholeness and health here viewed as synonymous, patients not in perfect health are viewed as less than whole. Nurses who wish to work with the "whole" person in this paradigm focus on integrating physical, mental, emotional, and spiritual care interventions in their plan to "fix" the patient. To truly care for the "whole" person, however, the nurse must function in a paradigm that views patients as inherently whole beings and healing as a natural process.

An Alternate Paradigm

Though not dominant in the healthcare industry in the United States, wholeness or healing paradigms are gaining wider recognition and application. One aspect of this shift is a greater awareness of energy as a dimension of human existence, a move beyond an exclusive force or the materiality of person. Beginning with Einstein, physicists have progressively substantiated that there is an essential connection among all forms of energy. It is becoming generally accepted that energy forms do not relate as independent entities one to the other, but rather as dynamic aspects of an interconnected web or whole (Capra, 1982). Martha Rogers' pioneering work in 1970 applied the concept of "energy fields" to nursing practice. Over 25 years ago, "Rogers introduced into nursing the concept that the fundamental unit of the living system was an energy field, coextensive with the environmental energy field" (Quinn, 1992). When Rogers first introduced her theory of nursing, it was considered quite revolutionary for its time. As advances in quantum physics, biology, psychoneuroimmunology, and other sciences as well as philosophy have become better known, her work has steadily been validated and expanded.

Building on Rogers' theory as well as the work of Bohm (1980) and Bentov (1978), Margaret Newman (Newman & Marchione, 1986) developed the theory of health as expanding consciousness. Newman defines consciousness as "the information capacity of the system (in this case the human being): that is the ability of the system to interact with environment. Consciousness includes not only the cognitive and affective awareness we normally associate with consciousness but also the interconnectiveness of the entire living system that includes physiochemical maintenance and growth processes as well as the immune system. This pattern of information is part of a larger, undivided pattern of an expanding universe" (p. 38). In this paradigm of health, illness is recognized as an opportunity for expanding consciousness. According to Rogers (in Newman & Marchione, 1986), "health and illness are simply expressions of the life process—one no more important than the other"

(p. 4). In this context, the nurse's focus is on recognizing life patterns and how they manifest in the patient's experience.

In this paradigm, the patient has the central role. The nurse and other providers are supports and guides. Nurse–client interactions are focused on recognizing life patterns, their meaning to the patient, and the patient's response and choices relative to these patterns. As Barrett describes it, "Nursing care is concerned with patterning the environmental field. The nurse, together with the client, patterns the environment to promote healing and comfort. Regardless of the practice modality being used, the nurse's objective is to pattern the client's environment to promote health and well being" (Barrett, 1990 referenced in Quinn).

The endogenous healing process is a natural phenomenon that moves one toward harmonious energy patterns and expanded consciousness. Scandrett-Hibdon and Freel (1989, pp. 66–67) have identified six assumptions relative to the endogenous healing process:

1. Human beings are whole with unique and varying patterns.
2. Changes are constant in the process of living.
3. Health is a process of becoming.
4. Disease can be viewed as a disharmonizing energy pattern.
5. Humans are consciously participating in the healing process.
6. Healing is a process in which humans attain harmony within themselves and the environment.

An example is useful in demonstrating the differences in these two paradigms. A woman named Sara is diagnosed with cancer. She seeks help from a provider who operates within the dominant paradigm of a health–illness dichotomy. Sara goes through a series of tests to pinpoint the extent and nature of her problem. A treatment plan is developed to specifically manage her problem in terms of eliminating or ameliorating the cancer. All provider and nursing activities would be focused on controlling the cancer. Sara would be expected to "comply" with the treatment plan. The nursing staff focus on her physical, mental, emotional, and spiritual needs as it relates to her experience of the problem of cancer. Sara's interactions with the nursing staff and other healthcare providers all center around managing the problem of her cancer and her responses to it.

Now let us assume Sara sought help from healthcare providers that operate within the paradigm of health as expanding consciousness. She undergoes a series of diagnostic exams that help identify the nature and the type of illness that she is experiencing. Concurrently the nursing staff explore with her life patterns that are being reflected in this state of illness. Sara would have the opportunity to discover how these patterns may be affecting her life—physically, mentally, emotionally, and spiritually. The nursing staff would create an environment focused on engaging her endogenous healing process. The nursing staff's interactions and energy exchanges with Sara would be recognized as part of this healing environment and consciously directed. Sara would help determine what she would like to repattern as part of her treatment plan in response to this illness episode. As you can see there are similarities and differences in practice reflected in these paradigms. Clinical interventions selected for Sara may have many similarities. However the caring dynamics and the transpersonal experiences would be quite different.

Nursing has the opportunity to play a key role in shifting the health-care paradigm. In fact, nursing theorists and researchers have been in the forefront of describing "wholeness" paradigms and researching practice modalities that focus on repatterning and healing. However, these concepts and modalities have been implemented on a very limited basis in the service arena.

Though nursing research has implicitly addressed the nurse's potential to facilitate healing outcomes, the underlying phenomena responsible for this process has not been definitively described. The absence of a conceptual framework for these phenomena limits understanding and the development of practices that purposefully employ the nurse as a therapeutic agent. It was from this perceived need that we developed our concept of *therapeutic capacity*.

THERAPEUTIC CAPACITY

The concept of therapeutic capacity proposes that the essence of nursing lies in creating a healing environment and in engaging the patient's consciousness in the healing process. Nursing practice includes and transcends clinical judgment, technical intervention, and caring dynamics. The transcending factor is the nurse's ability to establish a channel of mutual consciousness that facilitates the patient's endogenous healing process. In our model, therapeutic capacity has three dimensions: clinical interventions, caring dynamics, and transpersonal efficacy. Clinical interventions are implemented in a manner consistent with the clinical setting and plan of care. The nurse–patient caring dynamics are appropriately responsive to the patient's personality, culture, and needs. The nurse's transpersonal connection with the patient evolves from a mutual process of pattern recognition and resonance.

The following diagram illustrates these dimensions:

$$(CI + CD)^{TE} = \text{Therapeutic Capacity (TC)}$$

where (CI) Clinical Interventions: Clinical judgments and techniques focused on resolving or managing specific health problems or enhancing health.

    (CD) Caring Dynamics: psychosocial, relational, and communication interactions focused on providing support and comfort.

    (TE) Transpersonal Efficacy: the ability to open a channel of mutual consciousness (shared corridor of consciousness) that facilitates the patient's endogenous healing process; multiplies the impact of clinical interventions and caring dynamics exponentially.

and therefore

$$\frac{\text{Therapeutic}}{\text{Capacity (TC)}} + \frac{\text{Open Client}}{\text{Energy Field}} = \frac{\text{Healing}}{\text{Encounter}}$$

Transpersonal efficacy is the *exponent* in therapeutic capacity. Transpersonal efficacy is defined as the ability to create a shared corridor of consciousness that facilitates the patient's endogenous healing process. To understand this aspect of therapeutic capacity we would like to describe what we mean by mutual or shared consciousness. As we begin to explore mutual (shared)consciousness, the focus is shifted from the behavior of the individual to the behavior patterns and processes occurring between persons. Traditional interaction research has provided little or no language and few strategies for empirically studying these processes. However, if we believe that health is expanding consciousness, it is essential to attempt to describe and study these processes.

In our framework, we propose that healing encounters occur when the patient and nurse "connect" through a shared corridor of consciousness. As interconnected energy fields, we share the same universal source of consciousness or ground of being. According to Bohm, "there exists in our universe an unseen multidimensional pattern that is the ground, or basis for all things; this is the implicate order. Arising out of the implicate order is the explicate order, a kind of precipitate of the implicate order. The explicate order includes the tangibles of our world. These tangibles—the things we can see, touch, hear, feel—are so much more real to us than the underlying unseen pattern that we think the explicate order is primary, the real thing." Actually according to Bohm, the implicate order is primary, the explicate order arises periodically from the implicate, like waves appearing and disappearing on the surface of the ocean. The explicate, whatever form it may take, is a temporary manifestation of a total undivided pattern" (Newman & Marchione, 1986 pp. 12-13). "Pattern recognition is the heart of human interaction. It is basic to responding to the individuality of another person and therefore, basic to the health professional's effective use of self and therapeutic interaction. What we sense in terms of pattern is a function of our own level of awareness, sensitivity to self, and point of view" (Newman & Marchione, p. 18)

The client's endogenous healing process is engaged by the transpersonal efficacy of the nurse to create a shared corridor of consciousness:

Client's Endogenous Healing Process	Shared Corridor of Mutual Consciousness	Nurse's Transpersonal Efficacy
Awareness	Attunement	Centering
Intention	Convergence	Intentionality
Alignment	Resonancy	Connecting
Repatterning	Synchrony	Repatterning

Transformational Healing

This diagram proposes a beginning framework for exploring observable process patterns indicative of expanding consciousness and transformational healing. Because process is an inclusive, overlapping, integral part of a functioning whole, there is no intent that these processes be viewed in a step fashion.

The endogenous healing process of the client indicated in the first column has been described by Scandrett-Hibdon and Freel (1989) as inherent in all humans. Healing is a movement toward wholeness. "The ultimate goal of healing, and often its parallel growth, is the uniquely human phenomenon of human evolution in consciousness. Evolution of consciousness is the expanding of awareness and understanding about the self and the environment. Growth is the exercising of free will and learning from the lessons of consequences. Being conscious involves the interplay of awareness, choice and growth. The outcome of each healing is perceived and determined by the human involved" (Scandrett-Hibdon, 1989, p. 67). While the healing process is internal, recurring behaviors are observable and these are listed.

Transpersonal efficacy describes nurse behaviors (in column 3) that are exhibited through a conscious process of centering, intentionality, connecting and repatterning. These abilities enable the nurse to create a shared corridor of consciousness.

Many authors speak to the importance of *centering* as a way of being in touch with one's spirit, of increasing self-awareness, as preparation for therapeutic touch and foundation for holistic nursing. It is our belief that centering is essential in expanding consciousness in healing encounters. Centering is the process of being present to oneself. It is the quieting of the mind, of going inside to that sacred space that we all carry inside, a moving to that deeper dimension of being. "If we all pay attention to the spaces between our thoughts, we notice an energy there. This is our unconditional nature which we can draw upon for healing" (Welwood, 1992, p. 38).

Intentionality is a critical idea that merits increased exploration in nursing. Bohm (1980) states that every action starts from an intention in the implicate order. Intention is the behavior that can move one into conscious relationships. Chopra (1993) indicates that "intention is the active part of attention; it is the way we convert automatic processes into conscious ones" (p. 19). We define intent as "one's focused will." Involving spirit, mind, and body. The nurse can center and intend to be present, to be a healing force for the patient.

There is an emerging awareness of the importance of *connecting,* of understanding unitive consciousness—that we are not separate, that we are all one. Physicists state that the universe is an inseparable whole, a vast web of interacting, interweaving probabilities. As we become increasingly aware of this oneness—this interconnectedness, we can view the nurse-patient encounter as a dynamic, open, ever-changing energy system. There is a continuous multilevel exchange of energy between nurse and client. "The nurse does have a profound effect on the patient and we need to assume responsibility for awareness of this effect" (McKinergin & Daubenmire, 1994, p. 76). Dossey states "When our focus is toward a principle of relatedness and oneness, and away from fragmentation and isolation, health ensues" (Dossey, 1982, p. 112).

Repatterning interventions are based on Roger's Principle of Integrality of the continuous repatterning of human environmental fields and may include specific clinical interventions, comfort measures, caring dynamics or just being with the patient in your wholeness and helping the patient to identify with his or her wholeness.

Describing the patient–nurse connection and interactions experienced in *a shared corridor of consciousness* is difficult. The following terms drawn from research in energy field phenomena have been selected to describe the process: attunement, convergence, resonancy, and synchrony. Attunement and resonancy are internal processes and can not be observed, but can be reported as experienced states over times. Convergence and synchrony are observable processes which occur between two persons as they respond to each other in an encounter and may provide insight into the shared consciousness phenomena.

In the *attunement* or induction phase there is a continuous multilevel exchange of energy between nurse and patient that continues throughout the encounter. The nurse perceives the patient's wholeness from a centered state and listens at both a higher and deeper level. There is a feeling of oneness with nurse and patient which creates a healing space for the patient to increase awareness, begin appraisal and become involved in his or her own endogenous healing process. Attunement is described by Rush (1981) as a model of healing:

> *Healing is a multidimensional attunement of all component systems in dynamic interaction and interchange that results in a harmonic patterning of these systems into an interacting process that occurs at many levels of organization within the body during healing. (p. 192)*

Convergence is defined as "a process of increasing similarity in behavior, literally duplicating the actions and speech patterns of each other in various degrees and ways" (Daubenmire & Searles, 1982, p. 301).

Rogers defines *resonancy* as a continuous change from lower to higher frequency wave patterns in human and environmental fields (Rogers 1970). In an encounter framework, resonancy can be defined in terms of the intensity, frequency, rate, and fruition of one person's patterns rhythmically matching the patterns of another person. There seems to be an energy vibration that creates a sense of connection and communion, a sense of presence and unconditional love, a shift of consciousness from hopelessness to hope and powerlessness to power.

Synchrony is defined as a state in which the nurse and patient are transformed into a new state which is more than the sum of individual behaviors, the state of the dyad described as one unit. The nurse and pa-tient are one system and would be measured or studied as one unit. There seems to be an opening of conscious awareness to literally feeling others. There is a sense of communion and oneness. It is an "I–Thou" re-lationship. "It is through relationships that we become whole" (Bren-nan, 1993, p. 179). When people are not within the same frequency rate or cannot synchronize harmonically, it is extremely difficult to commu-nicate. "When two people do commune, the fields affect each other in a beautiful way. The pulsation of one field cause changes in the other which then build and create new changes in the first" (Brennan 1993, p. 180). It is at this level that there is the most potential for transforma-tional healing. Each encounter is an opportunity to heal and be healed

"We believe that nurse-patient relationships developed under stress have the potential for being intensified in time in either a positive or negative way. Relationships which might take days, weeks or months to develop under other circumstances are developed very quickly in the hospital or primary care setting" (Daubenmire & Searles, 1982, p. 309). Are there ways, then, nurses can become more conscious of their effect in these rela-tionships and intentionally develop healing encounters which have the po-tential to expand consciousness and evoke the endogenous healing process of the patient?

Based on literature reports and our own experiences, we propose that healing encounters between the nurse and patient can be described in two categories. The encounter may occur at a time when the patient is highly aware of his or her pattern, is open, resonates with the energy pat-tern of the nurse, and responds to the environment therapeutically. Under these circumstances, the patient may have a dramatic shift in pattern with only one encounter with a therapeutically capable nurse. More com-mon, however, is the cumulative impact of a series of healing encounters. In these instances, patients gain awareness, focus intention, align and repattern as a result of numerous encounters with a therapeutically capa-ble nurse or several therapeutically capable nurses. The power of this syn-chrony is achieved through shared states of consciousness.

As the exponent of therapeutic capacity, transpersonal efficacy cre-ates the critical variance in nursing practice. Clinical interventions and caring dynamics can be employed in the dominant paradigm of medical management as well as a healing paradigm. To facilitate healing, how-ever, the nurse and client need to connect through a corridor of shared consciousness.

$$\begin{array}{c}\text{Therapeutically}\\\text{Capable Nurse}\end{array} + \begin{array}{c}\text{Open Client}\\\text{Energy Field}\end{array} = \begin{array}{c}\text{Healing}\\\text{Encounter}\end{array}$$

Healing encounters provide the energy and awareness necessary for repatterning and expansion of consciousness.

SUMMARY AND IMPLICATIONS

Historically nursing theories and models have emphasized either a science or caring focus. After the introduction of Martha Roger's theory, a number of nurse researchers investigated and demonstrated the potential of energy field therapies. The most widely referenced of these efforts have been in the area of therapeutic touch. Krieger and her protégés have demonstrated that nurses who consciously intend to heal can do so by following a four step procedure which culminates in the transmission of "energy" between the nurse and client (Krieger, 1979). This process has been described and examined as a phenomenon discrete from other nursing efforts. Our review of the literature revealed that most theories, models and research, focus on one dimension of nursing and rarely describe the relationships among the dimensions. This conceptual framework proposes the integration of scientifically based clinical interventions, caring dynamics, and transpersonal efficacy. In order to be effective, we believe nurses need to be competent and effective in all of these dimensions.

In the discipline of nursing, most theoretical examinations and developments are being done within academic settings with limited testing in practice. In the meantime, the average nurse practices using principles taught in his or her basic educational program or by following examples of more experienced nurses in clinical settings. In academic programs, nursing students are either exposed to a wide range of theorists and directed to select a theory they feel most comfortable using in their practice or to combine principles from multiple theories. Some are taught a particular theory or model that has been selected by their faculty. Rarely do they have the experience of seeing their selected model practiced consistently in the clinical area. This ambiguity has created barriers to nursing achieving its full professional potential.

According to Kuhn (1970), it is common for developing disciplines to propose multiple theories. As the theories are subjected to rigorous testing "one paradigm gains almost universal acceptance" (Bramlett, Gueldner & Boettcher, 1993, p. 23). In this search, healing and nursing's role in the process can be a force for integrating important theories and principles.

Kritek (1994) identifies healing as a central nursing construct inherent to professional nursing's metaparadigm. This metaparadigm identifies four essential elements in any theoretical conceptualization of nursing: the nurse, the patient, the context and health. In our conceptual framework, healing involves the nurse and the patient interacting in a given context in response to a health experience in which the nurse works in a pattern of mutuality with the patient, facilitating healing in response to a patient's elicitation of nursing involvement and expertise. Nurses employ clinical intervention and caring dynamics skills while using their transpersonal efficacy to open a corridor of shared consciousness. The goal is to engage the patient's endogenous healing process. The use of healing as a central construct provides a way of integrating scientifically based clinical interventions, caring dynamics, and transpersonal efficacy. The question of finding ways of helping nurses to expand their therapeutic capabilities requires a significant increase in the collaborative and unified efforts among researchers, practitioners, and educators.

REFERENCES

Barrett, E. A. M. (1990). Health patterning with clients in a private practice environment. In E. A. M. Barrett (Ed.). *Visions of Rogers' science-based nursing.* New York: NLN Press.

Bentov, I. (1978). *Stalking the wild pendulum.* New York: E.P. Dutton.

Bohm, D. (1980). *Wholeness and the implicate order.* London: Routledge & Kegan Paul.

Bramlett, M. H., Gueldner, S. H., & Boettcher, J. H. (1993). Reflections on the science of unitary human beings in terms of Kuhmn's requirement for explanatory power. *The Journal of Regerian Nursing Science, 1*(1):22–35.

Brennan, B. A. (1993). *Light emerging: The journey of personal healing.* New York: Bantam.

Capra, F. (1982). *The turning point.* New York: Simon & Schuster.

Chopra, D. (1993) *Ageless body, timeless mind.* New York: Harmony.

Daubenmire, M. J., & Searles, S. (1982). A dyadic model for the study of convergence in nurse–patient interactions. In M. Davis (Ed.) *Interaction rhythms.* New York: Human Science Press.

Dossey, L. (1982). *Space, time and medicine.* Boston: Shamhala, p. 112.

Gerber, R. (1988). *Vibrational medicine.* Santa Fe, NM: Bear & Co.

Krieger, D. (1979). *Therapeutic touch: How to use your hands to heal.* Englewood Cliffs, NJ: Prentice Hall.

Kritek, P. B. (1994). *Healing, a central nursing construct.* Unpublished Doctoral Program White Paper, The University of Texas Medical Branch School of Nursing, Galveston, Texas.

Kuhn, T. (1970). *The structure of scientific revolutions.* Chicago: University of Chicago Press.

McKinergin, M., & Daubenmire, M. J. (1994, March). The healing process of presence. *Journal of Holistic Nursing, 12*(1) 65-81.

Newman, M. (1982). Time as an index of expanding consciousness with age. *Nursing Research, 31*(5): 290-293.

Newman, M. (1987a). Nursing's emerging paradigm: The diagnosis of pattern. In A. N. McLane (Ed.), *Classification of nursing diagnoses: Proceedings of the seventh conference.* North American Nursing Diagnosis Association, pp. 53-60. St. Louis, MO: Mosby.

Newman, M. (1987b). Patterning. In M. Duffy & N. J. Pender (Eds.), *Conceptual issues in health promotion. Report of proceedings of a Wingspread Conference,* pp. 36-50. Indianapolis: Sigma Theta Tau.

Newman, M. (1990). Newman's theory of health as praxis. *Nursing Science Quarterly, 3*(1): 37-41.

Newman, M. (1994). *Health as expanding consciousness,* 2nd ed. New York: NLN Press.

Newman, M., & Marchione, J. (1986). *Health as expanding consciousness.* St. Louis, MO: Mosby.

Parse, R. R. (1987). *Nursing science: Major paradigms, theories and critiques.* Philadelphia, PA: Saunders.

Pettigrew, J. (1990). Intensive nursing care: The ministry of presence. *Critical Care Nursing Clinics of North America, 2*(3): 503-508.

Phillips, P. (1993). A deconstruction of caring. *Journal of Advanced Nursing, 18*: 1554-1558.

Quinn, J. (1984). Therapeutic touch as energy exchange: Testing the theory. *Advances in Nursing Science, 6*(2): 42-49.

Quinn, J. (1989). Therapeutic touch as energy exchange: Replication and extension. *Nursing Science Quarterly, 2*(2): 79-87.

Quinn, J. (1992). Holding sacred space: The nurse as healing environment. *Holistic Nursing Practice, 6*(4): 26-36.

Rogers, M. E. (1970). *An introduction to the theoretical basis for nursing.* Philadelphia, PA: F. A. Davis.

Rush, J. E. (1981). *Toward a general theory of healing.* Washington, D.C. University Press of America.

Scandrett-Hibdon, S., & Freel, M. (1989). The endogenous healing process: Conceptual analysis. *Journal of Holistic Nursing, 7*(1): 66-71.

Welwood, J. (1992). The healing power of unconditional presence. *The Quest,* 35-40.

CHAPTER 6

A Healing Parable

MARY ANNE HANLEY, MA, RN

I had just returned home from three weeks of intensive Therapeutic Touch course work. Returning to the "real" world is never easy. As I decided to turn off the phone at midnight Diane called, "It's Shawn. He's in Connecticut. They're airlifting him to the hospital. Can you drive us?"

We were directed to a waiting room. Institutional green, it was the basic color in the older part of the hospital. The hospital was familiar; Diane and I had been students here. We experienced a sense of dislocation. We were in the wrong room.

Chaplains, nurses, residents, neurologists, and others stopped to provide detailed information, thinking that we understood. All Diane wanted to do was to see her son, Shawn. "Wait until he is cleaned up," they said.

As we sat waiting for dawn and news about Shawn's condition, Diane talked about feeling powerless to help her son. What do you do when you are a nurse; when your child has died or is near death; when your reality is turned upside down in the space of one phone call? You wait. You try to remember what you learned in school and hope that your friends can remember everything else. You hope they will remember what the doctors and nurses say—that they will ask the questions you forget to ask. You pray those caring for your son have the skills and knowledge to bring him back to life.

The Neuro-ICU was large. The nursing station, like the pupil of an eye, was in the center of the unit. We passed through the double doors, passed by the nourishment kitchen, to the second bed on the right. Shawn's face was abraded, scabs already forming in long thin lines. His hair was shaved close in some places, long in others. Sutured lacerations were bloody and tender. A silver spike extended into and out of his skull. Monitors were blipping and bleeping. Lights were blinking on and off, all at eye level.

We were shocked at our first sight of Shawn. His eyes were closed, puffy, and turning purple. His lips were compressed and unspeaking.

The tracheotomy was very high in his neck. Oxygen was being forced in and out of his lungs by the ventilator. Intravenous lines providing fluids and medication to battle infection and to create calming compliance with the mechanisms supporting his life were secured in place with tape. His hands were restrained at the wrists. Shawn had a severe closed head injury.

As soon as I had hung up the phone after speaking with Diane, I started to treat him energetically. I did this by directing universal life energy to Shawn, by thinking of him as healthy and whole. Now, we were face to face. When I first assessed his energy field, it resembled the snow you see on television after the channel goes off the air at night. There was no logic to the pattern. The area over his chest was especially active, the air vibrated erratically.

Our first objective was to release this volatile energy and underlying superficial congestion. During the first two days following the accident, we used Therapeutic Touch primarily for this purpose. Later, Therapeutic Touch was helpful in restoring pattern to his extremely disordered energy field.

We observed the monitors over time. His vital signs were labile, initially. As we treated Shawn, these stabilized, his pulse steadied, blood pressure leveled out, intracranial pressure normalized, and PO^2 saturation was greater than 95 percent. We closely monitored these symbols of his progress.

As time went by, we used Therapeutic Touch to direct healing energy to Shawn and to provide a healthy energy field to support his healing. Therapeutic Touch also helped us to manage our stress and anxiety. Knowing that we could assist Shawn at the energetic level was important to us. Still, there were moments when we were not certain that we were achieving our goal.

We talked to Shawn continuously. Intellectually, we knew that people in comas hear what is said to them. When Shawn did not respond, Diane struggled with the fear that Shawn could not hear her, let alone understand what she said. She began to doubt that he knew she was present with him. She felt powerless to help him. Diane would rub Shawn's feet and back thinking that she was helping herself more than she was helping him.

On the third day, Shawn began to surface. While his level of consciousness was higher than on previous days, he was still comatose. He began fighting the ventilator. This required increasing amounts of medication, which we believed would be detrimental in the long run. As I was treating Shawn during this time, I described the rhythm of the ventilator as the action of his scuba gear's air compressor and regulator. I encouraged him to allow the compressor and regulator to work for him. After several minutes, he quieted down and stopped resisting the ventilator.

A day or two later, as he was being weaned from the ventilator, his PO^2 decreased and Shawn had to be ventilated. Diane and I used a foot massage technique called reflexology with him. The massage stimulates various areas of the body and creates an overall relaxation response. We focused on the areas of his feet that correspond to the lungs. Shawn's PO^2 increased with the massage. The relaxation response could have accounted for the initial increase in oxygenation. However, PO^2 levels of greater than 95 percent persisted and he was weaned ahead of schedule.

Three weeks after the accident and his brief stay in the Neuro-ICU, Shawn told his mother about a scuba trip he had taken earlier in the month. He insisted that he had been "down under," in Australia with his stepfather. Diane was relieved to learn that, on some level, Shawn had understood what we said to him while he was in the coma and he knew that she and his stepfather were with him in the hospital.

All who cared for Shawn were surprised at his relatively short hospital stay, considering that upon his arrival at the hospital he was assumed to be dead. Shawn was moved out of the ICU nine days after the accident; two weeks later he was discharged to a rehabilitation program. We were not surprised. While numerous factors contributed to his recovery, including caring, skilled and knowledgeable healthcare professionals, the complementary modalities that Diane and I used, Therapeutic Touch, guided imagery, visualization, reflexology, and meditation, were significant factors in Shawn's healing journey.

As Diane and I helped Shawn and one another through this crisis, we were affirmed in our ability to help others, with loved ones in comas, to communicate through the perceived reality of waking consciousness to the open and vast reality of the universal consciousness. In fact, our sense of contribution and being able to assist in his return to health reflected our own healing, moving from feeling helpless and powerless to having a sense of control and connectedness with Shawn and each other.

Shawn's recovery has not been without problems. Therapeutic Touch was helpful during his periods of excitation and agitation, helping him to relax and focus his attention on the present rather than on random and distracting thoughts.

Six years later, the healing continues.

CHAPTER 7

Healing and the Human Spirit

B. J. LANDIS, PHD, RN, CFNP

A powerful association exists between the human spirit and healing that warrants closer attention from health professionals in general and nurses in particular. Spirituality and healing are expressly important to the discipline of nursing because both are embedded within two of nursing's metaparadigm concepts: person and health. Nursing interventions directed at improving the patient's spiritual well-being also improve the capacity for healing and movement toward health and wholeness. Ideas put forth hopefully will stir an interest in widening nursing's knowledge base of human spirituality, particularly in the healing experience.

Initially, I discuss the human spirit as a facet of the holistic person, identifying Spiritual characteristics and dimensions. I then address the concept of healing as an innate human process with movement toward individual wholeness and health. Finally, I discuss the human spirit and healing in the context of the discipline of nursing.

THE HUMAN SPIRIT

Spirituality is often equated with a religion or doctrinal belief, but spirituality and religion are not synonymous. Rather, religious activities serve as a vehicle for some people for the expression of their spirituality. Although my particular perspective is from a Christian paradigm, there are numerous others. Regardless of how individuals choose to acknowledge and express their spirituality, all concur that a dimension of reality exists beyond the material reality we are so familiar with, the world of the human spirit. For these spiritual systems, there is a focus on a divine object, whether an unconscious god, a created being, a supreme value, a philosophy, or a personal God (Ellison, 1983; Fish & Shelly, 1978; McGlone, 1990; Moberg, 1984; Stoll, 1989). Our belief systems differ and consequently, we express our humanity in different ways. Nevertheless, we share in common a human spiritual dimension.

Within my personal belief framework, I view humans as multidimensional yet holistic beings, consisting of biophysical, psychosocial, and spiritual components. Some other belief systems also view humans in a similar manner. However, to provide a conceptual basis for our discussion, this particular model of the human person is presented to explicate my conceptualization. The model is shown in Figure 7.1. The human spiritual component is represented by the innermost circle, surrounded by

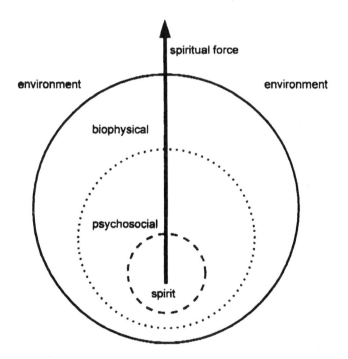

Model of Human Person

Spiritual components include: God-consciousness, Meaning and Purpose of life.
Psychosocial components include Intellect, Emotion, Will and Moral Sense. Personality.
Biophysical components include: 5 Senses, World Consciousness
Adapted from Stallwood & Stool, 1975

FIGURE 7.1. Conceptualization of a Human Person.

the psychosocial component shown as the middle circle, and finally, the biophysical component which is the outermost circle. The three components are interconnected and function together to form the whole person that interacts within the context of environment. Because of this holistic nature, our sense of spiritual well-being affects our psychosocial well-being. Likewise, our psychosocial well-being affects our spirit. These two inner parts of the human are intricately intertwined. Spiritual well-being also affects and is affected by our physical well-being (Stallwood & Stoll, 1975).

The spiritual component, our innermost being, represents our ultimate concern and provides the capacity for God-consciousness, however God may be defined. The psychosocial component includes our emotions, intellect, will, and moral sense. There is a dynamic interaction and interdependence among these four areas. The psychosocial component encompasses our individuality, self-identity, and personality. The biophysical component includes the physical body seen and experienced by others. It puts us in touch with the world through our senses (Moberg, 1984; Stallwood & Stoll, 1975; Stoll, 1989). The physical body is the visible expression of the whole person in the context of environment. Because we are made in the image of our Creator, every human being has inherent worth and dignity.

The human spirit, although empirically indefinable, is conceptualized as our inner-most resource (Ellison, 1993). Within the spirit are two dimensions—a vertical component representing a religious orientation related to God or a higher power and a horizontal component representing an existential orientation related to sense of purpose and satisfaction in life. The vertical and horizontal dimensions are interrelated, bi-directional, and interact together to form our human spiritual component (Stoll, 1989).

The vertical or religious orientation refers to a transcendence in relationship with a higher power or God, not necessarily defined by a particular religion. The religious orientation reflects a generic view of religion that simply recognizes a healthy relationship of person to God or higher power and is a direct consequence of our rational spiritual nature. This orientation represents our ultimate concern, addressing such issues as life's purpose. It is thus, the basic value around which all our other values are focused. It is our central philosophy of life and consequently, guides our behavior (Fish & Shelly, 1978; Moberg, 1984).

Humans need to experience God or a higher power as the source of meaning and purpose for life, love, forgiveness, and hope (Fish & Shelly, 1978). In a humanistic framework, the individual may choose values that transcend and become the supreme focus of life or the higher power motivating a life style toward fulfillment of these goals. Religious growth for the Christian would be a deepening personal relationship with Jesus Christ. The Jew would grow toward keeping covenant with Jehovah. For the Buddhist or Moslem, growth would be toward emptying oneself through meditation to discover the divinity of self (Carson, 1989).

The horizontal or existential orientation of the human spirit refers to a sense of purpose and satisfaction in life. This dimension represents a satisfaction with self, others, and the environment. Religious practices are expressed through this dimension. The existential orientation is our transcendent or ultimate link with others and with our environment. This dimension allows others to influence our spirit while the religious dimension allows the divine to influence our spirit.

The human spirit has been characterized by four distinctive attributes (Banks, 1980). These characteristics give us some understanding of how the spirit functions holistically. First, the spirit is a unifying force that synthesizes the total personality and transcends the physical and psychosocial constituents. This spiritual energy force is essential for human wholeness and well-being.

Second, the human spirit enables and motivates us to find meaning and purpose in our lives and to relate to God. Frankl (1959) believed that the search for meaning is a primary force of one's life. We search for meaning for life in general and for meaning in suffering in particular. In order to find meaning in suffering, we must have a reason and purpose for living. Belief that God or a higher power is in control or influences our circumstances, brings meaning and purpose to our life situations and mediates our sense of powerlessness. I can recall numerous times when clients have moved beyond or "transcended" physical handicaps and suffering to experience spiritual and emotional health and growth. The key seems to be maintaining one's deepest spiritual commitments and the ability to interpret suffering within the context of a deeper positive meaning (Ellison, 1982; Frankl, 1959).

Third, the spirit transcends the person and provides a common bond among humans. This transcendent bond allows us to share ourselves with others. When our love and relatedness needs are met, we experience feelings of self-worth, joy, security, belonging, hope, and courage (Fish & Shelly, 1978). Indeed, our deepest and most endearing life events are shared with significant others via the human spirit. Through this transcendent bond we experience love, forgiveness, and hope (Carson, 1989).

Fourth, the spirit acknowledges the supernatural and is based on individual beliefs and perceptions. This spiritual quality enables us to discern experiences that can not be explained or understood with our intellect alone (Carson, Soeken, & Grimm, 1988; Moberg, 1984). We appraise religious and supernatural experiences through this spiritual attribute.

Overall, we need to establish and maintain a dynamic relationship with God or higher power (through our vertical dimension) and from that relationship experience meaning and purpose in life, love, forgiveness, and hope (through our horizontal dimension). In summary, we are complex, holistic human systems who need to live in harmony with God or higher power, ourselves, and others. We need an ultimate meaning and purpose for our lives. We need harmonious relationships from which we can experience love, forgiveness, and hope. With this conceptualization of the human person, we can now consider how spirituality, in my paradigm, relates to healing and health.

HEALING

"Healing" is indeed a familiar term among healthcare professionals, but its meaning is complex. For example, heal and cure are often used interchangeably. Yet these phenomena are no longer viewed as synonymous. The term "cure" refers to alleviation of symptoms and focuses on a disease process while the term "healing" refers to movement toward wholeness and focuses on the person with the disease. Cure uses outside agents to manipulate the body in order to reduce symptoms of disease. Healing refers to our natural human capacity and focuses on that which is impeding our wholeness (McGlone, 1990).

The approach to cure is treatment while the approach to health is healing. Treatment modalities are mechanistic and symptom oriented, arise from professional authority, and are crisis oriented. The goal is the absence of signs and symptoms of disease. In contrast, healing modalities are holistic, require self-responsibility, and are long-term. The goal is experiencing full health and wholeness (Dacher, 1993). Thus it is possible for one to be cured without being healed and consequently, one may be healed without being cured. For example, the process of accepting one's physical limitations, and even death, may be accompanied by a profound personal healing (McGlone, 1990).

The healing experience, like any experience, is difficult to explain. However, it is an active process of mobilizing one's inner resources toward achieving balance and wholeness. Thus everything necessary for healing lies within the human person. But, as yet science cannot explain extant healing, what the actual force behind it is, or how it can be activated

(McGlone, 1990). My position is that the human spirit is the source of our healing and the innate spiritual force is the energy that permeates our psychosocial and biophysical components promoting their healing and wholeness. Consequently, one's level of spiritual health or well-being determines the energy that is available for holistic healing and health. Spiritual well-being can permeate our entire being bringing harmony, wholeness, healing, and health. Thus, one's spiritual well-being is a major factor in the healing process.

The concept that disease is the result of an imbalance of energy is the basis of many ancient healing practices. The two major Eastern systems of medicine—Ayurveda and Chinese—both have a holistic approach to illness and focus on balancing energy movement to promote healing and health (Martin, 1989). Even though these practices existed long before the birth of Christ, they are still practiced today all over the world. The ministry of Jesus related an incidence of healing that involved energy flow. The woman with an issue of blood was seeking healing from Jesus and merely touched the hem of his robe. Instantly, her "issue of blood" was dried up, she was healed and Jesus replied, "Someone touched me; I know that power has gone forth from me" (Luke 8:46).

Nursing is also familiar with the idea of energy related to healing. Nightingale, our first theorist, recognized that each individual had "vital natural powers for the reparative process" (Chinn & Jacobs, 1987, p. 44). Likewise, Martha Rogers, a contemporary nurse theorist, viewed the unitary human being as an energy field with energy extending beyond the discernible body (Heliker, 1992). Today therapeutic touch, a well-known treatment modality, is used by nurses throughout this country. The basis of therapeutic touch is the idea that human beings are energy systems and that energy extends beyond the individual. When therapeutic touch is used there is an interaction of energy between practitioner and client that seeks to bring about balance and harmony to the client's energy field, promoting healing (McGlone, 1990).

Cognitive perceptions of life events are assigned meaning based on our deepest beliefs and values that are formed and reside within the human spirit. These beliefs and values are explained through our intellect and experienced through our emotions within the psychosocial component. Recent research supports a mind-body link suggesting that our thoughts, emotions, and attitudes exist not only in our mind but are also reflected in the physiology of our body and its healing capacity. Psychoneuroimmunology is the study of these physiologic connections. The brain changes our thoughts, attitudes, and perceptions into nerve impulses and bioactive chemicals. These chemical messenger systems activate the hormonal and immune systems. Consequently, immune system competence can be negatively affected by emotional stress. Accordingly, the immune system can be positively affected by feelings of health and well-being. For instance, the herpes virus is an example of this mind-body connection. Persons exposed to this virus remain infected their entire life. However, activity of the virus, whether it remains dormant or active, is thought to be directly related to immune system competence (Criddle, 1993; Dacher, 1993; McGlone, 1990).

Thus, our thoughts, emotions, and attitudes are significantly influenced by our level of spiritual health reflected in our sense of spiritual well-being. Not only is there a mind-body connection but there is a spirit-mind-body connection to healing and health. With these thoughts in mind, we can consider healing and the human spirit in the context of nursing.

HEALING AND THE HUMAN SPIRIT IN THE CONTEXT OF NURSING

The discipline of nursing posits a holistic conceptualization of the person that focuses on human responses to actual and potential health problems. Nursing therapeutics incorporate modalities that recognize the client as the central force in the healing process and work to facilitate progression toward desired human wholeness and health. Therefore, nursing practice includes both curative and healing interventions.

The therapeutic nurse-client relationship, a foundation of clinical practice, is an interactive human process that seeks to facilitate movement of the client toward wholeness and well-being. This relationship operates in the existential domain of the spirit because it is experienced through the transcendent attribute that provides the common bond between humans. Nursing care includes interactions directed at fostering the client's sense of competence, self-determinism, and self-worth that promotes a sense of spiritual well-being that in turn fortifies the innate spiritual energy. Utilizing one's spiritual energy to vitalize the psychosocial and biophysical components would enhance the natural healing process and move one toward wholeness and health.

In addition to person and health concerns, nursing care involves attention to environmental factors that promote or inhibit healing. Because healthcare is provided in multicultural environments, there are differences in culture, religion, life styles, and philosophies among nurses and their clients. Nevertheless, ensuring a healing environment that allows for distinctions of religious beliefs and spiritual expression is an important therapeutic nursing intervention. Therefore, when curative agents are employed to treat disease and illness along with healing modalities that promote healing and health, a therapeutic synergism is achieved that maximizes movement of the client toward both cure and healing. This is the desired goal for nursing practice and indeed, should be for all health-care practice.

Nevertheless, most of nursing literature assumes humans as biopsychosocial beings. Noticeably the human spirit is omitted. Spiritual attributes, if acknowledged at all, are subsumed as psychosocial phenomena. Ignoring the effect of the human spirit on the physiologic and psychosocial functioning of the individual, prevent nursing from adequately attending to this vital human capacity for healing.

From this discussion, it appears to me that nursing should explore more fully the human spiritual dimension related to the healing experience. Such exploration should have an aim toward identifying nursing therapeutics that improve the client's spiritual well-being and ultimately healing and health for all those seeking nursing care.

REFERENCES

Banks, R. (1980). Health and spiritual dimensions: Relationships and implications for professional preparation programs. *Journal of School Health, 50,* 195–202.

Carson, V. (1989). Spiritual development across the life span. In V. B. Carson (Ed.), *Spiritual dimensions of nursing practice* (pp. 24–51). Philadelphia & London: W. B. Saunders.

Carson, V., Soeken, K., & Grimm, P. (1988). Hope and its relationship to spiritual well-being. *Journal of Psychology and Theology, 16,* 159–167.

Chinn, P., & Jacobs, M. (1987). *Theory and nursing* (2nd ed.). St. Louis, MO: C. V. Mosby.

Criddle, L. (1993). Healing from surgery: A phenomenological study. Image: *Journal of Nursing Scholarship, 25,* 208–213.

Dacher, E. (1993). *PNI: The new mind/body healing program.* New York: Paragon House.

Ellison, C. (1993). Spiritual well-being: Conceptualization and measurement. *Journal of Psychology and Theology, 11,* 330–339.

Fish, S., & Shelly, J. (1978). *Spiritual care: The nurse's role.* Downers Grove: InterVarsity Press.

Frankl, V. (1959). *Man's search for meaning.* New York: Simon & Schuster.

Heliker, D. (1992). Reevaluation of a nursing diagnosis: Spiritual distress. *Nursing Forum, 27*(4), 18-20.

McGlone, M. (1990). Healing the spirit. *Holistic Nursing Practice, 4*(4), 77-84.

Martin, J. P. (1989). Eastern spirituality and health care. In V. B. Carson (Ed.), *Spiritual dimensions of nursing practice* (pp. 113-131). Philadelphia: W.B. Saunders.

Moberg, D. (1984). Subjective measures of spiritual well-being: A neglected subject in quality of life research. *Review of Religious Research, 25,* 351-365.

Stallwood, J., & Stoll, R. (1975). Spiritual dimensions of nursing practice. In I. L. Beland & J. Y. Passos (Eds.), *Clinical nursing* (3rd ed., pp. 1086-1095). New York: Macmillan.

Stoll, R. (1989). The essence of spirituality. In V. B. Carson (Ed.), *Spiritual dimensions of nursing practice* (pp. 4-23). Philadelphia: W. B. Saunders.

CHAPTER 8

The Ethnocultural Context of Healing

JUDITH C. DREW, PHD, RN

The healing initiatives of nursing in modern society are challenged by the pluralistic, ethnocultural premises upon which many individuals base their health and illness needs and practices. While each person's ways of explaining, understanding, and healing health problems are unique, they are guided by shared systems of common sense knowledge that are structured according to cultural beliefs and propagated by an ethnocultural network. In recent years, the increased interest in relationships between ethnicity, culture, and healing has been attributed to the shift in American population demographics and a decline in the acceptance of theories that suggest sameness through assimilation (Fandetti & Gelfand, 1983).

Basic to common sense knowledge systems are the shared beliefs of a culture that individuals use to interpret life events and guide behaviors, including those related to health, illness, and healing (Garfinkel, 1960; Helman, 1984; Schutz, 1943). The culturally constructed common sense knowledge systems that provide individuals with rules for interpreting the world are based on normative structures held by a group and are used to sanction one's competence for membership in the group (Garfinkel, 1960; Schutz, 1943). Furthermore, the role of culture in influencing health, illness, and healing is understood when the meanings and interpretations of behavioral standards are attached to particular social relationships and institutional settings (Kleinman, 1978). For example, the key aspects of an individual's cultural background that influence beliefs and behaviors about health, illness, and healing (Kleinman, 1980; Kub, 1986) may be found among several dimensions of ethnicity. Network composition, language use, lifestyle habits, and religious expression are just a few of the dimensions of ethnicity that frame the social and institutional relationships within which a culture is contextualized and perpetuated (Clinton, 1982).

While healing relationships require that attention be given to the cultural context of health and illness, many nurses lack an understanding of the influence of ethnoculture on health beliefs and practices (Fong, 1985). Even though many individuals may renounce a conscious identification with their ethnic heritage and appear to have assimilated into the majority culture, they may still retain beliefs and values of the aggregate group (Greeley, 1974) and may pass those standards on to their children. It is imperative that we begin to understand our clients' health, illness, and healing beliefs and behaviors from their own perspectives by discovering and describing the cognitive structures through which their perceptions are filtered (Geertz, 1973).

Positive healing interactions between clients and providers require an understanding of cultural knowledge systems and the roles they have in the development of an individual's responses to health and illness events. It has been hypothesized by many researchers that the different beliefs and knowledge systems used by clients and providers to explain and manage health, health problems, and illness realities contribute to conflicts and misunderstandings that interfere with healing outcomes (Allan & Hall, 1988; Angel & Thiots, 1987; Apple, 1980; Blumhagen, 1982; Cheung, 1987; Eisenberg, 1977; Helman, 1985; Kleinman, 1988; Mechanic, 1972; Stein, 1986; Zola, 1983). Kleinman (1986) suggests that the barriers to healing relationships can be minimized by studying and understanding cultural systems of knowledge consisting of systematically linked beliefs and behaviors sanctioned by shared meanings, values, and norms.

The purpose of this chapter is to offer a theoretical perspective on the significance of cultural knowledge systems as cognitive schemes that represent common reference points used by individuals to judge the appropriateness of their health, illness, and healing decisions and actions. Healing is understood as a phenomenon experienced, acknowledged, and appraised by individual clients in the context of their beliefs about health and illness and in their explanatory models for each experience and expected outcomes. The following sections will identify the role of culture in health and illness experiences, discuss the roles of health and illness ideologies in healing actions or choices, and explore proposed relationships between explanatory models of illness causation and healing alternatives.

CULTURE IN HEALTH AND ILLNESS

For purposes of this paper, culture is defined as a learned and shared system of symbolic meanings that shape social reality and personal experiences. Several authors have concluded that cultural factors are the major determinants of whether or not a health condition will be recognized as a problem and what kind of action will be taken (Angel & Thiots, 1987; Cheung, 1987; Eisenberg, 1980; Geertsen, Klauber, Rindflesh, Kane, & Gray, 1975). Others have emphasized the influence of sociocultural factors acting together on the processes of symptom recognition, affirmation, and help seeking. Across several models of health and illness discussed in the literature, culture mediates the recognition and conceptualization of symptoms, the vocabularies for communicating health problems, the modes and content of illness expression, and the range of healing alternatives available to a group (Mechanic, 1986). In essence, culture provides the foundation for cognitive structures that mediate the interpretation of physical and emotional states by the individual (Angel & Thiots, 1987; Fabrega, 1974; Kleinman, Eisenberg, & Good, 1978).

Basic to these cognitive structures are beliefs or ideologies which are organized into interpretive schemes for the purpose of ascribing meaning to life events. Cultural rules that are evident in norms and values also serve to guide the behavioral expression and are used as criteria to construct an experiential reality. The ideologies of the culture and the interpretive schemes woven from them influence many aspects of health behavior by enabling the recognition of health status, attaching significance to a health problem, ascribing meaning to health and illness events, contributing to explanatory models of causation and expected healing outcomes, and identifying acceptable behaviors related to seeking help. In essence, this process begins to elaborate for the individual and the provider the sociocultural context within which health, illness, and healing events are recognized, interpreted, understood, and managed (Harwood, 1981; Kleinman, 1980).

DIFFERENT REALITIES OF CLIENTS AND PROVIDERS

Clients and professional providers view health, illness, and healing from different perspectives (Allan & Hall, 1988; Angel & Thiots, 1987; Apple, 1980; Blumhagen, 1982; Cheung, 1987; Eisenberg, 1977; Helman, 1985; Kleinman, 1988; Mechanic, 1972; Stein, 1986; Zola, 1966). In essence, the two have different cultures and cognitive systems of knowledge. Modern, scientific medicine has historically based its perspective on the necessities of scientific rationality, objective and quantifiable measurement, mind-body dualism, and disease-cure relationships (Helman, 1984). This perspective represents the cognitive, interpretive model used by this discipline to construct a reality which excludes phenomena outside of its frame of reference (Allan & Hall, 1988; Eisenberg, 1977). Fabrega and Silva (1973) have speculated that the medical perspective assumes that diseases are universal in form as well as in progress and content. In this context, the subjective symptoms of the client achieve significance, meaning, or are made real to the provider only when they can be explained by objective, physical facts (Good & Good, 1981; Taussig, 1980).

While individual professionals across several disciplines may employ a variety of perspectives in their repertoire of interpretive models (Helman, 1984), some have been accused of giving only superficial attention to sociocultural factors in the search for causes of physical or emotional complaints (Allan & Hall, 1988; Good & Good, 1981). While nursing's holistic philosophies have directed its practitioners to explore the cultural meanings of the experience for the client, illness and healing remain elusive constructs for researchers and providers (Drew, 1996). This difficulty may have it roots in the cognitive knowledge systems that have predominated in our educational programs and have therefore defined our cultures as providers.

In contrast to the paradigms of most professional providers, the concept of illness, rather than disease, is central to the layperson's subjective response to being unwell. It includes the meaning and significance of the experience for the individual constructed according to common sense knowledge and supported by cultural norms (Eisenberg, 1980; Harwood, 1981; Helman, 1984; Kleinman, 1980). The significance of exploring the lay perspectives of health, illness, and healing is to further clarify the beliefs and cognitive structures from which clinical realities are constructed by our clients (Roberson, 1987). A new understanding may shorten the distances between lay conceptions of what it means to be ill and the healing initiatives of providers (Tripp-Reimer, 1982; Weidman, 1979; Weiss, 1988).

HEALTH AND ILLNESS BELIEFS: COGNITIVE CONTRIBUTIONS TO HEALING SCHEMES

The sets of beliefs in cultural knowledge systems represent the basic truths and values shared by group members (Black, 1973). Beliefs are the basic guidelines for perceiving, interpreting, organizing, and understanding meaningful experiences. Beliefs also serve to guide behavior and provide strategies for solving problems and making choices among alternatives for action (Black, 1973; Goodenough, 1957; Spradley & McCurdy, 1972; Young & Garro, 1982).

Health beliefs form the basis of the reasoning process used by individuals to link plausible explanations for causes of an illness with alternative solutions for the health problem (Billig, Condor, Edwards, Gane, Middleton, & Radley, 1988; Kleinman, 1980; White, 1982). Health beliefs are basic to the formulation of explanatory model propositions which assist the individual in constructing the illness reality and plausible healing alternatives. Although illness realities are thought to change and evolve during one's life experiences with illness (Kleinman, 1980), several researchers have found that basic health beliefs, even after one is exposed to Western biomedical models of disease, remain unchanged (Blumhagen, 1982; Greenfield, Borkan, & Yodfat, 1987; White, 1982). Models of healing are also embedded in health beliefs and must be elicited within the context of the common sense system of knowledge.

Health ideologies also establish the framework for the continuous evolution of criteria used by individuals to recognize health and health status deviations. They form the basis of the reasoning process used by individuals to link health outcomes with actions, phenomena, lifestyles, and behaviors. For example, health beliefs are instrumental to the individual's definition of health and what it means to be healthy, performance of behaviors that maintain health, and selection of healing alternatives that can be used to restore health (Drew, 1990).

While health ideologies exist independent of and prior to a given episode of illness (Kleinman, 1980), time and experience with an illness are necessary to work the set of beliefs into a functioning set of causal propositions that explain etiology, give direction to behavior, and offer options to achieve healing (Blumhagen, 1982; Chrisman, 1982; Good & Good, 1981; Kleinman, 1980; Young, 1982). Furthermore, the social process of becoming ill and assuming a sick role is culturally sanctioned (Blumhagen, 1982; Chavez, 1984; Cheung, 1987; Helman, 1984; Kleinman, 1980) in that illness is defined as syndromes from which members of a group suffer and for which their culture provides an etiology, a diagnosis, preventive measures, and regimes of healing (Rubel, 1977).

Illness beliefs form the cognitive basis of the reasoning processes used by individuals to link plausible predictions about illness causation with potential actions perceived to alter or control threats to health. They are revealed in an individual's statements about the conditions, actions, or situations they think contribute to their susceptibility or vulnerability to illness (Drew, 1996). Together, health and illness beliefs represent a set of common sense structures in the cognitive knowledge system used by individuals to understand and interpret health and illness experiences. Although there is agreement amongst many researchers that health is a more elusive concept than illness, the cognitive and behavioral structures supporting the cognitive interpretation of health are of critical significance to the individual's determination of what it means to be ill and to the selection of healing strategies.

Health and illness ideologies prepare individuals to react in culturally salient ways to the life changes presented by an altered health status. The subjective illness reality which is based on the syncretic meanings of the symptoms and causal propositions for the dysfunction, guides the expression of acceptable behaviors and the selection of alternative choices for healing. In responding to an episode of illness, the individual formulates the meaning of the experience through interaction within a sociocultural context. More specifically, the recognition, interpretation, significance, treatment, and evaluation of the experience evolves from interaction with the family and the social network mediated by the cognitive and behavioral standards of the ethnic aggregate. During this process, the individual integrates views in part idiosyncratic and in part acquired from the health ideology of the popular culture to construct a subjective illness reality that includes strategies for healing (Kleinman, 1980). Healing in this context is a means, not an end. Healing facilitates the return from an illness role to the culturally sanctioned productive and prescribed role usually performed in a relative, functional health state.

EXPLANATORY MODELS OF ILLNESS: CULTURAL ANSWERS TO "WHY"?

The fact that people search for answers to the "whys" of illness indicates a search for meaning beyond cause and a guidepost for healing. White (1982) refers to explanatory statements as central organizers used to reason about illnesses and give direction to healing actions and behaviors. Explanatory models are made up of common sense causal propositions formulated from beliefs about health and illness in the larger cultural knowledge system of ethnic groups (White, 1982). These central organizing themes are developed by individuals through interaction with their sociocultural environment, and are used to structure healing responses to an illness experience. Explanatory models assist the individual in making sense of the illness experience by linking the individual's syncretic belief system with culturally sanctioned actions to express and resolve the health problem (Blumhagen, 1982; Good, 1977).

Eliciting the explanatory models of our clients gives us insight into the cultural beliefs the client holds about the illness, including the personal and social meaning attached to the health problem and the rationale for the client's choice of healing actions. Differences in explanatory models between professionals and their clients influence the interactions between them and the ability to develop acceptable strategies to promote health and healing. Explanatory models (EMs) provide a sense of order in an otherwise disruptive state of illness and are therefore important components of common sense models of illness and healing (Kleinman, 1988).

Since EMs also serve as interpretive operators, they characterize the meaning individuals attribute to the illness as they try to explain it to themselves and others (Kleinman, 1980). However, the extent to which illness phenomena can and need to be explained by the individual is influenced by the beliefs one holds about those phenomena in the first place. That is, in most cultures, demonstrating competence as a member of the collectivity is dependent upon invoking socially appropriate causes to explain given events and the choices for healing. Inappropriate explanations would be attributed to cognitive incompetence (Locker, 1981). Explanations offered for illness experiences must fit with common sense ideas about typical causes, effects, healing strategies, and the links between them.

Individuals typically choose EMs from a set of causal relationships sanctioned by cultural rules and supported by the social network. It should be acknowledged that certain cultures are known to recognize certain causal agents while rejecting others. However, the significance of the EMs in explaining the illness to others is that they represent interpretive frames used by individuals to construct the definition of a situation and plan an orientation to action (Good, 1986). According to Good (1986), "culturally-grounded illness theories shape its members' illness behaviors and choices they make among therapies" (p. 163).

CULTURAL PRESCRIPTION FOR SICK ROLE AND SANCTIONS FOR HEALING

Assessments and appraisals of signs and symptoms, learned within a socio-cultural context, constitute prime elements in acknowledging the presence of illness in the self or in another, and play important roles in acting out the illness and in making decisions to seek help for healing. Illness behavior refers to the individual's total response set of cognitive perceptions, interpretations, and meanings attached to a particular health problem. In essence, illness behaviors are the individual's operationalization of cognitive beliefs about health and illness, and the theoretical propositions of explanatory models which have constructed the illness reality for the individual.

Although illness behaviors are culturally sanctioned, they represent the individual's subjective interpretation of the meaningful experience which influences evaluations of the illness and its impact upon patterns of daily living, attainment of appropriate care, and healing outcomes. One type of illness behavior is the sick role. Determining sick role behavior is part of a temporal process influenced by the cultural salience of an individual's definitions of health, appraisals of well-being, identification of links between symptoms and illness, explanations of illness causation, and evaluations of outcomes of actions taken to seek healing. Common sense knowledge continues to influence the individual throughout the determination of sick role behavior by illuminating relevant courses of action and conduct that allow those experiencing illness to be recognized as competent members of their collectivities (Campbell, 1975; Cicourel, 1973; Dingwall, 1977; Jones, Wiese, Moore, & Haley, 1981).

The congruence between one's cognitive beliefs and those of the social network also influence the expression of sick role behaviors and healing choices. For example, the process of defining oneself as ill begins with a self-diagnosis confirmed by significant others, based on the implicit standards of what it means to be well (Angel & Thiots, 1987; Eisenberg, 1980; Helman, 1984). A person is defined as ill when there is agreement between self-perceptions of impairment and the perceptions of those around the person (Helman, 1984; Weiss, 1988).

The social, ethnic, and cultural values upon which the illness judgment is based focus on the experience of discomfort, failure to function in expected roles, and a change in physical appearance. Whether or not a symptom is recognized as significant or normal is also influenced by the occurrence, persistence, and prevalence of the symptoms amongst group members (Angel & Thiots, 1987; Helman, 1984). All of the judgments about persons who are sick influence the healing initiatives taken by the individual (Drew, 1996). If sickness is not recognized or acknowledged by the social network because its presence is evaluated by norms that differ from those of the prevailing culture, then the sanctions for expression of sick role behaviors and actions necessary for healing may be withheld.

According to Parsons (1951), Levine and Kozloff (1978), and Zola (1966), a change from the well role to the sick role must be acknowledged and recognized by the individual as congruent with the social network's expectations before comfort with the role can be achieved. Cowie (1976) found that shared knowledge about the way familiar or known illnesses manifest themselves is critical to the way the individual compares the present, active experience to what has been known before. Such previous and vicarious experiences can have significant impacts upon the healing choices made by those who are considering seeking help for their illness.

SEEKING HEALING: RESPONSES TO ILLNESS REALITIES

People who become ill make choices about whom to consult for healing. Jones et al. (1981) found that the meanings people attached to various symptoms and illnesses are the key factors in considering the implications for healing. The significance of cultural ideologies of health and illness to sick roles and healing choices are documented in the literature as supporting the reasoning processes which link culturally salient interpretations of illness with potential solutions for health problems (Chrisman, 1977). Many researchers agree that another critical determinant of a person's symptom related behavior is the interpretation of the subjective meaning of the illness experience (Bishop, 1987; Fabrega, 1974; Mechanic, 1979). Specifically, attitudes toward healing alternatives have been shown to vary according to one's subjective, sociocultural interpretation of the symptoms (Bishop, 1987; Cheung, 1987; Sharp, Ross, & Cockerham, 1983; Zola, 1973). Mechanic (1982) has suggested that one's attention to symptoms and actions taken to seek help for healing are a function of learning based in the family and the culture.

The individual, in seeking help to achieve healing, establishes a therapeutic network that may include informal and formal relationships with several types of healers. Within the context of this healing network, the client makes choices for treatments using previous and vicarious experiences, and common sense knowledge that addresses the significance of the symptoms, the explanatory models of cause, course, and duration, and desired outcomes of treatment (Blumhagen, 1982; Chrisman, 1977; Kleinman, 1980; Young, 1982). Different types of healers may be used concurrently or in sequence, and the network of potential consultants may range from members of the nuclear family to lay healers and licensed professionals (Angel & Thiots, 1987; Friedson, 1961; Helman, 1984; Kleinman, 1980; Mechanic, 1982; Roberts, 1988).

To understand the factors that influence the selection of healing strategies, one must understand the cognitive beliefs, explanatory models, and illness realities interacting within the cultural healthcare system of identified groups. According to Kleinman (1980), cultural healthcare systems represent the ranges of scientific, popular, and folk beliefs and practices used by individuals and groups in the recognition, interpretation, and management of illness realities. Cultural healthcare systems are made up of individuals experiencing and treating illness and the social institutions mediating the interaction between the recipients and providers of care (Kleinman, 1980).

The popular sector of cultural healthcare systems is made up of informal healing relationships that occur within one's own social network. While the family is at the nucleus of this sector, most healthcare takes place between people linked by kinship, friendship, residence, occupation, or religion (Helman, 1984). Within this sector, both the recipient and the provider of care share similar assumptions about health and illness, misunderstandings are rare, and the healer's credentials are based on experience rather than professional education and licensure (Chrisman, 1977; Kleinman, 1980).

The folk sector of cultural healthcare systems includes the interaction between a client and sacred and secular healers. Most healers share the same basic cultural values, beliefs, and world views about health, illness, and treatment as their constituents, and family members are included in the diagnosis and treatment of the individual. The holistic approach of healers in this sector includes the analysis of the client's relationship with other people, with the natural environment, and with supernatural forces (Helman, 1984). Treatment rituals and recommendations are prescribed to correct the imbalance and promote healing. Healers have little formal training although some have served an apprenticeship with another healer. Most are believed to receive healing powers through family position, inheritance, signs, revelations, or gifts (Helman, 1984; Lewis, 1988).

The professional sector of cultural healthcare systems is made up of organized health professionals who are formally educated and legally sanctioned (Kleinman, 1980). Unlike in the popular and folk sectors, the client and the provider typically differ in their social and cultural values, beliefs, and assumptions in the professional sector. Based on these differences and the unfamiliar surroundings and rules of the institutions in the professional sector, the client-provider relationship frequently is one of mistrust, suspicion, and conflict.

Some researchers hypothesize that the degree of congruence between the cognitive beliefs and explanatory models of healthcare system sectors is a primary determinant of whether or not people, once believing themselves ill, choose healing treatments in sectors other than their own (Friedson, 1961; Kleinman, 1980). Yet, others have found that accessibility of healthcare services has a major role in determining the healthcare seeking choices of individuals regardless of the incompatibilities in ideologies between the provider and the client (Young & Garro, 1982).

Given the individual's perceived needs for healing and the viable choices one has to achieve healing, cognitive schemes based on common sense knowledge will continue to direct the health and illness behaviors that sanction membership in a cultural group. Priorities for healing will be determined by the individual, within a sociocultural context that provides guidelines for judging the appropriateness of behaviors and actions.

SUMMARY

Explanatory theories of health, illness, and healing have made important contributions to understanding the client's perspective on these life experiences. Many disciplines, such as nursing, anthropology, and psychiatry have made important contributions to the development of theories about the influence of ethnic culture on health and illness beliefs and behaviors. Culturally sensitive healing can be advanced by reviewing and understanding the substantive theoretical concepts identified and linked to diversity of need, expectations, roles, and desired outcomes among and between ethnic groups and cultural healthcare systems.

Several researchers have shown that variations in explanatory models between clients and providers in different sectors of cultural healthcare systems are sources of conflict, misunderstandings, and barriers to effective healthcare (Angel & Thiots, 1987; Blumhagen, 1982; Chavez, 1984; Mechanic, 1979; Tripp-Reimer, 1982; Weiss, 1988). Although unintended, provider ethnocentrism communicates to the client that their perceptions, knowledge, and experiences have little significance and that their cultural health beliefs and practices should be disregarded (Weidman, 1979). Changes made in the ways we interact with clients must continue, and we must sustain the goals of working to promote health and healing from the viewpoint of the client. We need to continue researching the factors that influence the individual's ability to acknowledge changes in health, cope with the meanings of illness, and select and use healing strategies that will effectively restore wholeness.

REFERENCES

Allan, J. D., & Hall, B. A. (1988). Challenging the focus on technology: A critique of the medical model in a changing health care system. *Advances in Nursing Science, 10*(3), 22-34.

Angel, R., & Thiots, P. (1987). The impact of culture on the cognitive structure of illness. *Culture, Medicine, & Psychiatry, 11*, 465-494.

Apple, D. (1980). How laymen define illness. *Journal of Health and Social Behavior, 1*, 219-225.

Billig, M., Condor, S., Edwards, D., Gane, M., Middleton, D., & Radley, A. (1988). *Ideological dilemmas: A social psychology of everyday thinking.* Beverly Hills, CA: Sage.

Bishop, G. D. (1987). Lay conceptions of physical symptoms. *Journal of Applied Social Psychology, 17*(2), 127-146.

Black, M. B. (1973). Belief systems. In J. Honigmann (Ed.), *Handbook of social and cultural anthropology.* Chicago, IL: Rand McNally.

Blumhagen, D. (1982). The meaning of hypertension. In N. J. Chrisman & T. W. Maretzki (Eds.), *Clinical applied anthropology: Anthropologists in health science settings* (pp. 297-323). Boston, MA: Reidel.

Campbell, J. D. (1975). Attribution of illness: Another double standard. *Journal of Health and Social Behavior, 16*, 114-126.

Chavez, L. R. (1984). Doctors, curanderos, and brujas: Health care delivery and Mexican immigrants in San Diego. *Medical Anthropology Quarterly, 15*(2), 31-37.

Cheung, F. M. (1987). Conceptualization of psychiatric illness and help seeking behavior among Chinese. *Culture, Medicine, & Psychiatry, 11*, 97-106.

Chrisman, N. (1977). The health seeking process: An approach to the natural history of illness. *Culture, Medicine, & Psychiatry, 1*, 351-377.

Chrisman, N. (1982). Anthropology in nursing. In N. J. Chrisman & T. W. Maretzki (Eds.), *Clinically applied anthropology: Anthropologists in health science settings* (pp. 117-141). Boston, MA: Reidel.

Cicourel, A. V. (1973). *Cognitive sociology.* Harmondsworth: Penguin.

Clinton, J. (1982). Ethnicity: The development of an empirical construct for cross-cultural health research. *Western Journal of Nursing Research, 4*(3), 281-300.

Cowie, B. (1976). The cardiac patient's perception of his heart attack. *Social Science & Medicine, 10*, 87-96.

Dingwall, R. (1977). *Aspects of illness.* New York: St Martin's Press.

Drew, J. C. (1990). *A nursing study of health and illness beliefs, explanatory models, and help seeking patterns among Franco-Americans.* Unpublished Doctoral Dissertation. Austin, TX: The University of Texas at Austin.

Drew, J. C. (1996). Cultural competence in partnerships with communities. In E. T. Anderson & J. M. McFarlane (Eds.), *Community as Partner* (pp. 138-161). Philadelphia, PA: Lippincott.

Eisenberg, L. (1977). Disease and illness: Distinctions between professional and popular ideas of sickness. *Culture, Medicine, & Psychiatry, 1*, 9-23.

Eisenberg, L. (1980). What makes persons patients and patients well? *American Journal of Medicine, 69*(2), 277-286.

Fabrega, H. (1974). *Disease and social behavior: An interdisciplinary perspective*. Cambridge, MA: The MIT Press.

Fabrega, H., & Silva, D. B. (1973). *Illness and Shamanistic curing in Zinacantan: An ethnomedical analysis*. Stanford, CA: Stanford University Press.

Fandetti, D. V., & Gelfand, D. E. (1983). Middle class white ethnics in suburbia: A study of Italian-Americans. In W. C. McCready (Ed.), *Culture, ethnicity, and identity: Current issues in research*. New York: Academic Press.

Fong, C. M. (1985). Ethnicity and nursing practice. *Topics in Clinical Nursing, 7*(3), 1-10.

Friedson, E. (1961). *Patient's view of medical practice*. New York: Russell Sage.

Garfinkel, H. (1960). The rational properties of scientific & common sense activities. *Behavioral Science, 5*(1), 72-83.

Geertsen, R., Klauber, M. R., Rindflesh, M., Kane, R. L., & Gray, R. (1975). A re-examination of Suchman's views on social factors and health care utilization. *Journal of Health and Social Behavior, 16*(2), 226-237.

Geertz, C. (1973). *The interpretation of cultures*. New York: Basic Books.

Good, B. (1977). The heart of what's the matter: The semantics of illness in Iran. *Culture, Medicine, & Psychiatry, 1*, 25-58.

Good, B. (1986). Explanatory models & care seeking: A critical account. In S. McHugh & T. M. Vallis (Eds.), *Illness behavior: A multidisciplinary approach*. New York: Plenum.

Good, B., & Good, M. J. (1981). The meaning of symptoms: A cultural hermeneutic model for cultural practice. In L. Eisenberg & A. Kleinman (Eds.), *The relevance of social science for medicine*. Boston, MA: Reidel.

Goodenough, W. H. (1957). Cultural anthropology and linguistics. In P. Garvin (Ed.), *Georgetown University round table on language and linguistics*. Washington, DC: Georgetown University Press.

Greeley, A. (1974). *Ethnicity: A preliminary reconnaissance*. New York: Wiley.

Greenfield, S. F., Borkan, J., & Yodfat, Y. (1987). Health beliefs and hypertension: A case control study in a Moroccan Jewish Community in Israel. *Culture, Medicine, & Psychiatry, 11*, 79-95.

Harwood, A. (1981). *Ethnicity and medical care*. Cambridge, MA: Harvard University Press.

Helman, C. (1984). *Culture, health, and illness: An introduction for health professionals*. Boston: Wright.

Helman, C. G. (1985). Communication in primary care: The role of patient and practitioner explanatory models. *Social Science & Medicine, 20*(9), 923-931.

Jones, R. A., Wiese, H. J., Moore, R. W., & Haley, J. V. (1981). On the perceived meaning of symptoms. *Medical Care, 19*(7), 710-717.

Kleinman, A. (1978). Clinical relevance of anthropological and cross-cultural research: Concepts and strategies. *American Journal of Psychiatry, 135*(4), 427-431.

Kleinman, A. (1980). *Patients and healers in the context of culture*. Berkeley, CA: University of California Press.

Kleinman, A. (1986). Illness meanings & illness behavior. In S. McHugh & T. M. Vallis (Eds.), *Illness behavior: A multidisciplinary perspective*. New York: Plenum.

Kleinman, A. (1988). *The illness narratives: Suffering, healing, and the human condition.* New York: Basic Books.

Kleinman, A., Eisenberg, L., & Good, B. (1978). Culture, illness, & care: Clinical lessons from anthropologic & cross cultural research. *Annals of Internal Medicine, 99,* 25-58.

Kub, J. P. (1986). Ethnicity: An important factor for nurses to consider in caring for hypertensive individuals. *Western Journal of Nursing Research, 8*(4), 445-456.

Levine, S., & Kosloff, M. A. (1978). The sick role: Assessment & overview. *Annual Review of Sociology, 4,* 317-343.

Lewis, M. C. (1988). Attribution and illness. *Journal of Psychosocial Nursing, 26*(4), 14-21.

Locker, D. (1981). *Symptoms and illness: The cognitive organization of disorder.* London: Tavistock.

Mechanic, D. (1972). Social factors affecting the presentation of bodily complaints. *New England Journal of Medicine, 286,* 1132-1139.

Mechanic, D. (1979). Correlates of physician utilization: Why do major multivariate studies of physician utilization find trivial psychosocial and organizational effects? *Journal of Health and Social Behavior, 20,* 387-396.

Mechanic, D. (Ed.). (1982). *Symptoms, illness behavior, and help seeking.* New York: Prodist.

Mechanic, D. (1986). The concept of illness behavior: Culture, situation, and personal predisposition. *Psychological Medicine, 16*(1), 1-7.

Parsons, T. (1951). *The social system.* New York: Free Press.

Roberson, M. (1987). Folk health beliefs of health professionals. *Western Journal of Nursing Research, 9*(2), 257-263.

Roberts, S. J. (1988). Social support and help seeking: Review of the literature. *Advanced in Nursing Science, 10*(2), 1-11.

Rubel, A. J. (1977). The epidemiology of a folk illness: Susto in hispanic America. In D. Landy (Ed.), *Culture, disease, and healing: Studied in medical anthropology* (pp. 119-128). New York: Macmillan.

Schutz, A. (1943). The problem of rationality in the social world. *Economica, 10,* 130-149.

Sharp, K., Ross, C. E., & Cockerham, W. C. (1983). Symptoms, beliefs, and the use of physician services among the disadvantaged. *Journal of Health and Social Behavior, 24*(1), 255-263.

Spradley, J. P., & McCurdy, D. W. (1972). *The cultural experience.* Chicago, IL: Science Research.

Stein, H. F. (1986). Sick people and trolls: A contribution to the understanding of the dynamics of physician explanatory models. *Culture, Medicine, & Psychiatry, 10,* 221-229.

Taussig, M. T. (1980). Reification and the consciousness of the patient. *Social Science and Medicine, 14B,* 3-13.

Tripp-Reimer, T. (1982). Barriers to health care: Variations in interpretation of Appalachian client behavior by Appalachian and non-Appalachian health professionals. *Western Journal of Nursing Research, 4*(2), 179-191.

Weidman, H. (1979). The transcultural view: Prerequisite to interethnic (intercultural) communication in medicine. *Social Science & Medicine, 13B*, 85–87.

Weiss, M. G. (1988). Cultural models of diarrheal illness: Conceptual framework and review. *Social Science & Medicine, 27*(1), 5–16.

White, G. M. (1982). The role of cultural explanations in somatization and psychologization. *Social Science & Medicine, 16*, 1519–1530.

Young, A. (1982). The anthropology of illness and sickness. *Annual Review of Anthropology, 11*, 257–285.

Young, J., & Garro, L. (1982). Variations in the choice of treatment in two Mexican communities. *Social Science & Medicine, 16*, 1453–1465.

Zola, I. (1966). Culture and symptoms: An analysis of patient's presenting complaints. *American Sociological Review, 31*, 615–630.

Zola, I. (1973). Pathway to the doctor-from person to patient. *Social Science & Medicine, 7*, 677–689.

Zola, I. (1983). *Sociomedical inquiries: Recollections, reflections, & reconsiderations*. Philadelphia, PA: Temple University Press.

CHAPTER 9

Toward an Ethic of Healing

PHYLLIS BECK KRITEK, RN, PHD, FAAN

If the human activity of thinking were a tour through a mansion, reflection on the multidimensional complexity of the concept of healing would reveal rooms as yet unexplored. Without such reflection, we may not discover this because within our culture we are acclimated to a fairly limited concept of healing, one that tends to focus on physical wounds. Stripped of the healthcare culture's more obtuse language system, the process seems quite linear, logical, and predictable: body part broke, ruptured, dysfunctional → fix it → healed. Indeed, that is the tradition of allopathic medicine in the United States, one that nursing has hastened to imitate in the development of its own science. We have sought comfort and certainty in the land of the logical positivist.

The fact is that much of the activity engaged in both by physicians and nurses is not grounded in "hard natural science." Few of our interventions have been subjected to rigorous clinical trials. We are more likely to engage in actions that have been tried with some "good results," and therefore incorporated into our lexicon of interventions. Thus our propensity for a simplistic linear model and our preference for attending to decontexted physical phenomena can lead us to decision making that has an aura of illusion, perhaps even delusion about it. We tend not to discuss this much or acknowledge it even to one another. Certainly we are reluctant to share this with our patients.

It thus seems somewhat inevitable that malpractice and wrongful action lawsuits have proliferated to the point of insanity. We in healthcare tend to describe this to ourselves as due to the inappropriate avarice of lawyers, but are loathe to note that we present to the public an aura of knowingness that is too often inflated and arrogant in nature. For the most part, had we the minds and hearts of the scholar, we would present our competencies as the best we're aware of today, likely to be improved upon tomorrow.

When our propensity for self-inflation is measured against the complexity of the concept of healing, the issues that emerge become even more troublesome. We in nursing posit that healing involves wholeness, integrity of the entire person, a balancing of all the forces and realities of the human, an integration of all dimensions of what it means to be human for this unique individual person. We further posit that there is an intrinsic capacity in the human to move toward healing, and that this essential or core capacity exists in each person. We acknowledge that the individual person has to seek healing, to activate this capacity, and that we, as health professionals, attempt to facilitate and enhance both the healing capacity and outcomes sought by the individual. We essentially posit that there is a power or force that exists in the other, and that enabling the activation and success of that force is our job.

This is not how we act, however. We are more likely to treat the individual patient as a "broken" or "dysfunctional" entity, even a thing, that has come to our shop to be fixed. We get out our tools, do the fix, tell the patients how to be, act, think, feel, function, and behave, and dismiss them. We call this the outcome. If we do this with a generous enough dollop of authority and self-assurance, we can even silence the nervous or frightened questions and concerns of the patient, enabling us to keep our illusion alive with greater assurance, since we are not distracted by the troublesome perspectives of the patient. While we give lip service to an ideal, we generally act quite differently.

We assume the good intentions of our belief system will carry the day, assume that we work in environments where our beliefs will be honored. Indeed, in nursing, we expend minimal energy creating the environments we wish to work in. We may focus heavily on the individual patient's environment, but are unlikely to create whole institutions or systems of care designed to optimize healing. We are more likely to expend considerable energy bemoaning the nature of our larger scale work environments and systems of care as nonhealing—ones determined and controlled by powerful others.

THE SEARCH FOR HEALING ENVIRONMENTS

The corporatization of healthcare and the economic patterning of managed care have made our propensities even more apparent. As a patient, one purchases the standard package for a given problem and is advised to stay within the confines of the normal curve for the process and the outcomes of this problem. Deviation from these norms will lead to troublesome conflict and loss of support, to say nothing of pain and suffering.

This is perhaps no where better exemplified than the dramatic move toward shortening the length of stay in hospitals. Nurses have accepted this norm and adapted to it without much question. Indeed, we have often congratulated ourselves publicly for our compliance. We have apparently felt it is inappropriate for us to question this normal curve laid over the individual needs of the patient, or to note that during longer stays we did many things of worth and value to patients that in a very short period of time were simply eliminated. They had never seemed the essential dimensions of the patient's experience, and hence could readily be deleted. Suddenly, patients need about 25 percent of what we once thought they needed in terms of nursing care. Now we send them home, sometimes with some advice to friends or family, sometimes with a prescribed number of visits for home care, sometimes with nothing at all. We know virtually nothing about the home they are returning to or the community, and say it is better for them to be at home to heal without any evidence that demonstrates that this is true.

Two hours after an operative procedure, most persons do not feel whole, integrated, balanced, nor are their families necessarily equipped to address the feelings they do have. Two days after a diagnosis with implications of a shortened life, it is more likely that one feels torn apart, fragmented, out of balance. Hence, the moment where healing processes might be activated often emerges for our patients in their transit home.

We seem reluctant to acknowledge this, making somewhat guarded observations about our inability to do anything about the system, the need to be fiscally responsible, the changing times, the demands of cost containment, down-sizing, re-engineering, and other current buzz words that explain our current behavior. In corporatizing the healthcare delivery system, we have effectively turned the human into a "thing." There is no mystery of individualism here; it is not in our pricing structure.

How do we humans heal under such conditions? Do we simply hope for the best and go on? Do we have the intrinsic ability to heal ourselves without help? These questions trouble me daily. The steady demise of the role of healer is obvious, and we are loathe to admit it, even to ourselves. We are now a clean, sleek corporate culture, fixing and mending an assembly line of broken humans, repairing and discharging efficiently and in a cost effective manner. It becomes harder and harder to find the human dimension, and therefore the healing dimension of current allopathic medical practices in the United States.

The Dilemma in a Larger Context

At a global level of inquiry and reflection, this pattern is even more disturbing to observe. We cherish the thought in the United States that we have the best healthcare system in the world, the most amazing and complex of gadgetry for fixing and repairing. I tend to describe this to myself as "in extremis" healthcare. If indeed we are seriously broken, there is surely no better place to get sophisticated and seemingly magical assistance in getting fixed. I would prefer being in this country for any trauma, burn, or cardiac event. We excel. We are less competent, however, in maximizing fullness of life, well-being, peace of mind, joy, or the capacity to love well. The intrinsic capacity of the human to heal when these central aspects of human possibility are disrupted is neither a value nor a manifest skill.

This is not so in other countries, and in the United States, we worry about our troublesome infant mortality rates, our cardiac disease and cancer rates, more recently the return of old scourges like tuberculosis, measles, and malnutrition, our suicide and trauma rates, our violence and homicide rates. We do not look like the healthiest nation in the world, despite our rich array of "in extremis" competencies. We appear more stressed than balanced, more despairing than joyful, more driven than peaceful. We find other nations wondering how we have become so misguided, and we merely respond with defiance. The lurking question emerges: Just how does healing look in this country of wealth, privilege, and strength?

We who lay claim to the public identity of "healthcare provider" are challenged by this set of observations. If indeed my goal as a healthcare provider is to enable the human faced with a health experience to sustain or regain a sense of personal wholeness, a perception of personal integrity, how then do I assure this in the healthcare culture we have created? A long look at Hippocrates admonition to "do no harm" brings me up short, and I cannot help but wonder how harmful to the human spirit the current practices actually are. Yes, they may be uncomfortable, but what does it mean to become a "thing" so completely that the central negotiation of seeking care is "what is covered" and "eligibility"? While there is no question that we needed to exercise a good deal more corporate competency, we seem to have swung the pendulum to the point of total depersonalization of the patient. If I, as a patient, seek healing, do I find current health practices conducive? Where do I find the assistance I need to heal? Is this simply no longer a service provided? Does the healthcare system even acknowledge that such healing is one of its responsibilities?

Many patients are expressing their concern through the use of alternative therapies. If the allopathic system cannot treat me as a human, cannot hear me out and see my concerns as unique and compelling, cannot give me the comfort measures I need to heal, is not willing to answer my questions or listen to my fears and anxieties, then I will find these services elsewhere because I need them. They are the services I need to heal. Indeed, some of the things done to me in allopathic medicine are so hurtful, intrusive, invasive, and depersonalizing that I can only heal if I seek these other services.

The often cited study by Eisenberg et al. (1993) informs us that about one-third (34%) of the citizens of this country sought alternative therapies in 1990. Of that group, 72 percent elected to not tell their primary healthcare provider in allopathic medicine about their decision. What is less often noted is that persons who go to alternative therapies are likely to go back, to have numerous return visits. Hence, the actual visits to unconventional therapies in 1990 (425 million) exceeded that to allopathic medicine (388 million), and were paid for out of pocket (average charge of $27.60), since insurers rarely cover these services. Apparently, the people who seek these services find them helpful; they return for more.

THE ETHICAL IMPLICATIONS OF CREATING A HEALING ENVIRONMENT

It is within the context of this morass of strange occurrences in healthcare that we conduct an enterprise labeled "healthcare ethics" or more often "biomedical ethics." Our dilemmas of choice tend to focus on the exact issues that emerge in "in extremis" care: life supports, informed consent, genetic manipulations, termination of life. And these issues are indeed compelling and important. Since we are so deeply committed to creating the technology that will somehow "conquer disease," we inevitably create the moral dilemmas that emerge as the technology emerges, or more often, well after the technology emerges.

We are far less likely to explore the moral dilemmas that face the healthcare provider as healer, one who assists others in activating their healing potential in order to seek wholeness. Thus, to know how and why to do the "good" in the care of a patient in a way that enhances healing is simply not a point of discussion. Indeed, much of our ethical debate focuses so completely on a rarely admitted concern with cost management that we are loathe to even acknowledge the economic dimension of our choices. It is perhaps inevitable that a culture so driven by wealth will reframe its sense of morality in the context of cost as a central variable. That the new models of healthcare do assure profits for some individuals, even if they are different than the prior individuals, is worth noting. Cost containment in this sense becomes simply a different funneling mechanism, with profits gleaned through changes in access and availability.

These concerns are often cynically dismissed, the musings of a person resistant to change, unable to adapt to the new corporate model, the need for fiscal responsibility. Hence, significant services that can and do promote healing are simply eliminated from the package deal, and those who nostalgically look backward are the albatrosses resisting change. We seem to have lost our moral compass, and our eagerness to look like we are adaptive and responsive, "going along with the changes," drives our decisions.

What do patients need from healthcare providers if they are to actually experience a healing outcome from a health event? Is it simple physical phenomena: the mended incision, the successful completion of chemotherapy, the institution of a new drug regime, the reactivation of daily functions, the improved mobility, the decrease of pain? Are we so comfortable in our materialism that comfort, nurturance, support, encouragement, suggestions for easing the process, listening, touch, being present, caring are no longer germane, the desires of a person who wants more than we are supposed to be providing? What is the "good" in this situation?

NURSING VOICES IN THE CREATION OF HEALING ENVIRONMENTS

Nurses are uniquely well equipped to address this question because the dimensions of healthcare listed, those that enable the healing process, have historically been the purview of nursing. Using a somewhat simplistic distinction, we have been fond of saying that we focus on *care* in contrast to those who focus on *cure*. It is our caring activities that create the conditions for healing in our patients. We acknowledge this daily and find our greatest satisfactions in this dimension of our work. We are very good at this work, and know our patients need it and benefit from it. We have not, however, successfully demonstrated that this healing process is an integral dimension of the services our patients seek, require, or deserve.

Bonhoeffer (1955) observes that "The ethical as a theme is tied to a definite time and a definite place. That is so because man [sic] is a living and mortal creature in a finite and destructible world and because he [sic] is not essentially or exclusively a student of ethics" (p. 264). He goes on to describe the tendency of the moralist to treat all moments of human existence as if they are fraught with moral choice. "They seem to imagine that every human action has had a clearly lettered notice attached to it by some divine police authority, a notice which reads either 'permitted' or 'forbidden'" (p. 264). He makes a case for confining ethical phenomena to their proper place and time in order to render them fully operative.

This advice seems germane to the dilemmas that characterize nursing's choices about healing in our current healthcare delivery system. The simple choices that one makes with each patient are important, but fail to confront the larger issue of what the healthcare delivery system is for, why it exists. If this latter question were answered differently than it has been to date, the assumptions we make in our daily choices would simply flow along these alternative parameters.

Nurses are eager to serve the patient in an ethical fashion; they are reluctant, often ill-equipped to enter the larger ethical debate that precedes the developmental shifts in the system. We nurses are more likely to adapt at the patient level to this year's cumbersome restraints than to enter the dialog concerning moral choice at the macrolevel. Were we to do the latter, we might find that the dilemmas we face could be eliminated, rather than circumvented. Health policy and the design of delivery systems, for most nurses, is something that happens "out there" by powerful others with the right and authority to make such choices.

Susan Sontag (1978) in her analysis of illness as metaphor deplores the "militaristic hyperbole" this culture uses in the description and treatment of cancer, treating it as an "absolute evil"; "implying either a fatalistic diagnosis or a rousing call to fight by any means whatever a lethal, insidious enemy" (pp. 85–87). Eleven years later, she wrote a comparable analysis focused on AIDS, noting "We are not being invaded. The body is not a battlefield. The ill are neither unavoidable casualties nor the enemy. We—medicine, society—are not authorized to fight back by any means whatever" (p. 183). Sontag's observations highlight the impact of the social construction of illness, and the moral dilemmas that ensue when we select a problematic metaphor. If disease is an enemy, and we are engaging in war against it, then the issue of healing is unlikely to emerge as a consideration.

Lakoff and Johnson (1980), in their powerfully useful book, *Metaphors We Live By*, observe that metaphors are culturally grounded, and that war is a central metaphor of our culture, as is "time is money." Not surprisingly then, we create a healthcare system where saving money is assured by decreasing time, and disease is an enemy to be met with warfare. In our culture, these are more intrinsic dimensions of healthcare than nurturance or listening, and policy follows metaphor. More troublesome, however, is the fact that the metaphor, once in place, determines reality. We trim our sense of what is to keep it congruent with the metaphor. As these authors note, "There are cultures where balance or centrality plays a much more important role than it does in our culture" (p. 24). If balance is the desired outcome of healing, the metaphors we use become deeply troublesome.

Hence, we find that those voices, such as nurses who are most committed to the healing dimensions of healthcare, are too rarely articulated or heard, and the voices that prevail create a system where money, time, and effective warfare shape the system of care. This system has variously been labeled objectivist, masculinist, analytic, and materialistic. What is clear, independent of the label applied, is that it reflects values and norms more often prescribed in our culture for and rewarded in men than those comparably emphasized for women. While the various women's movements have created substantive shifts, and the actual variance with genders is greater than the variance between genders on most measures, the reality of a male-controlled healthcare delivery system in the United States is a given.

Feminist ethicists, a group that should conceivable be of interest to nursing which is a discipline with a 96 percent female membership, attend to such issues. Jaggar (1991), in a comprehensive analysis of the complexity and diversity inherent in feminist ethics, notes that there are two approaches to ethics that all those described as feminist share: "The first of these is that the subordination of women is morally wrong; the second is that the moral experience of women should be treated as respectfully as the moral experience of men" (pp. 97–98). Creating a healing environment for those who need one is clearly, in our culture, the purview of women and is shaped by the moral experiences of women.

If indeed the prevailing definition of "healing outcomes" denies the reality of specific outcomes of interest to the patient, if it excludes the recognition, attention to, and funding of healing modalities that lead to wholeness, balance, integrity, and a sense of wellness in the patient, and if these have historically been the purview of nurses, and therefore women in healthcare, then the troublesome moral dilemma of simple elimination or denial of these dimensions is a problem of significance, a moral dilemma that all nurses might wisely attend to and address. And in the main, we have not.

THE DEFAULT OPTION RESPONSE OF NURSES

Rather than crafting our own careful statement of healing, creating metaphors that acknowledge its reality, challenging existing metaphors that deny or distort human needs, we have continued our alignment with what exists and adapted to the shifting sands of the system. Many of our therapies are inherently violent or toxic. While for centuries acupuncture has been used successfully as an anesthesia for surgery in China, we continue to use relatively toxic chemicals when we have a far less intrusive alternative available. We elect to chemicalize much of our healthcare, so that a drug such as Prozac becomes a solution to a myriad of complex life problems. If there is something noxious in the body, we add an additional noxious force to fight the original problem. It is rarely a peaceful system of care, and it is therefore rarely a healing system of care. The outcome of warfare is victory, not healing.

What do we actually know of the body's potential to heal itself, of the importance of self-integration and personal integrity on the outcome of our interventions? Given our current moral debate in healthcare, this question will not be readily answered. It will largely be one of continuing to introduce amazing technology and assessing its impact. The alternative therapies will continue on their paths, the traditions of allopathic medicine continue on theirs. Nursing, a discipline that has historically served both masters, one more overtly than the other, is uniquely placed to identify and bring into the dialog a richer and more balanced perspective on the nature of healthcare. While we may craft bridges between these two worldviews, at some point we will simply need to face the fact that each operates out of a specific paradigm or worldview, each embraces distinctive metaphors quite unlike the other's.

Over the years, I have been repeatedly assured that the reason nurses do not exercise moral agency is that no one thinks we have the right to do so. I have been startled at the number of times people thought I didn't have this right, which I consider a responsibility. I have also often paid dearly for continuing to operate as if I did have moral agency as an intrinsic dimension of my humanness and my role as a professional nurse. Being a moral agent is not easy or casual under these contextual conditions. As Gruen (1986) states in his seminal work on the betrayal of self through the fear of autonomy, "in this resides the real meaning for the growth of our consciousness; to endure in the struggle for our own reality in the face of the ubiquitous pressure to conform to a distorted and diminished reality" (p. 29).

What if the nursing practice councils of emerging healthcare networks published and disseminated white papers articulating the values and beliefs about healing environments for patients as envisioned by nurses? What if nurses crafted clear statements about the role of the nurse in patient healing and shared these with managed care administrative centers, following this document with a request for a formal meeting with the administrators where dialog would clarify the commitments of each? What if nurses elected to publicly and collectively speak out concerning the substantive philosophical and ethical differences they discover between the discipline's moral stances and those of other groups in healthcare?

What if the public knew? Would they recoil or rejoice? Patients are eager for advocates, and in a united stance, we might make a difference. While we slog through lobbying efforts at the national, state, and local level, we are often accused of self-interest. It might be in our self-interest to begin at the grass roots of ethical choice, thinking globally but acting locally, with a clear statement of our beliefs, values, convictions, and commitments. Why doesn't society know about these? Have we embraced political negotiation without first carefully attending to the challenge of articulation, of having voice in all arenas, of telling our story clearly and courageously? Can we create healing environments without doing so?

CONCLUSION

We humans have need for a more robust definition of health and of healing. If indeed we succeed in finding more wisdom in our search for these definitions, we will certainly unveil truths that challenge existing moral choices made in healthcare. We will introduce new considerations into our definition of the "good" that incorporate the rights and the healing potential of the patient, the importance of a noncontrolling healthcare provider, the acceptance of the patient's moral agency, and the forces for self-healing too often trapped inside frightened and suffering patients. Sharon Welch (1990), the feminist ethicist who views her ethics as one of risk puts it well, "When we begin from a self created by love for nature and for other people, choosing not to resist injustice would be the ultimate loss of self" (p. 165).

REFERENCES

Bonhoeffer, D. (1986). *Ethics.* New York: Macmillan.

Eisenberg, D. M., Kessler, R. C., Foster, C., Norlock, F. E., Caulkins, D. R., & Delbanco, T. L. (1993). Unconventional medicine in the United States. *The New England Journal of Medicine, 328*(4), 246-252.

Gruen, A. (1988). *The betrayal of the self: The fear of autonomy in men and women.* New York: Grove Press.

Jaggar, A., M. (1991). Feminist ethics: Projects, problems, prospects. In C. Card (Ed.), *Feminist Ethics* (pp. 78-104). Lawrence, KS: The University Press of Kansas.

Lakoff, G., & Johnson, M. (1980). *Metaphors we live by.* Chicago: University Press.

Sontag, S. (1989). *Illness as metaphor and AIDS and its metaphors.* New York: Doubleday.

Welch, S. D. (1990). *A Feminist ethic of risk.* Minneapolis, MN: Fortress Press.

SOME CORE COMPONENTS OF HEALING

PHYLLIS BECK KRITEK, RN, PHD, FAAN

The thoughtful reader, having reflected on the essential nature of healing, will now be given an opportunity to explore some of healing's core components. Part Two provides a more focused exploration of some critical dimensions of healing processes, and demonstrates the robustness of the concept of healing in the inclusion of the multiple facets of nursing's work.

One of the more troublesome aspects of professional nursing's struggle toward an understanding of our discipline, which is both scientific and humanistic in nature, is a persistent confusion about the multivariate nature of the field of study and our work. We have a difficult discipline to describe. While other disciplines cast careful boundaries around what they will and will not include within their domains, we in nursing have insisted on a holistic perspective, yet find ourselves amazed at the complexity this stance commits us to exploring. It may be that we simply have not found a way to make sense of the devaluation of nursing in our culture, and drift toward an agreement of that perception.

I am always somewhat amazed when a nurse scholar defensively declares disappointment or disgust that our science is so minimally developed, pointing to the work of other disciplines as the preferred stage of development and excellence. While these nurses may not be attending to the limited time thus far invested in creating a systematic body of knowledge, or perhaps are frustrated by the oppression undergirding the delays we experience, a more disturbing dimension exists; their reluctance to embrace the inherent complexity of nursing, and thereby acknowledge that we have set ourselves a difficult task. Embedded in the complaint they raise is the subtle but effective voice of the self-hating oppressed victim. And like all victims, they disdain their colleagues whom they see as beneath them; they implicitly define these persons as less able than themselves. This behavior also reflects a willingness to participate in the expression of social norms and standards that are dismissive of nurses, when they might more wisely question them.

Several years ago, while trying to draw pictures of taxonomic trees for the incipient nursing diagnoses crafted by the North American Nursing Diagnosis Association, I had one of those amazing "aha!" experiences that told me this world of nursing, as unveiled by our limited construct delineation, was a good deal more complex than we realized, that our theories were often incomplete in acknowledging interactive effects and sources of variance, and that we had a long road to walk precisely because we had chosen a much longer and more difficult road. It had a comforting effect on me, but it has been less clear to me how I might share this insight.

Part Two of this book helps me. Each of the authors provides a snapshot exploration of one critical aspect of healing processes. While not exhaustive or comprehensive in scope, they do provide a surprising range of options and outcomes possible if one does nursing from a perspective of healing processes. They reveal the promise of the concept itself.

In Chapter 10, Peggy Standard explores a process of assisting persons who have experienced family incest and seek, through survival and recovery, to heal from the experience. Describing the work she does with such persons, she focuses on healing an emotional wound and describes the process as one of self-discovery and empowerment. In this process, she serves as guide and supporter who facilitates the process, assisting her patients to discover changes in self-perception that lead to empowerment. Such empowerment provides the strength needed to make changes in one's life. She describes this as a healing cycle, a description used by others who work with incest survivors.

Peggy uses the metaphor of a journey with her clients, and as a nurse psychotherapist views herself as a pathfinder. She describes a process she gradually developed from the first experience she had with an incest survivor in the early 1980s when everyone knew far less about the nature and extensiveness of family incest. Her primary source of learning was her clients. In her paper, she describes the actions of one guide assisting in the healing process for persons struggling with family incest. She emphasizes self-reflection and self-expression, including the active use of journal writing and drawings (useful examples are provided) through the various stages of the cycle. She describes this work as one of activating the healing potential in the other. Peggy's paper shows how the nurse can play a central role in the healing process by serving as guide, pathfinder, and catalyst of healing potential. She demonstrates the possibilities available to us if we elect to see healing as a central construct of our discipline. She concretizes the ideas described in Part One, and does so with a clear description of one healing process created by a nurse.

So does Corinne Opperman in Chapter 11. She describes her paper as a description of a "reflective spiritual philosophy about my experiences of self-healing from the grief of loss through the death and dying of loved ones." Exploring three experiences of the dying process and the death of loved ones, she describes her struggle to stay whole as a person and competent as a professional nurse while providing supportive care for the person dying and for this person's friends and family. She notes that many nurses facing this challenge tend to give priority to the needs of others over themselves, and hence are ill-equipped to sustain the effort or are personally depleted because they fail to attend to self-healing during the process, something she views not as an option but as a responsibility. She hopes to stimulate reflection in practicing nurses concerning this dilemma and the potential of constructive options available to them. She gives particular emphasis to the role her personal spirituality played in crafting her self-healing process.

Corinne describes wholeness as "a person's sense of integrated peacefulness," a wonderful example of the diversity of descriptions that can emerge from a careful exploration of what healing means to oneself, and hence, self-healing. She narrates the story of the dying process and death of each person, observing that the nurse guides the process for those others who are on this journey with the patient, and hence creates an opportunity for interactive relationships that mutually occur among the participants, often healing them, decreasing their fear of death, and creating new supportive relationships. From her three experiences, the first providing a beginning understanding of her self-healing, she amplifies from subsequent experiences and crafts a model of self-healing as an evolving process. She notes that the patient is the person who controls the process and that the patient's belief system guides the nurse's response. In her discussion, she shares her perceptions of enabling factors for furthering her self-healing as expressed within her belief system. Through her stories, she demonstrates the need for nurses to find a careful balance of self-healing and participation in the healing processes of others.

Chapter 12 demonstrates yet another way that understanding healing changes the way we think and act as nurses. It is co-authored by a faculty member, Barbara Carnes, and a student who completed the BSN completion program at our school, Rebecca Harbin. The paper is written in the first person and tells of Rebecca's compelling struggle to seek healing and the lessons she has learned along the way. It concludes with a poem that expresses the wisdom she has acquired in the process thus far.

Her story is one of abuse—the mental, emotional, and spiritual damages—and her decision to confront this unfinished business. She describes the various defenses she used and their self-destructive nature, defenses that collapsed when she was sexually assaulted by her boyfriend's friend, who was HIV positive. It is a triumphant story of self-confrontation and personal courage. She aptly uses the metaphor of a festering boil and gives a detailed account of treating this boil by seeking a process of healing. It is a personal and powerful story that demonstrates how understanding healing processes provides one with the template needed to pursue wholeness and integrity. She also candidly honors her own woundedness and describes the power of being a nurse as a stimulus to self-healing. She provides a wonderful example of the human spirit as described by B.J. Landis in Part One.

Susan Scoville Baker, in Chapter 13, provides an excellent example of the ethnocultural context of healing described by Judy Drew in Part One. Susan's paper is one of those that pulls you up short by asking you to re-image a set of familiar ideas as she describes survival as health, an intrinsic capacity for healing. Building on an experience she had in Brazil as a curriculum consultant for a group of Brazilian nursing faculty, she walks the reader through a reflective analysis of a "theory of nursing for desperate times."

Honoring the context of this nursing faculty, she listened to the faculty describe their desperate economic conditions; some had not been paid for months. Brazil was caught in a cycle of escalating inflation, accompanied by pandemic violence and robberies, displacement to less adequate living conditions for most people, a well-founded fear for their personal safety and a steady erosion of quality of life. These nurses defined health as "survival." Susan wanted to make sense of their message, and the paper records her process of thinking this through.

She notes that health can be viewed as a starting point for humans, not an outcome. Health can be seen as a resource inherent in humans that can sustain us through a myriad of environmental, developmental, and situational challenges. During such challenges, health may be best demonstrated by the will to live, to survive. In delving into another culture, these nurses assisted Susan in expanding her understanding of healing processes; she admires her Brazilian nurse colleagues who are committed to assuring survival for their patients. She also discovers the enriching impact of difference and diversity: it expands your worldview and enriches it, a central premise of this book.

In Chapter 14, Doris Campbell guides us through an analysis of a component of the healing process that we all tend to agree is valuable but one which we fail to address consciously in many situations: sleep. Doris' chapter provides a much needed example of focusing on a normal human process to better understand its healing potential and its impact on the individual seeking healing. She explores both the physiological and psychological dimensions of sleep to demonstrate the multitude of ways sleep can serve as a healing activity.

Focusing on the physiological, she traces the history of acknowledging the restorative powers of sleep, its role in attaining and maintaining equilibrium. She notes that sleep is a key ingredient in mending tissue, and due to the active phases of sleep, the enhancement of growth that can actually include creatively solving our problems as we sleep. Some of the psychological effects of sleep were implicit in many of the ideas presented in Part One. The author notes that dreams are essential for healthy functioning, that sleep gives us an opportunity to review and re-integrate our life experiences and consolidate our memories. She notes that sleep is an essential dimension of integration.

This description shows the innate potential of the human to activate healing through a natural cyclic process we call sleep. It also shows that those human processes that integrate and synthesize our life experiences further the healing process. The example of sleep proves a useful one in beginning to understand the human process of healing. As Doris notes, it gives us the opportunity to increase our self-knowledge, modify our behavior, and enhance our relationships. It is a thought-provoking window on healing, especially since the commitments of Nightingale so ably chronicled by Poldi Tschirch seems, in relation to sleep, to be too often honored in the breach in current healthcare environments. Perhaps a reflective awareness of this core component of healing would bring us back to a greater respect for our patients' inherent resources and how we might best further their access to such resources.

In the final chapter in this part of the book, Barbara Mason provides an analysis much like Doris', with some of the same implications and impact. She explores the use of reminiscence as a healing therapy for older adults. Both Barbara and Doris give us explicit snapshots of the human's natural capacity for integrative activity and note the neglect of both in our current health practices. In discussing reminiscence, the review of past experiences, she demonstrates that this is an activity appropriate and necessary for one's final stages of life, where we survey and re-integrate life's events as we face the imminence of death. She describes this integration as normal and healthy but poorly understood and often dealt with insensitively or labeled as senility. She notes that enabling reminiscence is therefore a "powerful tool for the nurse." She describes involving students in both learning about and experiencing directly the meaning and power of reminiscence and describes the impact of her own efforts to do this with her students. She observes that the students may actually benefit as much from this as the elderly persons, perhaps even more. She discusses the importance of accepting silences and emotions, and observes this process as one of importance to the wellness and development of elderly persons. She closes with a germane quote from Kovach who describes reminiscence as helping us to "pull together the elements of our existence into a coherent whole."

This quote is powerful precisely because it demonstrates the essential nature of this intervention in facilitating healing, described as a process toward wholeness and integration. Mason demonstrates that healing can reframe a human behavior from one of diminishment to one essential to healing. She shows us that our understanding of healing might reframe much of our practice, and help us discover when we indeed function as a healing presence and when we fail to do so.

Part Two provides an opportunity to experience a variety of perspectives on nursing behavior that emerges from an understanding of healing. Implicitly, it asks us to return to our roots and remember what we are about. If we indeed are in the business of enabling healing in our patients, then essential dimensions of healing cannot be ignored or overlooked. Refocusing our nursing practice as a healing practice may aid us in establishing care priorities. Healing is a complex business, and requires steady awareness and a consciousness of our intentions, as Phyllis Waters and Jean Daubenmire have already advised us in Part One. There are no simple answers and we would be wise to reflect on that fact if we wish to describe our work as healing.

CHAPTER 10

The Journey of Self-Discovery in the Healing of Invisible Wounds

PEGGY L. STANDARD, RN, MSN, MA, LPC, LMFT

In the early 1980s in my practice as a nurse and family therapist, I received my first referral of "family incest" from Child Protective Services. Like many other healthcare professionals, I had no idea how to treat such an "enigma" and I certainly did not perceive it being a problem of such societal magnitude. Baffled, I consulted with colleagues only to discover that most of them were just as perplexed. So I turned to the survivor to learn, and I listened and observed as both children and adults began to reveal their stories. I perceived that the pain of this assault had been profound and that the wounds it had left on the souls of these individuals, although invisible, were deep and festering. Nevertheless, I also witnessed the resiliency and the intense need to overcome; and it is from these stories that I began to believe that it is the nature of human beings to seek survival and recovery—to heal.

The healing of a wound that is invisible to the healer may seem intangible; yet, the healing of an emotional wound is a natural process much like that of healing a physical wound. In a healthcare context, the healing process is described as occurring from within an organism even though the origin of the assault may be external. Physiological activity occurs from within the body that mobilizes healing agents; consequently, medical interventions focus on efforts to support and reinforce these natural internal healing processes. The earlier the wound receives therapeutic attention, the sooner the healing process is supported and the less likely

---

The specific therapy process introduced in this chapter is one of many therapeutic approaches used to promote the healing of invisible wounds brought about by emotional trauma. This approach, although unique in many ways, shares many common elements and techniques that other approaches have also discovered to be useful. While this approach may not be appropriate to use with all survivors, it is a therapeutic process that has, for some, successfully facilitated the healing journey.

avoidable complications will ensue. Like a physical wound, invisible wounds heal through support of the individual's natural internal healing powers; and it is through the process of self-discovery and empowerment that these internal healing powers can be activated.

The power to heal is within oneself. Everything needed to discover meaningful answers, to challenge one's shame-based identity, to recognize one's self-worth, and to heal the festering wounds are defensively stored within the survivor. The clinician, as a guide and supporter, facilitates the journey of self-discovery as it progresses through various stages of the natural healing process. As this journey creates opportunities for re-evaluation, healing changes that occur in the survivor's self-perception may ultimately lead to a greater sense of empowerment. Empowerment awakens the survivor's inner resources generating the strength to make positive personal life changes.

The healing process is not to be overly simplified, for the complexity of the work and experiences that occur through each of its phases is intense. Although the healing of invisible wounds is a highly individualized process, certain experiences are predictable and tend to progress through an identifiable "healing cycle." Various clinicians, including Courtois (1988), Kritsberg (1993), and Laidlaw, Malmow, and Associates (1990) have theorized stages of the healing process in the surviving adult that generally involve three to five stages. The names of each stage may vary; however, certain elements in the healing process are congruent: exposure of the wound, remembering and/or an intense reliving of the trauma, catharsis, externalizing the pain, re-evaluation of the trauma and its effects, grieving, and integration of the experience into a higher level of well-being. Through my experience as a clinician, I have come to believe that self-discovery is a continuous process; a process that transcends through all phases of the healing cycle strengthening the sense of empowerment that, in turn, fuels healing.

When trauma is experienced, survival defenses, such as repression, denial, and dissociation, are developed that help the survivor continue to function in the world, despite the profound pain that exists. Unfortunately, these same defenses, while protecting the survivor from the pain of the trauma, also restrict life's vitality and limit access to emotional resources. According to Rieker and Carmen (1986, p. 360), the adaptive survival strategies employed by the victim later form the core of the survivor's psychopathology. This results in observable secondary consequences: emotional numbing and/or flooding, nightmares, compulsive-addictive diseases, intimacy dysfunction, offender behaviors, multiple personality disorders, and physical illness, among others (Kritsberg, 1993, p. 57). The invisible wound, however, enveloped by denial of its existence and sealed with a repression of painful feelings and emotions, continues to fester. As a result, healing is prevented and past experiences continue to control unconsciously the present and future. This unconscious "survival dance," as I refer to it, continues until the survivor is able, with support, to expose the wound, deal with the pain, and integrate the trauma into conscious living.

True healing begins with exposing the wound. Rather than continuing to experience the pain of the trauma through secondary consequences, the survivor begins to search consciously for the source of the pain to explore the wound. At the same time, the protective defenses that were developed to prevent an encounter with overwhelming feelings become more permeable and the survivor begins to experience a cleansing catharsis of repressed painful feelings.

A critical task for the clinician is to create a safe environment for the ventilation of painful feelings and to encourage this expression, in order to validate the individual's capacity to survive. Once I have established a trusting relationship, for example, I find it helpful to introduce the healing process as a journey—a sometimes difficult and painful journey that takes one's self-perception from that of a helpless victim to an empowered survivor. I also suggest that this journey be recorded in a creative journal that serves as a tool both for gaining self-understanding and a positive self-concept through self-reflection and expression. Thoughts, feelings, pains, and fears are written down and drawn to record the words and images of the inner world. Because the journal is private and confidential, it provides for the individual a safe place to release painful feelings, recall memories, and further explore the impact of the trauma. Spontaneous creative drawing and reflective writing provide an avenue to learn about oneself and to gain insight into life's experiences. Continued encouragement and acceptance of the expression of contained emotions is very important as well, and especially to further the survivor's acceptance of those feelings, and ultimately of him or herself.

Since creating a safe environment is crucial to the progression of the natural healing process, I ask the survivor to create a safe place to store the journal, to imagine this place, and then to draw it (Figure 10.1). This process structures the imagination somewhat by providing a visual representation of safety. By symbolically placing the journal in a safe place the survivor will hopefully experience some transference of that sense of safety for him or herself.

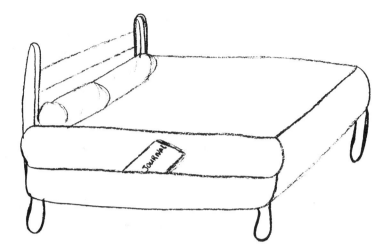

FIGURE 10.1. The survivor imagines a safe place to store the journal and then draws this.

As the wounds are exposed, intense emotional reactions and overwhelming feelings can emerge, which often precipitate the fear of losing control; that is, of his or her sanity. In assisting the survivor to prepare for those inevitable times, I use an intervention I refer to as "the container," a technique modified from the work of Jan Ellis (Laidlaw, 1990, p. 247). In implementing this technique, I ask the survivor to visualize a container, one with a locked opening to which only the survivor holds the key. This container should be attractive and strong enough to securely enclose intense feelings, including rage, guilt, shame, sadness, confusion, betrayal, loss, pain, and fear. I then ask the survivor to draw this container in the journal so that it is readily accessible, yet safely secured. The container will help to secure as many feelings as needed until the survivor, with support, consciously chooses to experience one of them. Figure 10.2 provides an example of this container drawing. According to Ellis (Laidlaw, 1990), the construction of the container is a symbolic act that represents the existence of boundaries and control of emotions (p. 247).

Once a safe environment has been created, it is time to begin the "journey of self-discovery" and to learn about the person within—a person who, on one hand is vulnerable with painful thoughts, feelings, and fears; while on the other, a person who brings strengths and power for recovery. I believe that drawing becomes a most significant resource for assessing the

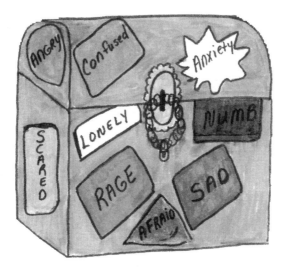

FIGURE 10.2.   In preparation for the journey, the survivor draws a container that will secure intense feelings.

full experience in that it is a tool for bypassing the unconscious protective defenses that often mask true feelings and concerns. Drawing combined with reflective writing and discussion, reveals a more total picture of the person within, including a portrayal of difficulties, obstacles, coping patterns, unconscious feelings and fears, strengths, and resources.

To initiate this process, I ask the survivor to draw a self-portrait in the journal and then to title the portrait. This reflective portrait reveals the survivor's conscious and unconscious perceptions of the person within. Most often, this initial self-portrait personifies a traumatized victim whose powerlessness and shattered self-worth is mirrored through vacant eyes and helpless features. Figure 10.3 shows an example of this picture. I then ask the survivor to reflectively record the story of the person in the portrait.

As the feelings begin to flow and the fear of losing control intensifies, I use relaxation exercises and the "container" technique in an effort to reinforce the survivor's ability to maintain some control while continuing to experience the feelings. Whenever the survivor feels too overwhelmed by fear, I reinforce safety by allowing the survivor to choose when it is time to enclose the feelings once again in the container. In doing so, I am

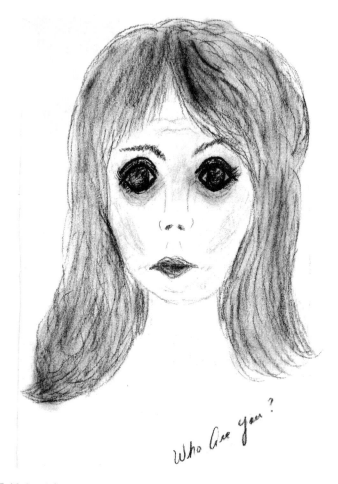

Who Are you?

FIGURE 10.3.   The survivor's initial self-portrait often personifies powerlessness and shattered self-esteem as mirrored through vacant eyes and helpless features.

hopefully encouraging and strengthening the survivor's conscious control of his or her own destiny.

As the healing process continues, I encourage the survivor to engage daily in relaxation exercises, followed by a quiet time for recording in the journal. The survivor may be led to record poetry, drawings, reflective writings, scribbles, or whatever, as long as the unconscious urges are al-lowed to guide the creativity. At each meeting, I encourage the survivor to share the journal experiences and process its contents along with the feelings being generated. As the journey of self-discovery continues, the pain is externalized as the protective defenses weaken, feelings intensify, and catharsis becomes a more powerful experience. This is the most in-tense phase of treatment and it is not unusual for the survivor to rage, sob, scream, or experience a re-emergence of nightmares, personal crises, or even self-destructive tendencies that require close monitoring. The survivor appears to be somewhat decompensating as he or she recon-nects with the feelings and re-experiences the trauma.

As the threatening feelings continue to emerge, there will be attempts by the survivor to once again cut off emotions. Most survivors will resist journalizing at this time. There are a few, however, who will experience a creative burst and use the journal to express their intense feelings through art and creative writing. The role of the clinician during this phase is to re-main unwavering and supportive; gently, yet firmly encouraging continua-tion of the healing journey. This approach is crucial even though the survivor often believes that true healing will never occur. The survivor vacillates between rage and despair and feels overwhelmed by the enor-mity of the healing task. It is important to remember that the clinician can never change or compensate for the survivor's past. Rather, the journey provides an opportunity to explore the past with a "pathfinder" whose task is to direct the life force through the darkness as the survivor's sense of personal empowerment becomes rooted and slowly begins to grow and strengthen.

Eventually, the despair and rage give way to grief as the survivor al-lows him or herself to mourn past losses. This grief is accompanied by an indepth re-evaluation of the trauma and its effects. As a part of this re-evaluation, the survivor will attempt to make some sense out of the cir-cumstances surrounding the trauma, becoming more aware of its after effects and the losses that resulted. Threatening feelings continue as the rage and intense grief manifest; however, the survivor now feels a greater sense of personal empowerment and is more willing to stay with the feelings and find closure.

I have been able to visibly witness the growth of personal empower-ment as the survivor begins to make small positive changes in his or her life, to be followed later by even greater, more impactful changes. Life's vitality is visibly returning as a sense of freedom envelops the spirit and

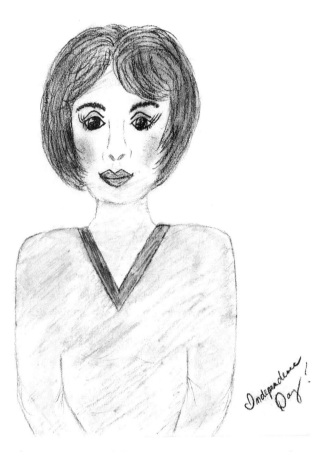

FIGURE 10.4. Integration of the traumatic experiences into living is solidified in the self-portrait of an empowered survivor.

the wounds cease to control feelings and actions. The survivor, who feels more in control, begins to make up for the losses of childhood and is now able to integrate the trauma experiences into living, not just surviving, as one's history and one's soul is reclaimed.

The final task is to help the survivor solidify integration of the trauma by providing a way for the survivor to visualize the healing and formalize the transition to health. As a final assignment, I ask the survivor to draw and title another self-portrait in the journal. Figure 10.4 exemplifies this final drawing.

This survivor, as portrayed, is then asked to write a letter to the first portrait validating its experiences, integrating the healing journey, and providing self-support and nurturance. The intent of this exercise is to connect the wounded victim to the now empowered survivor so, at those times in the future when the memories will again invoke intense feelings, the victim of the past can rely on the strength and nurturance of the survivor in the present to sustain emotional well-being. The empowered survivor now becomes his or her own resource for continued recovery. To formalize the transition to health and to close this chapter in the journey for self-discovery, I ask the survivor to plan a ritual. This unique ritual is a symbolic representation of whatever the survivor feels is needed for closure. One essential component of this ritual to be included, however, is a reading of the closing letter.

Dear Little One,

During these past few months, I've come to know you well. Rarely does a night go by that I don't see, but for a moment, those sad and frightened eyes. God knows those eyes have seen and endured things that no child has ever deserved. And from those eyes the tears flowed until there could be no more tears. The pain, oh, the unbearable pain! It was then that you locked them in your heart and sealed them forever, so you thought. Little did you know that they would always have complete control of your life. Little One, you are truly a survivor; you are stronger than you think. You protected us the only way you knew how. You helped me to forget the things I could not yet face, and because of your strength, we now have a chance to truly live.

I can't honestly say that I don't fully understand it all, but I know now that we, together, can face the pain. It's time now to live. It's my turn to care for you—to keep you safe, to love you, and to teach you how to live and enjoy life through me. Part of me is excited at new possibilities, yet part of me is still frightened of the journey. Nevertheless, I believe now that I am strong enough to do this for us. As difficult as it may be, I am asking you to trust that we shall overcome. You are my soul mate, Little One. I have missed you and I need you so that I may, once again, become whole.

—Independence Day

REFERENCES

Butler, S. (1985). *Conspiracy of silence. The trauma of incest.* Updated. San Francisco: Volcano Press.

Courtois, C. A. (1988). *Healing the incest wound: Adult survivors in therapy.* New York: W. W. Norton.

Kritsberg, W. (1993). *The invisible wound: A new approach to healing childhood sexual trauma.* New York: Bantam Books.

Laidlaw, T. A., Malmo, C., & Associates. (1990). *Healing voices: Feminist approaches to therapy with women.* San Francisco: Jossey-Bass.

Reiker, P., & Carmen, E. (1986). The victim-to-patient process: The disconfirmation and transformation of abuse. *American Journal of Orthopsychiatry, 56,* 360–370.

CHAPTER 11

Self-Healing: A Right and a Responsibility

CORINNE M. OPPERMANN, RN, MSN

From the grief of loss through the death and dying of loved ones a reflective, emergent spiritual philosophy of self-healing can arise. The experience of having three loved ones die from incurable illnesses over a period of several months has taught me as much. During these periods of grief from the impending loss of a loved one, I struggled to remain personally whole and professionally competent as a nurse. It seems strange to express the obvious. However, as a nurse, I had consistently placed the needs of others as the priority, sometimes at the exclusion of my own. Like many of my colleagues, I have faced the grief work of self-healing during periods of full-time employment in nursing practice.

Managing full-time employment and supporting a loved one who is dying is not the unique or exclusive domain of nurses. Our domain is the manner in which we engage in our healing practice. By this I am referring to our compassionate and therapeutic ability to fully support the healing process of the dying loved one, together with the loved one's family and friends. The energy required to engage in this process, while concomitantly experiencing grief is enormous. I have often felt the challenge was insurmountable. Is it possible to do the work of self-healing and remain competent in nursing practice? I believe that it is not only possible, but that it is a personal and professional responsibility.

I have defined self-healing as the ability to feel the pain of loss while continuously moving toward a state of wholeness in body, mind, and spirit. Wholeness refers to a person's sense of integrated peacefulness. Competency refers to the nurse's ability to adequately perform the responsibilities associated with one's practice while remaining therapeutic and humanistic.

Recognizing that the practice experiences of nurses who read this paper may range from novice to expert (Benner, 1984), with life experiences which span wide variations, it is imperative to state there is no single prescription for self-healing. Each of us enters into the self-healing process at different developmental and maturational levels both personally and professionally. I have practiced nursing in a variety of settings over the past 25 years. The critical events of loss discussed herein span a period of 12 years.

PHILOSOPHY AND THEORETICAL FRAMEWORK

The philosophy in this chapter reflects my belief in the spirituality of persons and the divine presence of the universe. It is congruent with Florence Nightingale's philosophy, "the laws of science are the Thoughts of God" (Macrae, 1995, p. 8), and "spirituality as intrinsic to human nature and compatible with science can guide the development of future nursing practice and inquiry" (p. 8).

Whereas the philosophy of this paper is significantly spiritual, the theoretical framework is grounded in humanistic nursing practice theory (Paterson & Zderad, 1988). "Humanistic nursing practice theory proposes that nurses consciously and deliberately approach nursing as an existential experience" (p. 3). The framework guides my exploration of the developing human potential for healing, both the loved one's and mine (the nurse), as it occurs in the unique domain of healing from loss through death (Paterson & Zderad, 1988). What is the meaning of dying to the loved one who is facing personal mortality? What promotes healing for the loved one and the loved one's family, friends, and the nurse as family or friend? Are there interactive healing relationships that mutually occur among those experiencing the healing process?

To report what I have come to know and understand about the interactive process of healing, a phenomenological description of each experience is provided. In compiling and synthesizing these experiences, I have developed a model for self-healing. Recognizing that the number of cases (3) is small, the utility of this model for others is uncertain. The model for self-healing and the practices that have promoted my self-healing following the loss of loved ones is shared in the hope that it will stimulate further exploration. Examples of healing practices gleaned from experiences are interwoven with stories throughout the paper to clarify its content. The stories are told with permission of the families (see note at the end of the chapter). The self-healing practices discussed herein are not all inclusive.

SELF-HEALING MODEL

In addition to reflecting a spiritual philosophy, model development was guided by the belief that personal and professional growth is an ever-evolving process. This process of personal and professional growth is critically affected by grief from the loss of a loved one through death. The model is cyclic in nature and reveals the interactive process of mutuality. Mutuality of growth has the potential for occurring through relationships developed among those engaged in the death and dying process. The key elements of the model suggest that it is the nurse who guides the process.

Although painful, the nurse receives the opportunity for growth by being open to the mystery of death and accepting the invitation of the loved one to share in the sacredness of the dying journey. Concomitantly, the following interactions are occurring and evolving. The nurse recognizes the importance of healing self and initiates the process through introspection. The nurse provides support and comfort for the loved one who is experiencing and guiding the dying journey. The nurse experiences and facilitates the healing relationships mutually evolving among family, friends, and the person who is dying. Mutuality of providing and receiving support and comfort is experienced by the nurse, family, and friends of the dying loved one.

The purpose of the model is to: (1) provide the opportunity for nurses to heighten self-awareness in recognizing the importance of self-healing from the grief of loss through the death and dying of a loved one, (2) to acknowledge the sacredness of experiencing a person's dying journey (Foos-Graber, 1992), (3) to recognize the impact of the interactive process of mutuality of support experienced among family members, friends, the loved one, and the nurse, and (4) to suggest that one's nursing practice may be enhanced through professional growth from contending with the pain of loss. What is not apparent in the model is the depth of growth that the nurse experiences. The depth is without an end and uniquely resides within each of us, varying among us. This cyclic model is depicted in Figure 11.1.

In describing the experience of self-healing phenomenologically, I have used the process suggested by Paterson and Zderad (1988). "The process of how to describe nursing events entails deliberate responsible, conscious, aware, nonjudgemental existence of the nurse in the nursing situation followed by disciplined authentic reflection and description" (p. 7). As one would expect, the first step to initiating self-healing is the recognition that it is an internally guided process; one that entails introspection, reflection, thoughtful deliberation, and evaluation. Although

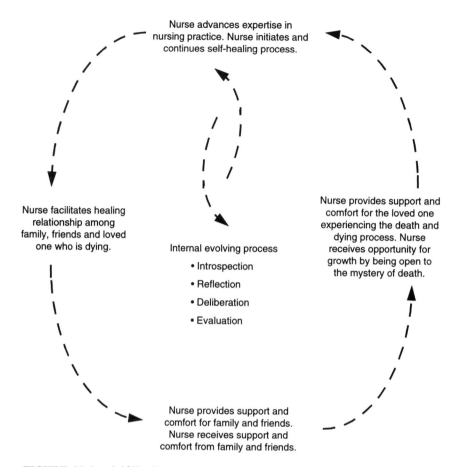

FIGURE 11.1.   Self-Healing: An Evolving Process.

internally guided, the self-healing process involves mutuality with others whereby healing connections are established. Self-healing is also an evolving journey without an end.

The following three stories provide descriptions of my experiences in traveling with loved ones through their journey. I have used the term deathing to describe the dying process. The foundation for my learning experience about self-healing begins with Katherine's story. The breadth and depth of my learning is further developed with Jane's and Norma's stories.

Opening up to the pain of death, our own or that of someone we love, is one of the most mysterious blessings of life. (Marianne Williamson, 1994, p. 116)

KATHERINE'S STORY

In 1983, I served as the director of nursing for the ob-gyn nursing service in a large university health science center in the southwestern United States. I was also one of two nurses within a large family. The first nurse in our family was dying. She was my husband's mother. The mother of five sons, mother-in-law of four, grandmother of 17, with two living sisters, a sister-in-law, and brother-in-law, she was the beloved matriarch of the family. Knowing that she was dying, Katherine was clear about her wishes to remain at home. She found comfort in the many visits of her family.

At this time, the Hospice program was in the early beginnings in our city. Although Katherine was informed of their services, she had decided who would be permitted to care for her and was not willing to allow any "strangers" into her home. Katherine was lucid, oriented, and in control of her dying process and it was like this until her death.

It was during Katherine's dying process that I first began to recognize my need to make room in my life for grieving. As a result of this experience, I became aware of the dangers of denying my need to grieve. By being open to the pain of Katherine's dying, I was given the opportunity to learn to self-heal.

Katherine was widowed and lived alone. Our family had ensured that she received visits or phone calls on a daily basis since the death of her spouse. Although some of the family lived within an hour or a few hours travel time by car, all, except our family and a sister-in-law, lived in another city. Holidays were celebrated by most members of the family at her home. As long as Katherine was able to manage the activities of daily living, the energy required in providing her support and comfort was minimal. During the last three months of her life, she became progressively weaker, requiring more assistance. The energy required to provide her care became intense.

The work responsibilities required in my role as nursing director and the increased family responsibilities in my role as the nurse member of the family were exceeding my supply of energy. I felt as though I were on a treadmill running full speed with an ever-decreasing energy level. It was during this time that I developed the self-awareness that I alone could make the choice of how to proceed. It was either stop and face the pain of the situation, or deny and collapse from exhaustion.

Prayer says something incalculably about who we are and what our destiny may be. (Larry Dossey, 1993, p. 6)

Where does one begin in seeking wise answers to difficult challenges in times of crisis? For me, the beginning and the end are the same—the alpha and the omega—a divine wisdom that, when sought, is found within. I found an answer through daily prayer and meditation. It is not my intent to provide advice on how to pray or even if one ought to do as I did. One's conversation with the universe is unique and personal. Whether one's religious belief and practices be Christian, Jewish, Hindu, Buddhist, Muslim, Jain, Confucian, Sikhs, Zoroastrian, or other, the opportunity to use prayer is present (Eck, 1993). And for some, who have no formal religious preference, spiritual communication with the universe remains an option. The use of prayer thus enabled me to find the courage to turn and face the painful truth of Katherine's dying and accept my limitations in providing her care.

Deathing has two aims: to make sure that the dying are comfortable and comforted as they die, and to help all of us prepare for the greatest adventure we will face since birth. (Anya Foos-Graber, 1992, p. i)

Having decided to face the overwhelming sense of pain that I felt and that of Katherine and family members, I began to recognize and accept Katherine's deathing process. I realized that I was then better able to hear her wishes and subtle directives. She was very clear on the importance of her being in her own home during this most intimate journey. And she was also very clear about whom she would allow to accompany her: the members of her family. With the knowledge and support of Katherine's oncologist, I prepared a nursing care plan for her home care with her participation. Katherine wished to provide the direction for the activities that were incorporated into the plan. Upon completion of this initial plan, I recognized that if Katherine's wishes were to be realized, I must accept my limitations, both personally and professionally, in providing her care alone or with minimal assistance.

An ordinary family: my family is ordinary, but we share love. (John Bruhn, 1980, p. 25)

My husband, Gus, is the first-born of Katherine's five sons and it was with him that I first discussed my concerns. After thoughtful deliberation, we decided to request a family meeting with his brothers. During the meeting, each brother received a copy of their mother's plan of care and each volunteered to assist with portions of this care. For example, this meant learning to prepare her favorite foods, assisting with her oral medication administration, managing oxygen equipment and administration, and rotating weekend coverage. During the weeks that followed, Katherine's grandchildren and sisters also took turns with providing her care. Her home became the central hub of family activity. During the weekdays, a long time family friend and household employee stayed with Katherine while Gus and I were at work. During the weekday evenings and nights, Gus and I took turns staying with Katherine. It was during these times that I began to keep a journal of activities and my inner thoughts which was beneficial in helping to revise Katherine's care plan to satisfy her needs. The journal assisted me in becoming increasingly introspective and aware of my own internal struggles and pain. As a result, I was able to release my feelings through writing, thereby remaining therapeutic for those around me. The practice of writing a journal during this experience was healing.

The process of humanistic nursing stemming from the nurse's authentic commitment is a kind of being with and doing with. It aims at the development of human potential through intersubjectivity and responsible choosing. (Paterson and Zderad, 1988, p. 20)

As nursing director for ob-gyn nursing service for seven years, I practiced humanistic nursing administration. Thus, while faced with the high-energy demands of guiding and participating in Katherine's care plan, I realized that I would not be able to expend the same high energy in my professional role. I prepared myself to resign my position and seek another position that would require less energy. In discussing this plan with the ob-gyn nurse management team, their response was a surprise. They requested that I reconsider this decision. They suggested that they felt prepared to assume more responsibility and were clear on the mission, standards, and goals of the nursing service. Further, they knew the parameters for their boundaries of decision making. They helped me to understand that they were ready to advance their growth, but were not yet ready for my departure as nursing director. I reflected on this communication. After thoughtful deliberation regarding their readiness and preparedness to assume more leadership and management responsibilities, I was able to accept their support. By so doing, we mutually experienced growth. They advanced their skills and knowledge regarding the humanistic practice of nursing administration. I was able to conserve the energy needed to initiate and continue my self-healing process while facilitating

Katherine's care. This shared experience has produced connections among us that endure.

> *The power of God is greater than death. (Marianne Williamson, 1994, p. 117)*

After three months of continuous care by family members, Katherine died. She remained in her home until her death. We knew that she had given us a great gift by inviting us to be with her on her deathing journey.

> *We release what was and make room for what shall be, we testify within our minds that life does not end but merely transmutes, that today we say goodbye and yet we also say hello. (Marianne Williamson, 1994, p. 283)*

Katherine's funeral services were planned by her sons, each suggesting certain prayers, music, and rituals that had been important to Katherine and thus were important to us as a family. We found comfort and healing in Katherine's memorial services.

Through reflection, I realize that Katherine taught us how to die. And in so doing, we advanced our knowledge of living. We are not the same. We have grown as individuals and in our relationships as a family. We are connected and these connections endure.

> *It is well to give when asked, but it is better to give unasked, through understanding. (Kahlil Gibran, 1923, p. 20)*

There are many ways that a loved one may be remembered following death. The practice of making donations to charities and organizations is one that serves to benefit many. Katherine's memory is perpetuated through the establishment of an endowed scholarship for nursing students. Initiated by her sons, most members of the family made contributions. I could sense her joyful spirit when the donations arrived from the grandchildren. The memorial scholarship endowment assisted each of us with our self-healing process and supported our celebration of Katherine's life. Since her death, three grandchildren and a daughter-in-law have entered the nursing profession.

The evolving process of my self-healing initiated during this journey continues. Although I have accepted Katherine's loss, there are times when some event or word will recall special memories of her. I pause to experience the feeling and sometimes tears flow.

Model Application

By being open to Katherine's dying process, I was able to begin the self-healing process while supporting Katherine's lead in her dying journey. This meant authentically being with her and with myself while not imposing my feelings upon her. To Katherine the dying process meant being with her family members as she grieved their loss at her impending death. Being with Katherine and providing care and support for her through her deathing process, provided her family with mutual comfort and support.

What were the key elements that I learned about the self-healing process from this experience? Through introspection, reflection, and thoughtful deliberation, I have identified these elements as: (1) use of prayer in self-healing; (2) recognizing and accepting Katherine's deathing process; (3) recognizing and accepting my limitations; (4) accepting the support of family, colleagues, and friends; (5) preparing and revising Katherine's care plan to provide for the continuity of her care by family members; (6) writing a journal to remain open to my feelings and empower myself to manage them; (7) participating in bringing closure to Katherine's death at her funeral service; and (8) celebrating Katherine's life through the perpetuation of her memory in the establishment of an endowed scholarship to benefit nursing students.

Several years after Katherine's death, Jane, a dear friend and nursing colleague, was diagnosed with an untreatable cancer and told that she had six months to live. She resigned her position as director of pediatric nursing and retired to her home. Jane had lived with her adoptive mother, Lua, who was planning early retirement from her supervisory position in surgery nursing service to care for Jane at home. Jane, Lua, and I had served together in administrative nursing positions in three separate hospitals at the same university health science center.

Through prayer we find what we cannot find elsewhere: a peace that is not of this world. (Marianne Williamson, 1994, p. 73)

JANE'S STORY

Shortly after Jane learned of the prognosis associated with her cancer, she requested that I visit her. It had been three years since my transfer from the nursing director's position to a faculty position at the university's nursing school. This first visit was difficult and painful for both of us.

Jane shared her feelings regarding the shock of the prognosis. "What am I going to do?" she questioned. For a short time, we sat in silence, holding hands. During this period of silence, I was able to center myself and prayerfully listen for guidance. Prayer "flows from one's true center" (Dossey, 1993, p. 23). "It is focused, authentic, genuine, and accepting of any outcome" (p. 23). I asked Jane if she would find it helpful if we prayed together. She replied that she would like to do so. Jane was our prayer guide. I could not presume to know how Jane should approach God in facing her mortality. Being authentically present with Jane as we prayed together provided me with a sense of peacefulness. At the conclusion of our prayers, Jane stated that she found comfort and hope in our prayers. She asked if we could do this again sometime. Thus our weekly prayer visits began and, over time, several of Jane's friends and nursing colleagues joined us. These prayer practices proved to have a reciprocal effect among those of us who participated. Jane lived for two years following her diagnosis. During this time, Jane used prayer as a part of her healing therapy. The healing power of prayer is discussed by Larry Dossey in his book *Healing Words* (1993).

And in the sweetness of friendship let there be laughter, and the sharing of pleasures. (Kahlil Gibran, 1980, p. 59)

Watching Walt Disney was among the pleasurable activities that Jane and I shared. We were both Disney fans and found laughter to be healing. Jane was also a fan of the Chicago Bears and Cubs and watched their games with great zest. Although I did not share this enthusiasm, I appreciated the opportunity to share experiences with Jane that brought her delight. Throughout her dying process, Jane retained her joy for living.

If you love, let these be your desires: to wake at dawn with a winged heart and give thanks for another day of loving. (Kahlil Gibran, 1980, p. 13)

Approximately eleven months before Jane died, her only child Kathleen became pregnant. Jane requested that our weekly prayer sessions center on her desire to see and hold her grandchild. During this period of anticipating the delight of being a grandmother, Jane began to reminisce about the many joyful experiences in her life. And in most, Kathleen, Steve, and Lua were the focus. Kathleen and her spouse, Steve, lived in the Midwest and frequently visited Jane.

A few days before the expected date of her grandchild's birth, Jane traveled to the Midwest via airplane. She was at the hospital when her granddaughter, Mary Jane, was born. Jane held her shortly after birth. Words cannot adequately describe Jane's exultation with this experience.

During Jane's dying process, I maintained a written journal of my observations and reflections of the meaning of being with a loved one as she faced her own mortality. Again, I experienced healing in writing about Jane's journey.

Nursing implies a special kind of meeting of human persons. It occurs in response to a perceived need related to the health illness quality of the human condition. (Paterson and Zderad, 1988, p. 24)

Following Mary Jane's birth and several weeks after returning home, Jane weakened. She was unable to walk or care for herself. Lua was providing complete nursing care for Jane with the help of a Hospice aide during the night. When Lua became very ill requiring hospitalization, Jane was transferred to respite care at a local hospital. The limitation on Jane's respite care was one week. Thereafter, she would be moved to a nursing home. Lua expressed grave concern that she would not be able to support Jane's wishes to die at home.

A special kind of meeting occurred among nurses in response to this concern that we perceived was of critical importance to Jane and to Lua. Members of pediatric and ob-gyn nursing services requested that I attend an emergency meeting to determine how to assist Jane and Lua during this crisis. After much discussion, the following plan was implemented.

Susan, a former member of Jane's nursing staff, who regularly visited her, obtained Jane's permission to request nursing volunteers for Jane's care. Susan wrote a letter to the nursing staffs of pediatric, ob-gyn, and surgery for this purpose. The response to the letter was notable. Nurses from the seven nursing services and the nursing school volunteered to provide Jane with nursing care at home. Within three days, the number of nursing volunteers was adequate to assist with Jane's care at home for a two-week period.

To provide for continuity of care, a written care plan was developed with Lua and Jane's guidance. Lila, a nurse manager, from ob-gyn nursing service prepared the comprehensive plan of care as well as the scheduling of nurses. Serving as consultant to Lila for this plan, my knowledge of the healing process associated with the care of a dying loved one was increased. This increased level of knowing served to enhance my nursing practice.

Shortly after Jane returned home, Lua was also discharged from the hospital. Lua, still recovering from her illness, was grateful to be at home with Jane. Eleven days into the implementation of Jane's plan of care, Jane died at home with Lua at her bedside. Some of their nursing friends were with them. We were open to the mystery of dying and to our truth in the meaning of self-healing.

> *Even the death of friends will inspire us as much as their lives. (Henry David Thoreau, 1817–1862)*

An article in the university newspaper (*Impact*, 1993) contained the following quotation: "Jane had the unique ability to touch the lives of those around her in a special way. She was able to share her journey of pain, suffering, and terminal illness in a way that facilitated the growth of her friends and colleagues as individuals and professionals," said Beverly McCormick, Nursing Care Coordinator at Hospice (p. 5). Closure was brought to Jane's dying process through our participation in her funeral service. Donations were made to the university's nursing school to establish a scholarship for nursing students in Jane's memory.

Model Application

Many of the self-healing practices employed during Katherine's deathing journey were also used during Jane's journey. The practices were expanded to include the healing impact of laughter and of sharing joyful experiences. I increased my knowledge and understanding of the healing process. The interactive healing process was guided and experienced by several nurses. The mutuality of the healing connections that occurred among Jane's family, friends, and colleagues endure. We are not the same. We have grown.

> *There are friends who sail together through quiet waters and stormy weather, helping each other through joy and through strife. (Mary Dawson Hughes in* The Poetry of Friendship, *1973, p. 40)*

NORMA'S STORY

Norma, a friend of 26 years, was also my neighbor and confidant. She was a brilliant professional woman, articulate in written and oral communication.

When she was diagnosed with a terminal illness, she wanted to remain at home until her death. The loss of Norma's presence in my life would be severe. If invited, I was prepared to provide support for her dying journey.

A dying person most needs to be shown as unconditional a love as possible, released from all expectation. (Sogyal Rinpoche, 1994, p. 175)

Norma's only child, Jean, made arrangements to stay with her and provide her home care through the direction of Hospice. During my visits with them, I admired the strength and courage of these two women. Together they were preparing for Norma's death. The rhythms of their relationship were in concert. They balanced love, endearment, pain, suffering, laughter, stress, joy, integrity, remembrances in remarkable ways. To be in their presence was to experience unconditional love. It was a privilege for me to be welcomed into this sacred chamber. It was very clear that throughout her dying process, Norma's first thoughts were in Jean's best interest and Jean's first thoughts were always in the best interests of her mother. Jean's authentic support of Norma released her to face her own mortality without preconceived expectations or conditions.

During the three months that Jean stayed with Norma, Jean and I took frequent walks together usually at the end of the day. Our discussions often focused on the principles of Zen spirituality that Jean was studying with a Zen master. I realized that in order to effectively support Jean I needed to familiarize myself with the meaning of Zen spirituality. To do so, I read *Healing Breath: Zen Spirituality for a Wounded Earth* by Rubin L.F. Habito (1993) and *Thoughts of the East* by Thomas Merton (1995). These books assisted me in developing an acceptance of the paradox of Zen as well as the practice of meditation. "The word Zen comes from the Chinese Ch'an, which designates a certain type of meditation, yet Zen is not a method of meditation or a kind of spirituality. It is a 'way' and an 'experience,' a 'life,' but the way is paradoxically 'not a way'" (Merton, p. 30). "Zen is consciousness unstructured by particular form or particular system, a trans-cultural, trans-religious, trans-formed consciousness" (Merton, p. 34). Although I did not understand the "meaning" or "lack of meaning" of Zen, I respected the importance of the Zen experience in Jean's life. And in so doing, I found the "way" to support Jean and Norma in the final days of Norma's dying journey.

If your last thoughts are of the light (by whatever deity's name or form) and /or an enlightened being you know and love, a perfect mirroring occurs-enlightenment. (Anya Foos-Graber, 1992, p. 213)

Frequently, Jean practiced visualizing the presence of a light merging with her mother's light, which is a practice done on behalf of a dying person. During the week preceding her death, Norma would speak to Jean of the beautiful light that she saw in her bedroom. Although these conversations brought comfort to Jean, she was becoming very tired as Norma's care increasingly required more of her energy. Jean had kept her vigil and recognized that she was near the point of exhaustion. This caused her concern because it was important to Jean that she be with her mother at the time of her death. As Norma's condition weakened, Jean agreed to my staying with them. During the times that I sat at Norma's bedside, I prayed and visualized Norma's spirit merging with the light. I experienced peace and a spiritual "oneness" with Norma.

Meditation practice can be essentialized into three crucial points: bring your mind home, and release, and relax. (Sogyal Rinpoche, 1994, p. 62)

It was late, during the night before Norma died, that Jean recognized there was no further action that she could take to improve her mother's comfort. She allowed herself to release intense pain with great heaving sobs and irregular breathing. I held her to provide comfort and love. After a while I asked her if she wanted to take the medication available to assist her with relaxation. She responded "no." When I inquired as to what would she find helpful, she stated that she wanted to meditate. She practiced Zen meditation for over 20 minutes. After this, Jean rested. It was an enlightening experience for me to be with this young woman as she found the courage to bring her mind home, and release, and relax.

The following afternoon, Norma died. A short bedside service was conducted before Norma's body was removed from her home. Four months following Norma's death, Jean and Michael hosted a gathering of family and friends to celebrate Norma's life.

Model Application

As shown in the three stories, the spirituality of the self-healing process is internally guided through the use of introspection, reflection, thoughtful deliberation, and evaluation. By meeting my responsibility to self-heal, I have grown spiritually and professionally. The interpersonal relationships and connections that were established throughout these deathing journeys endure. Most importantly I have learned not to fear death. By so doing, I am better able to be with those who are dying and provide comfort and support for those who are grieving.

I am a philosopher studying my own mind . . . I essay to write my seeing and hearing and touching. (Alice Koller, 1990, p. 41)

I am a nurse studying the art, science, and spirit of self-healing from the loss of a loved one through death. In order to remain whole as a person and competent in nursing practice, I believe that it is my responsibility to engage in practices that support self-healing. Through my use of introspection, reflection, thoughtful deliberation and evaluation, a model was developed to guide the personal and professional growth of the nurse during the process of self-healing. The model identifies the interactive healing relationships mutually occurring among humans who are engaged in a loved one's dying journey.

According to Carper (1978), personal knowing is one of "four fundamental patterns of knowing" (p. 13). The science of phenomenology (Streubert & Carpenter, 1995) was used to describe my particular experiences with self-healing from the loss of loved ones through death and dying.

By being with and exploring the meaning of dying with loved ones, who are facing their own mortality, it is most important that the nurse accept, without judgment, the way each chooses to travel the dying journey. This is particularly important when the nurse has different religious and/or spiritual preferences from the loved one(s). The use of introspection helps to clarify one's own religious and spiritual truth while respecting and supporting that of the dying persons. Respecting the loved one's truth about the mystery and meaning of departure from one's body during the time of death is of critical importance to the loved one and to the self-healing process of the nurse.

ACKNOWLEDGMENTS

This paper is dedicated to Phyllis Kritek, my mentor for this publication. Katherine's Story is dedicated to Katherine and Mary Rose. It was written with the permission of Gus, IV, K. Robert, Theodore Joseph, John Conrad, and Joseph Kay with acknowledgment of ob-gyn nursing colleagues:

Cheryl, Vador, Lila, Marcia, Leelamma, Helen, Phyllis, Sandra, and Rose. Jane's Story is dedicated to Jane, Lua, Kathleen, Stephen, Maryjane, Mark, and Patrick, and Beverly of Hospice of Galveston County and nursing colleagues of UTMB Galveston Nursing Services. It was written with the permission of Lua and Kathleen. Norma's Story is dedicated to Norma, Jean and Michael, and Barbara and Binna of Hospice of Galveston County. It was written with the permission of Jean.

References

Bartlett, J. (1980). *Familiar quotations* (15th ed.), 6th printing. Quotation from Henry David Thoreau, 558, No. 13. In E. Morison Beck (Ed.). Boston: Little, Brown.

Bearly, B. S. (1973). *The poetry of friendship.* Kansas City, MO: Hallmark.

Benner, P. (1984). *From novice to expert.* Menlo Park, CA: Addison-Wesley.

Bruhn, J. C. (1980). *Being me is being human.* Galveston, TX: Author.

Carper, B. (1978). Fundamental patterns of knowing in nursing. *Advances in Nursing Science, 1*(1), 13-2.

Dossey, L. (1993). *Healing words: The power of prayer and the practice of medicine* (1st ed). New York: Harper.

Eck, D. L. (1993). *Encountering God: A spiritual journey from Bozeman to Banaras.* Boston, MA: Beacon Press.

Foos-Graber, A. (1992). *Deathing: An intelligent alternative for the final moments of life.* York Beach, ME: Nicholas-Hays.

Gibran, K. (1980). *The prophet* (104th ed.). New York: Alfred A. Knopf.

Halbito, R. L. F. (1993). *Healing breath: Zen spirituality for a wounded earth.* New York: Orbis Books.

Koller, A. (1990). *Working: The stations of solitude.* New York: William Morrow.

Macrae, J. (1995). Nightingale's spiritual philosophy and its significance for modern nursing. *Image: Journal of Nursing Scholarship, 27*(1), 8-10.

Merton, T. (1995). *Thoughts on the east.* New York: New Directions.

Paterson, J. G., & Zderad, L. T. (1988). *Humanistic nursing.* New York: NLN Press.

Powledge, M. (1995). Steinbach scholarship for nursing established. *UTMB Impact, 17*(5), 5.

Rinpoche, S. (1994). *The Tibetan book of living and dying.* In P. Gaffney & A. Harvey (Ed). New York: Harper.

Streubert, H. J., & Carpenter, D. R. (1995). *Qualitative research in nursing: Advancing the humanistic imperative.* Philadelphia: J. B. Lippincott.

Styles, M. M., & Moccia, P. (1993). *On nursing: A literary celebration, an anthology.* New York: NLN Press.

Williamson, M. (1994). *Illuminata: Thoughts, prayers, rights of passage.* New York: Random House.

CHAPTER 12

A Healing Journey: The First Steps

REBECCA A. HARBIN, RN, BSN, CEN

BARBARA A. CARNES, RN, CS, PHD

We happened to be sitting next to each other for our final lunch before leaving an Elisabeth Kübler-Ross, Life, Death, and Transitions Workshop. We discovered that we were both nurses, one a faculty member, the other a diploma graduate wishing for a BSN. "What is stopping you from getting your degree? Five years from now you'll be five years older whether you get it or not." Two years later we came together again, this time as student and faculty in one of the required courses in the BSN completion program. The student spoke of her healing as part of her class presentation, the faculty member invited her to share her healing journey with others. This paper is a result of our coming together to explore and to share our stories of healing. Since only one of us lived this particular story, this paper is written in first person. In the process of our exploring and sharing, we each moved farther along in our own healing. Perhaps we didn't just "happen" to be sitting next to each other at lunch; we continue to wonder and to treasure the gift we have become to each other.

Living the healing experience is a lifelong, interdependent process. In this paper, we will explore the lived experience of a healing journey. The journey is in process; it has begun, but it is not yet finished.

Healing involves one's whole being. It covers a variety of levels—physical, emotional, mental, and spiritual. All these levels intersect and each has an impact on the other. Physical injuries are obvious, and with attention, will heal leaving only a small scar. Often, there are emotional or mental injuries that occur simultaneously. Sometimes, the emotional or mental injuries occur and there are no concrete signs of damage. Too often, we bury these emotional or mental injuries thinking that they will just go away or that they are just a figment of a fertile imagination. This is a fallacy. By ignoring or burying the injury, one seeds the fertile field of an emergent boil. Too often this occurs in our society. "Be tough," "Pull yourself up by the bootstraps," "Brush it off." These clichés all fertilize the seeds of anger, rage, guilt, and shame. The mental, emotional, and spiritual damage associated with unfinished business does greater harm than any physical injury ever could do; the longer it is ignored, the more it festers.

Unfinished business can become a painful, purulent systemic infection. It directs attention away from the original wound; inducing pain in another area diverts attention away from the original source. By the time the decision to do something about the pain is made, the whole being can be infected. The infection rages throughout the body, festering, fermenting, and growing as it kills the spirit, the inner peace, the person. Healing will not occur unless the individual deals with the emotional and mental aspects of the wound.

All wounds must be examined. Acknowledging, observing, and understanding the wound contributes to its healing. An action plan must be developed after examining the options. This is often not a one shot deal. The immediate relief associated with the incising and draining of the wound is often followed by the filling of the newly created hole with more pus leading to even more pain. This procedure must be repeated until new, healthy tissue fills the hole.

Examining the wound's impact on the past, dealing with that impact, and learning to choose its impact on the future contribute to healing. Developing and implementing a plan of action takes mental, emotional, and spiritual work. These have been the most draining and painful steps in my journey thus far. It is possible to learn from the past to prevent recurrence of the injury in the future. The result of this work is growth and wholeness. The exudate can be used to fertilize flowers, vegetables, and fruits for the self, the birds, society, and all of nature.

My journey began in childhood, when I was about three or four years old, and there have been many twists and turns along the way. There was a lot of physical and emotional violence in my family. There were many secrets, and secrets kept me sick. I had asthma as a child; I had to be intubated several times. At ten years of age, I was writing about suicide and people dying. I tried to kill myself to get my parents' attention and the help I needed. I've been in depression all my life. I was taught that my family was like an island with little or no need for help from outside. My boundaries were breached in childhood, or maybe, I didn't know my boundaries. I wanted to trust my family; I wanted to believe them, but was told that I was a failure. My fear kept growing and growing. I was in pain.

Many of us who have been abused would rather die than feel the pain. Pain is a sign that something needs to change. My healing began when I recognized that I needed healing. I had to become aware of this need and I had to begin to take care of it. Sometimes, I dream that one day I will be healed and that when that day comes, I will be able to say, "Look what I did!" I also dream about being healed and living out in the country, growing my own food, and taking care of people in a clinic. There are other times when I believe that I'm unworthy of being healed. There are other times when I wonder about my ability to care for myself. I need to face the fear and figure out where that comes from. I need to know the fear, face it, and decide what to do about it. I believe that my physical, spiritual, and emotional beings are all connected and that I became physically ill because I didn't have the skills I needed to recognize and to deal with the emotional and spiritual wounds of my physical abuse. That is something with which I still need to deal.

As I was so young, and our family rule was isolation, I was a lonely traveler on this journey toward healing. I chose paths that looked promising; those that led to what I understood to be goodness, comfort, health, and love. Often, based on my brief experience of living, the path I chose led to even more injury rather than healing. There was a hole, an emptiness, inside me. I tried to fill the void with everything that offered to ease or to distract my attention from the emptiness and pain. Whenever the air would blow against my wound, I would medicate. This "medication" took the forms of unhealthy eating, drugs, sex, relationships, and high-risk behavior. At times, it seems like my whole life has been one self-destructive act.

I buried myself in relationships that I thought would prove to me that I was a lovable, valuable, and worthwhile being. These relationships always involved men who had problems that were consuming them. I didn't believe that I was worth saving, but I thought that maybe I could save them by giving up myself. Saving "others" was a legacy of my childhood fantasies. I knew that love could change them. I believed that if I could "love" them enough to save them, then maybe they would love me and I would be able to feel what love was. I had never felt loved unconditionally; I had always equated love with sex. I attempted to do that with others.

For a while, I thought that I had found the answer, but as each relationship escalated into abuse and violence, I learned nothing that advanced my knowledge of love. I never gave up; I kept searching. I repeatedly ended up in life-threatening relationships. At one point, I attempted to save a felon after his release from jail. That experience left me physically, sexually, emotionally, mentally, and financially bankrupt. I was devastated.

For the next five years, I continued my search for answers and for love, always in life-threatening relationships. I was dead inside. Nothing I did filled my self. This was a hole from which I couldn't escape. My final downward spiral into the black abyss began when I met a man whose friend sexually assaulted me. This "friend" was HIV-positive. Eventually I called my mom. She helped me get into therapy. Without my usual coping mechanisms, I ended up in seclusion in a psychiatric unit.

It was not until I gave up my long-standing belief that I didn't need help that I got help. I have discovered that when I have a failing attitude, when the negatives make up my inner core, I can't heal—the negatives knock out the positives and I just stagnate. It is impossible to find healing without direction. Finally, I made the choices to fill the emptiness with my higher power. I do not believe that I made this healing choice on my own. One night I hit a brick wall, fainted, and when I came to, I was seeing stars. One of those stars spoke to me, saying, "Wake up, stupid." When I "woke up," and turned my life over to a higher being, I started healing.

There had been many injuries in my family. I held on to the learned anger for a long time. I was ill and just didn't see it. In 1991, I followed a path that led to my coming together with an aunt to heal our relationship. My aunt is the person who has helped me to fill in the blanks of my past; ours is one of my most valued relationships. If I hadn't been open to this opportunity, I would not have grown as much as I have. That is what hate and anger does. They keep us from growing.

I have found other new paths that have led to growth. I discovered a wonderful healing process which was developed by Elisabeth Kübler-Ross. Her Life, Death, and Transitions Workshop provided me a safe, non-threatening environment with an abundance of unconditional love in which to begin the process of grieving the losses and the unfinished business associated with my childhood abuse. The Kübler-Ross process empowered me, and I began to feel and to deal with the unfinished business of my childhood. My higher power continued to guide me and to strengthen me with a willingness to delve even deeper.

Following a near-death experience when I was twelve years old, I had promised God that if I were allowed to live, I would become a nurse and give Him one year of my life. I kept that promise. I did become a nurse, but I enjoyed it and continued long after that first year. In my recovery, I began to view my nursing career as a healing path. The value that I placed on my nursing career contributed to my recovery. I didn't want to mess up that opportunity. If it hadn't been for my wanting to continue in nursing, I probably wouldn't have listened to the star. Writing this paper, talking about, and sharing my experience are all part of the healing process. I know my buttons have been pushed during this process. Frequently, this has been a signal to me that there is something that I need to hear. When I have listened, it has helped.

Often I have wanted to get into "my old shoes," but I'd be honest with myself, and realize that back then, there was only emptiness and darkness. Dishonesty and my dwelling on my past kept me caught in the quicksand of the great abyss, that place where I am a human doing, not a human being; that place where I am only an empty shell of flesh. I have come to realize that the memories can't kill me unless I allow them to. As a child, I survived the reality of the abuse. I can look at that experience and accept it for what it was. I realize that I have earned the wisdom that I gained from that lesson. No matter how terrible things appear, if I get in there and start working, they are only half as big as I assumed. Our minds protect us, but they also can exaggerate a past experience. As a child, everything is bigger than we are. If I have unfinished business from childhood, the memory will remain on the measuring scale of childhood. The size of it will continue to overwhelm me. I must remember that I have choices now. I am able to control my being. I don't have to allow anyone else to control me. If I do that, then I become the victim. I believe that these roadblocks were set up to see if I would give up or if my faith would fail. I choose to accept these challenges.

I must be 100 percent honest with myself if I want to grow, to become whole, to live life to its fullest. I have that choice. No one else can make that choice for me. I can free myself from my past, from my abusive, self-destructive ways, or I can stay there. It's my choice. I have to forgive myself and my parents and then move on. I still have days and weeks of deep depression, but I have been blessed with the willingness and the desire to understand my warning signs. When I start engrossing myself in work, acting out sexually, binge eating, isolating myself, or when I am irritated, angry or sleepless, I realize that I haven't been honest with myself or that there is something that I need to deal with. I tend to procrastinate; procrastinators want to make everything perfect. I'm learning to "just do it,"

I can always go back and fix it if it isn't right. There is no substitute for time and proper care of a wound. Gentle loving care is invaluable in healing. It takes a little more time to be gentle, but in the long run, every second invested in being gentle, is worth it.

Healing is never complete. To live we chance injury and insult; to heal begins with an injury or insult. I believe that one begets the other. Without injury healing cannot occur. If healing cannot occur, then growth won't occur. Without growth, we stagnate. To stagnate is to die. To die is not living. Injury is intrinsic to living. Healing enriches the process. If we say positive instead of negative things to each other, then we will start growth. It's a lot easier to receive lemonade than lemons. We love to squeeze those lemons on those sores, then we say, "No pain, no gain." I would see others out of control and tell them that; I didn't think that they knew about me. It is so easy to point the finger at others. When things are uncomfortable for us, we want to look at others. When I get angry about something that someone does, those are my buttons, that is myself talking to me. Until I took responsibility for myself, I couldn't heal. I believe that healing is a life-long, circular process. Every day has become a period of growth—every minute an opportunity for new birth and letting go of my past dishonesty. Healing one area gives the insight, strength, and the courage to heal the next wound, and the process continues. Once the cycle is complete, healing is complete. Life as we know it on this planet ceases. We continue on to our eternal life in heaven where we live wholly and completely, happily ever after.

I still become physically ill when there is something amiss emotionally, spiritually, or mentally. As a child, I was willing to die for my parents, believing that I had to give my life so that someone else could live—to sacrifice myself for others. I am not willing to do that now. Fear is what motivates people to do violent acts. I believe that the people in my life were motivated by fear—fears of rejection, abandonment, infidelity, and failure. Additionally, they feared not being loved and their not being good enough. I realize that I can be happy and not hurt my parents by doing that. I know that I don't have to wear my little clown mask just to make them happy.

In my future—in the next six to twelve months—I see freedom, growth, and finally being happy. I'm learning what makes me happy and I am finding the strength to do it. It is comforting to know that I am never alone in this journey; it is just a matter of remembering that. Despite the setbacks, tears and pain, I choose to live, to feel, to risk. I choose to continue my healing journey and my family has joined me in this endeavor.

THE REUNION

Rebecca Harbin

I came here with some fear
It had been so many years.

It was only a matter of time
all those fears did pass me by
I was willing to do my best and try.

I wanted so to bridge
the years that had past
And nurture relationships
that would last.

Knowing I have found
a place (I've always had
but never fully realized)
I belong
I will continue to make
these bonds grow strong.

I can finally take off
my hunting boots
for I have found
my long lost roots.

CHAPTER 13

Survival as Health: An Intrinsic Capacity for Healing

SUSAN SCOVILLE BAKER, PHD, RN, CS

When I speak of "survival as health," people initially respond with shock, and say things like: "It's much more than that" . . . "What a hopeless outlook" . . . "No!" . . . and even, "Maybe it's actually 'healthier' not to survive under some circumstances." Obviously, I need to try to explain more clearly.

CONCEPT ORIGIN

The concept of "survival as health" was elaborated for me during a curriculum consultation I did with nursing faculty in Brazil. I was asked to lead a seminar on "nursing theory." Initially the faculty were resistant to attending; then they were outraged at my approach. Rather than presenting an array of North American theories of nursing, which I knew they would necessarily find incompatible with their reality, I chose to follow a discovery-learning model to help them construct a nursing theory that would apply to their own desperate circumstances.

At this time in Brazil (1992), inflation was skyrocketing, many hospitals and universities were on strike, and many nurses, including faculty, had not been paid in months. They were living with the reality of whole middle-class families being forced to move into one room in another family's home—and of the transformation of the "favelas" (slums) into refuges for the middle class. The poor had been displaced even from the favelas to the streets or to cardboard shanties under overpasses and bridges. The desperate economic conditions had led to rampant rates of assault and robbery, and marked changes in lifestyle to cope with fear for personal safety. More and more families had moved from their elegant homes to the security of guarded high-rise condominiums. Leaving these secure compounds and walking or driving around the city had become a high-risk activity.

Overcoming their resistance to the participatory learning activity I proposed, these Brazilian faculty began to define the central curricular constructs of person, environment, health, and nursing from an experiential rather than a theoretical base. They described "people" as isolated individuals within a divided society, lacking support, assistance, or protection. They defined the "environment" as hostile and threatening, describing as evidence the number of friends and acquaintances who had been victimized by crime. The only environment they considered amenable to a person's control was that individual's own internal environment. They were emphatic about this distinction between internal and external environment, emphasizing the importance of having some measure of control over some aspect of life.

Their fear and lack of control of the external environment made their attention to their inner environment of paramount concern. "Health" was defined as "survival" in the face of strong threats to life and safety and the grim outlook of these faculty toward any possible dramatic shift in their society. They held, however, a tragic hope that the situation had become so intolerable that it would have to improve.

Once I relate this story of the origin of the concept "survival as health," I find that many people from diverse cultural backgrounds share the perceptions of the Brazilian nurse faculty. "Well, it's not just them, you know. We all live in desperate times. Let me tell you how it is for me . . ." And, saying this, people are apt to share one of those stories of random violence we read daily in our newspapers or see reported with graphic detail on the evening news. Indeed, during this same consultation visit in Brazil, I could personally validate the universality of crime, violence, and vulnerability. At midday, I was walking down the main street of a major city with two Brazilian nursing faculty when a youth ran up, bumped me and grabbed a gold pendant from my neck. My Brazilian colleagues were mortified, but I was quick to assure them that I was all right; in fact, a similar event had happened to me near my own hometown in the United States not long before.

The main difference, it seemed to me, was the very different attitude taken by the police in those two cities. In the United States I had been told, "You know that the criminals are all out on the street now. You cannot continue to live life the way you used to." In Brazil, the police did not blame me, but shared information on the very clever strategies of the thousands of children making their living on the streets. Given some inkling, then, of the universality of this concept of "survival as health," we are challenged to relate that concept to healing and nursing.

HEALING AND HEALTH

At the outset, it may be difficult to find any health in the construct of healing, even though the origin of the two words is one and the same. Suddenly one day in a flash it came to me—perhaps I had been thinking backwards all along, believing "health" to be an outcome measure, the result of good genes, a nurturant or at least benign environment and good habits of living. Maybe in some contexts it is, but if you see health as the outcome of healing, then you must presuppose that individuals are intrinsically somehow "unhealthy," therefore they must "heal" in order to have health. I have colleagues who will argue quite eloquently that this is in fact so, challenging me with the query, "Who among us is NOT wounded?" But to me it seems a flawed and prejudicial view. In particular, it seems to hearken back to a traditional hierarchical concept of the healthcare relationship, in which the provider has maternalistic or paternalistic power over the recipient of care and somehow even controls access to the desired outcome of "health." Another problem with health as an outcome is that, even if one problem or deficit is "healed" and thus presumably made "healthy," the same individual may have any number of other unmet needs and thus remain in more respects "unhealthy" than "healthy."

If the relationship is reversed, however, health becomes the cause and healing the outcome. When I started thinking of health as a precursor to healing rather than its outcome, a new relationship emerged, in synchrony with my belief that healing depends on the innate capacity, behavior and determination of the individual, much more than on the skill or knowledge of any caregiver. Consider health then as an innate quality or a complex of qualities, the sum of which is a level of strength greater than whatever insult or injury occurs to that individual. In this formulation, health is the force that makes healing possible, probable, or perhaps even inevitable.

SURVIVAL, HEALING AND HEALTH

Does health as potential move us toward a model of health and survival that will help inform this construct of healing? One common reaction to discussions of "survival as health" is a shocked statement " . . . but health is much more than merely survival!" Survival is, however, in this context a triumphant state. There is nothing "mere" about it. Consider some of the survivors nurses meet—severely emotionally damaged children whose parents have committed physical, emotional, and sexual atrocities on them; women who have attempted suicide on command from their husbands; survivors of rape, natural or manmade disasters; inner city children who have witnessed the murders of close friends; prisoners of war who have endured unthinkable tortures.

THE QUESTION OF LEVELS OF HEALTH

What would constitute a model of survival as health? One possibility might be levels of health, with survival as the first level. If we think of health as stages, rather than a continuum, we should be able to define and describe the levels, each with its own particular unique characteristics. The problem with stages of health is that these stages, their characteristics and needs, start sounding just like Maslow's (1962) needs or Erikson's (1964) tasks rather than a unique paradigm. Also, any model based on stages must address the fact that such stages are seldom as linear as they appear. People, particularly those who seek help from mental health professionals, seem repeatedly to revisit earlier stages to resolve unmet needs or contend with unresolved developmental tasks.

Are there any levels here—are there differences in this quality of health as you progress through the life stages? Or are there, perhaps, quantitative differences in an essentially constant trait? Perhaps it will help to examine what might be required for survival at various developmental stages. Erikson defines tasks within each stage; are there in fact any different tasks involved in traversing the spaces *between* the developmental stages? Perhaps it will help elaborate the concept of survival as health if we can identify what is needed at these transition points between one life stage and the next.

For example, let us consider some of what happens between the developmental stages of childhood and adolescence. At the outset, there is rebellion as the young person seeks to establish a clear separation from the parents and their domain. Increasingly the adolescent is linked to peers and their expectations. To accomplish this transition, the child must move beyond home and family to establish an independent identity.

The problem with this formulation is that this description could just as well describe the tasks that lie within the stage of adolescence as it does those involved in the transition into it. Is there a difference if we consider some of the qualities required for survival during adolescence? A short list would certainly include a strong self-image, values, and a sense of responsibility, problem-solving abilities, and resources including allies.

Are there similar needs at all of these junctions between developmental stages? Let us consider the qualities needed for survival of the passage between the adolescent and young adult stages of life. A sense of self continues to be a basic need, along with expanded life skills and the means to make a living. Looking just at these two lists of needs, there is much more similarity than difference, despite the use of a slightly different vocabulary.

The proposal that there might be "levels of health" that correspond to and promote survival during the life stages weakens steadily on close examination. There appear to be few differences in the needs between the different stages. Most needs can be derived from Erikson's (1964) or Sheehy's (1977) formulations. Perhaps a concept of health as quality or potentiality can better be used to help inform or elaborate these life stage theories, rather than positing its own set of stages or levels.

SURVIVAL AS THE MANIFESTATION OF HEALTH

Rather than as stages of health, let us consider survival as an ongoing manifestation of the innate quality "health." In this model, survival fills in between the stages of growth and development and defines the journey from one stage to the next, with "health" as the resource base, energy boost, or impetus that an individual uses to traverse this gap.

Crisis theory may be useful in explaining this process. The transition from one developmental stage to the next has long been identified as a "developmental crisis." Many of the factors identified by Caplan's (1964) theory and Aguilera's (1990) paradigm of crisis intervention fit well within the domain of health. Among the factors they identify as important to a positive outcome are past success with handling crises, a support system, and a positive balance of strengths over stressors.

Perhaps survival as health could be portrayed as the "escalator of life" that moves from one stage to the next. The escalator might be seen as running along underneath the life stages, with the stages sitting on the steps along the way. Thus a person's ability to ascend any of these stair "risers"

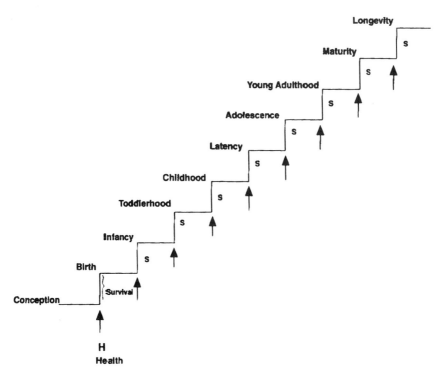

FIGURE 13.1.   An escalator model of survival as health.

between one developmental stage and the next reflects the ability to survive that particular developmental challenge or crisis.

HEALTH AND HEALING

Let us reconsider this model, emphasizing the concepts of nursing care and healing. If health is at the core of healing, it is its foundation, not its objective, a precursor rather than an outcome. What gives one person the capacity to heal and not another? As a corollary, what gives one person the capacity to facilitate healing and not another? Let us first re-examine health as the capacity to heal, in order to understand the helper's role in changing the odds and give an individual a better chance for survival.

How can we explain why healing can occur at some times and not at others? Recently my old dog died. He had suffered from chronic health problems for years, but finally they overtook him and he began to withdraw and finally staggered into the bedroom where my daughter and I were getting ready for work and school, lay down, breathing rapidly, stiffened, and stopped breathing. I have been with other elderly animals who died the same way—they began to fade away, becoming shadowy presences who didn't even always come for meals, then quite suddenly they began to look extremely frail and within a short time died peacefully and quickly with no struggle.

It is a great relief when an animal dies this way, taking away the human caretaker's painful duty to decide when the animal's suffering should be ended by euthanasia. I have made this decision at times also, after much soul-searching about whether my decision was based more on the animal's needs or my own. The difference in the quality of the animal's death is dramatic. I have held euthanized animals as they died; even with the most humane methods they show a continuing struggle for survival.

Is this evidence that what I call "health" is some force for life that must be present at some minimal level for a creature to continue breathing even without any additional insult or challenge other than continuing to draw breath? I am reminded of the number of long-time spouses who die within a very short time of each other, and the number of people who die within a short time of their retirement.

HEALTH AND THE WILL TO LIVE

In this context, then, is "will to live" synonymous with "health"? It would explain a lot of the situations in which people seem to die spontaneously when they no longer see a reason to live. It also may help explain a phenomenon observed with patients undergoing cancer treatment. Seemingly a host of factors enters into the success or failure of cancer treatment, one of the most important being the individual's attitude toward the illness. Those who believe they are doomed probably are. On the other hand, those who are determined to win, who use guided imagery and other positive strategies to take control, who are active against the disease, have much better prognoses than those who accept the fatality of their disease. As Betty Rollin (1976) pointed out in her account of her experience with breast cancer, some studies even show that angry, difficult patients have better treatment outcomes than "pleasant," compliant ones. These differences in survival may well be manifestations of the same kind of "health" or life force seen in my dogs; when that energy is finally gone, so is life.

Psychological Survival and Mental Health

It may also be helpful to apply the concept of "survival as health" to a psychological challenge rather than a physical one. Let us consider the experience of divorce. Certainly there is no really glorious outcome possible, but survival of the experience is much more than just getting through it. There is real triumph in getting beyond the many stumbling blocks and potholes that line the way, keeping sight of the overall goal and dealing with each obstacle as it comes along.

Physical survival is easy to validate. You are alive or not, or in a better or worse general physical state. On the other hand, how do you know that you are surviving emotionally? Clearly you are surviving a serious life stress emotionally if you meet some basic criteria: you are not obviously ill, either physically or mentally; you are functioning in your job and other daily activities; and you are enjoying your friendships with others.

A Model of Survival as Health

In addition to developmental stages, an array of other challenges await on life's path, somewhat like a video game. Survival involves getting through, past, over, or around them. An individual's survival is dependent on sufficient resources, including the inner strength which I call health. One representation of these resources is the phenomenon of "stores," special repositories of strength and added healing potential which can be drawn on when needed. The use of "stores" in healing is illustrated in the clinical story "Are You a Witch?" in this book.

Instead of the original escalator model proposed for survival as health, let us consider a video game model, or perhaps a combination of the two, with the stages remaining there in orderly fashion, while at the same time unexpected boulders or bottomless pits may suddenly appear in the way or meteors may fall from the sky. This amplification of the model includes not only added challenges to the traveler's survival, but also the opportunity for added resources to restore strength or provide a bridge to help the individual get past the next obstacle.

I like the way some video games allow you to build up your resources as you move through the challenges. You have the opportunity to barter and exchange for resources you need, but you also must continually evaluate your "stores" or resources and perhaps take time out to replenish them rather than continue on your quest or attain the next goal you

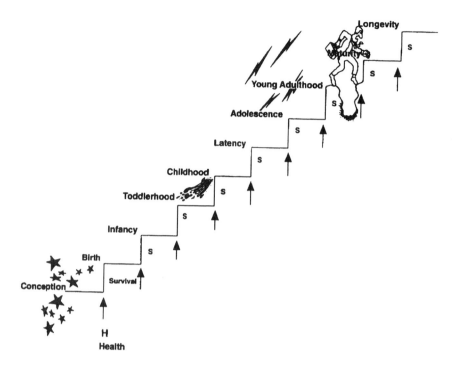

FIGURE 13.2. A videogame amplification of the model of survival as health.

desire. Eventually, also, you do use up all your powers or fail to anticipate an unexpected challenge, resulting in your annihilation.

Once again we are reminded of Aguilera's paradigm for crisis intervention. The difference between the model of survival as health and Aguilera's paradigm is that the model of survival as health is a directional one—it does not include an alternative "down escalator" to chaos and destruction. On the contrary, basic to this model is the underlying philosophy of developmental psychotherapy, that everyone has developed to a certain place and no farther because of some unmet need or some incomplete work from an earlier stage. Discovering these needs and identifying correctly the level of successful developmental achievement of the individual forms the foundation of the therapeutic endeavor.

This video game formulation of the model provides a framework for the role of helper, who can either substitute for, augment, or help individuals discover and use the "stores" they need to deal with their life challenges. Thus, the work of the nurse in this model is to help the individual

identify where on the escalator they have a solid grounding and to proceed from there. The helper might also be able to help other people fore-
see and avoid or at least minimize some of the hazards that lie ahead.

THE NURSING ROLE IN SURVIVAL AS HEALTH

Returning to the origin of the concept "survival as health" with the nursing faculty consultation in Brazil, I have struggled for months to understand their definition of nursing as "cuidado demais," literally translated
as "too much care." How could one care "too much"? Finally, in a moment
of revelation, I remembered that Brazilians are given to overstatement.
Thus, they will often use this sort of expression to refer to a person or
thing that they especially enjoy. For example, in Portuguese I might say "I
like mint chocolate chip ice cream too much." But in hearing this a Brazilian would not consider it a judgmental statement. They would understand
me to mean that I particularly like that flavor of ice cream.

Brazilian nurses don't think that nurses care more than they should,
just that they must care a great deal in order to overcome the tremendous
obstacles to survival in contemporary Brazil. They also believe very
strongly in nursing as a calling; nurses are especially chosen for having
the potential for this kind of caring. Being called to nursing also implies
that the individual has an extra measure of those potentialities I have call
"health" so that they have energy beyond that necessary to their own survival, energy which is available to assist others to overcome a wide array
of challenges and crises. In particular, within this model, nurses also
have unique traits which allow them to break through the isolation which
surrounds imperiled individuals and assist them in marshaling the resources needed for survival.

SUMMARY

The concept of "survival as health" underlies a theory of nursing for desperate times. Rather than health being an outcome of healing, it suggests
that health may describe a composite of qualities that sustain people in
the face of an array of environmental, developmental and situational
challenges. The model reveals its origin in Erikson's developmental theory and Caplan's crisis theory by emphasizing that the key to survival of

a developmental or situational crisis requires a preponderance of positive factors over stressors.

In the model of survival as health, visualized as an escalator or a video game, the role of nursing is to help other people identify just where they were standing on the escalator the last time they felt wholly integrated and strong. With the support and added strength of the nurse, people gather up whatever possessions they may have lost along the way or replace them with the alternative resources they need to attain the next step and beyond.

REFERENCES

Aguilera, D. C. (1990). *Crisis intervention: Theory and methodology* (6th ed.). St. Louis: Mosby.

Caplan, G. (1964). *Principles of preventive psychiatry.* New York: Basic Books.

Erikson, E. H. (1964). *Childhood and society* (2nd ed.). New York: Norton.

Erikson, E. H. (1968). *Identity, youth and crisis.* New York: Norton.

Maslow, A. (1962). *Toward a psychology of being.* Princeton, NJ: Van Nostrand.

Maslow, A. (1970). *Motivation and personality* (2nd ed.). New York: Harper & Row.

Rollin, B. (1976). *First you cry.* Philadelphia: J. B. Lippincott.

Sheehy, G. (1977). *Passages: Predictable crises in adult life.* New York: Bantam.

CHAPTER 14

Healing Power of Sleep

DORIS CAMPBELL, RN, MSN, ANP

> Now I lay me down to sleep
> I pray the Lord my soul to keep
> If I should die before I wake
> I pray the Lord my soul to take
>
> Anonymous, *New England Primer* (1781)

Sleep has been a mystery from ancient times. Its value has rarely been questioned, albeit never given the credit that it is due. That it promotes healing of the body and mind has been generally accepted. The answer to the question "What happens when we sleep?" has been asked and researched by the sages of ancient times and the present day scientists with their advanced technology. Sleep is instinctive; protective as well as renewing. We can readily identify the results of its deprivation. We say to our children when they are cranky that what they need is a "good night's sleep." By definition, sleep is a cyclical alteration of reversible unresponsiveness to the environment accompanied by complete change in multiple systems (Swik, 1992). We view sleep as an essential component of health. Our well being and quality of life are intimately dependent on the restorative powers that stem from effective sleep. When ill, the need for sleep to restore health is not questioned, although it is often disrupted in the interests of "care."

ANCIENT BELIEFS

The concerns about dying in one's sleep and of losing one's soul are echoes from the early Romans and Greeks (Hansen, 1987). During sleep, the soul was believed to wander the world over, experience magical insights, or become the prisoner of a god. If awakened too quickly, death could result because the soul did not have enough time to return to the body. The dichotomy of the sleeping situation was expressed in the *Iliad*

157

where sleep and death are seen as twin brothers. Cicero claimed that sleep was the image or brother of death (Dannenfeldt, 1986). Sleep was seen as the friend of man, while death was his fierce enemy. Other ancient authors personified sleep as a winged bird or an infant who carried a stalk of poppy from which a sleep-inducing liquid dripped.

Sleep is a major component in many fairy tales. Sleeping Beauty was doomed to sleep for one hundred years. Snow White fell into a deep sleep because her beauty threatened the queen. Rip Van Winkle and Goldilocks and the Three Bears had heroes who fell asleep.

RELIGIOUS BELIEFS

Sleep or the notion of rest is a common component of ancient religious ceremonies. The Egyptians had a religious service in which they sang a hymn to waken the sun from sleep. The grave or coffin was seen as a bed with the body positioned as in repose. The funeral service today still maintains this symbolism.

Sleep was an enigma that early man could not fathom. Thus a belief system was developed to explain the unexplainable. In some belief systems, to be asleep was to be powerless and helpless. Gods were depicted as having many eyes so that one was always open. Thus because one eye was open, the god was never totally asleep or without power. Elijah was a prophet for God. Elijah told believers of Baal to prove the existence of their god by having him ignite a fire under a prepared sacrifice. When the fire failed to appear and the sacrifice was not burned, Elija claimed that their god must be asleep, that is, powerless (I Kings 18:27-28, as cited in Hansen, 1987).

Lack of sleep was accompanied by unusual behaviors as well. In some religious groups, sleep deprivation was imposed for as long as three days in order to "transcend the normal bodily processes and to achieve heightened consciousness" (Hansen, 1987). In both the Christian and Taoist communities interruption of sleep was incorporated to attain this "out of body" experience. In the 16th century, many feared a person could become evil because "evil spirits entered his body while he was asleep."

ANCIENT PHILOSOPHERS

Hippocrates, the Western "father of medicine" identified sleep as an essential component of wellness and made some astute observations with specific recommendations about ensuring restful (healing) sleep. For example, he recommended that the temperature of the environment should be neither too hot nor too cold. In addition, he suggested that some treatment was indicated if dreams were contrary to the personality of the person. Lack of sleep occurred with old age and with pain and distress, a view not too far from our findings today (Dannefeldt, 1986, p. 435). Aristotle saw sleep as healing because it brought about an equilibrium in the quantity and quality of the "humors" and therefore was beneficial to the total well-being of the person. Writers of the Renaissance period recommended that lying down to sleep soon after a big meal or when hungry was not desirable either. Napping during the day was discouraged, but when ill, sleep was advised because of its recognized benefit to healing (Dannefeldt, 1986).

Another scholar of ancient times was Avicenna, a Muslim physician and philosopher. Avicenna wrote a twenty-volume encyclopedia, as well as a very important Canon of Medicine when he was only 21 years old. Avicenna commented, "sleep is the rest and quietness of the powers of the coulee, of mooing and of senses, without which man cannot live" (William Bullein, as cited in Dannefeldt, 1986, p. 422). Besides healing the body, Avicenna also noted the psychological advantages that result from sleep. When he was tired by his work, he would have a glass of wine and go to sleep. Upon awakening, he inevitably found the solutions to problems that had troubled him prior to his rest.

This experience of solving problems in sleep has been documented by others as well. It is reported that the concept of the benzene ring structure appeared in a dream to its discoverer Kekulé von Stradoits. In the dream, he saw snakes grasping tails in the formation of a ring. On awakening, he applied this to the way that the benzene ring was formed. The sewing machine was invented subsequent to a dream of a spear with a hole in its tip by Elias Howe.

SLEEP CYCLES

NREM

Today we understand that sleep is a cyclical process of biochemical and musculoskeletal changes that contribute to the healing of mind and spirit as implied by the ancient philosophers. We now know that there are two categories of sleep: the first is termed Non-Rapid Eye Movement Sleep

(NREM) and is marked by increasing physical relaxation and slowing of brain waves. There are four stages in this category. Stage I lasts for about 1 to 2 minutes and accounts for about 5 percent to 10 percent of the total sleep cycle. Stage I is the lightest period of altered consciousness and arousal is quite easy to accomplish. Pulse rate slows, respirations decrease, and muscle tone is minimal. Stage II, known as transition sleep, continues on this downward scale with a little deeper relaxation lasting about 5 to 10 minutes. Stage III, the transition stage to deep sleep is marked by delta brain wave activity (versus the alpha wave activity of Stage I and Stage II) and makes up about 20 percent to 50 percent of the EEG sleep record. Other physiological systems slow down as well, and the person at this point, becomes more difficult to arouse. In Stage IV, the body is completely relaxed and basal metabolism slows. Slow brain waves make up about 50 percent of the EEG readings during this stage. This period lasts about 5 to 15 minutes. Eye movement is not observed (Barkauskus, Allen-Stollenberg, Bauman, & Darling-Fisher, 1994).

REM

In 1923, a physiologist-physician, Dr. MacWilliam, studied blood pressure and heart rate during sleep and determined that there were two periods (or categories) of sleep. One he called undisturbed sleep, when blood pressure and heart rate were lowered. As discussed earlier, this is termed NREM Sleep. The other period he described as disturbed sleep because of the reported dreams and nightmares and the tumultuous changes in the blood pressure and heart rate. He connected these findings of disturbed sleep with its wild fluctuations in vital signs to cerebral and pulmonary hemorrhage, angina, and sudden death (Hemenway, 1980). As early as the 1800s, it was reported that the most common time for death was between 4:00 A.M. and 7:00 A.M.

We can validate these findings with our technology today. We know that during non-REM sleep, blood pressure and heart rate are decreased and muscle relaxation is maximized; the REM stage of sleep is identified by rapid conjugate eye movements, muscle twitching, and the highest thresholds of arousal. Blood flow to the brain doubles, oxygen consumption peaks, ADH increases while urine output decreases. The physiological state is similar to that of a person who is awake. This period of the sleep cycles is termed paradoxical because of these findings. Due to the eye movement and pupil size change during this stage it is also called the Rapid Eye Movement (REM sleep).

During REM sleep, the EEG shows activity, there are irregularities in the heart rate and respirations, the blood pressure oscillates, basal metabolism rates increase, and there are periods of apnea. This latter finding results in anoxia that may precipitate or contribute to some of the sleep disorders and crises associated with sleep. First and second degree A-V block are related significantly and consistently to the REM stage of sleep (Hemenway, 1980). Dr. MacWilliam's predictions of angina and sudden death have been currently supported by the studies conducted in sleep labs with more sophisticated instruments than those available in his time (Hemenway, 1980). Arrhythmias have been documented by different researchers. Rosenblatt reported an increase in premature ventricular contractions during the period of REM sleep and in the transition to wakefulness (Hemenway, 1980). Nevins (cited in Hemenway), in a larger study of the relationship of AV block to REM sleep, found a significant positive correlation. Documenting fluctuations in blood pressure, Roughgarden (cited in Hemenway) reported angina attacks in about 25 percent of his sample resulting from the increased and fluctuating blood pressure during the REM phase of sleep. While the poet saw sleep as something that "knit up the raveled sleeve of care," the more scientifically oriented writer saw sleep as the "diastole of the cerebral beat" (Hemenway, 1980, p. 453).

PHYSIOLOGICAL ACTIVITY

Many other active processes occur during sleep; some are healing, and some are dangerous to life. Scientists have explored many of the biochemical changes that occur during a 24-hour cycle, providing insight into the active processes that occur in sleep. They have learned that many of these processes are associated with repair and/or healing. Their findings support our belief that sleep is an important function, and that nurturing it is consistent with health.

Studies about cellular and intracellular activity during sleep have unveiled more about the healing that occurs with sleep. As mentioned earlier, there is a cycle or rhythm to the secretion of hormones, enzymes, and minerals in our body. These are coordinated and sometimes dependent on the circadian rhythm of the sleep-wake cycle. The role of the somatomedins (SM) and growth hormones (GH), including their actions and interactions, have been a major focus of the current study of sleep.

The somatomedins are endogenous peptides produced throughout the body, especially in the liver. They are dependent on and mediate growth hormone activity. They stimulate DNA synthesis and the proliferation of many types of cells. They are responsible for the growth of cartilage, skeletal tissue, and protein synthesis.

The growth hormone (GH) is a large peptide produced by the anterior pituitary gland with the primary functions of sparing protein and stimulating protein synthesis (Lee & Stotts, 1990). For example it is an initiator in the chain of many cellular activities. In addition, this anabolic hormone modulates somatomedin secretion. It also stimulates the liver to secrete factors that mediate growth. Fasting, hypoglycemia, exercise, ingestion of proteins, ovulation, and deep sleep stages stimulate the secretion of the growth hormone (Lee & Stotts, 1990). GH is stimulated by prostaglandin secretion, so that when damage to tissue occurs, repair or healing of damaged tissue is enhanced. This is accomplished through the interaction of GH and SM where, in the chain of interactions, SMs stimulate the DNA synthesis necessary for cell formation and growth. GH is also stimulated by psychological stress (Lee & Stotts, 1990). GH increases during Slow Wave Sleep (SWS) which occurs during Stage III and IV of sleep (Adams & Oswald, 1983). GH is suppressed by glucocorticoids and alcohol consumption.

Children and adolescents have longer periods of Stage IV sleep due to the interaction of the growth hormone with serotonin. Infants, with their rapid growth rate, sleep longest of all age groups. The elderly on the other hand, may have no GH secretion during sleep. Stages III and IV for them are shortened. Added to our current understanding of the relationship between the lack of GH secretion and SWS, the complaints of poor sleep by the aged may be understood.

Other hormones that interact and react to GH are insulin, thyroid, and serotonin. These hormones stimulate amino acid uptake in tissues and promote RNA and protein synthesis (Adam, 1980). The level of free fatty acids in the blood also rises during sleep. Freeing of these fatty acids provides a source of necessary elements for the construction of ATP (adenosine triphosphate), the power for most cellular activity, which Adam terms the"energy charge."

Adam (1980) hypothesized that the sleep/waking rhythm influences fluctuations in energy charge. This in turn influences the metabolic balance so that degradative processes are stimulated during wakefulness and restorative or synthetic processes are stimulated during sleep. Guttes and Guttes (1959) found that the energy charge and synthetic processes are heightened in a unicellular organism with enforced restriction of motion. In the sleeping human being, work decreases, ATP and the energy charge in cells increase, degradation is decreased, oxygen consumption is decreased, and synthesis is stimulated. Other studies also report variations in protein synthesis and ATP levels to support this hypothesis. Catecholamines, which are catabolic, are at higher levels during the day than during the night (Adam & Oswald, 1983). Thus we see that the rhythm of secretions supports and is dependent upon our sleep-wake cycle.

The advantages of sleep to the physical aspects of healing are well documented. A complete sleep cycle takes about 90 minutes. There are about five or six cycles per night. In the first cycle of the evening, the individual moves through Stages I, II, III, and IV and then has a short period of REM. He then cycles back through Stage IV, III, and II. The individual moves from Stage II to REM, returns to Stage II and thence to Stages III, IV. The NREM period of the cycles becomes shorter and there are longer periods in REM sleep as the sleep period continues. The physical repair so essential to function occurs in Stage IV early in the portion of the sleep period, and decreases in length towards the early morning hours. We see again how this is to the advantage of the young with their considerable construction of new tissue for growth and repair of the damaged tissue.

Understanding the physiology of sleep becomes important to nursing practice. If our goal is to facilitate the healing process, then our patients should have as few interruptions in their sleep period as possible. This hearkens back to the Renaissance period where sleep was a recognized therapy when a person was ill. Besides the physical advantages of sleep, we need to understand that sleep also contributes to the psychological health of our patients.

PSYCHOLOGICAL HEALING POWER OF SLEEP

"Sleep that knits the ravelled sleeve of care"

Studies have determined the psychological healing powers of sleep. The activity of the brain when individuals learn has been widely documented (Fishbein, 1981). Now, it is apparent that this "learning" occurs in sleep as well during the period known as REM sleep. This period of the sleep cycle was discussed earlier as being one of extreme and sometimes erratic activity in the brain, as well as in other systems. Storage of new information depends on some activation of the brain at critical times. Fishbein (1981) reports that consolidation of new information continues during paradoxical sleep. When subjects were deprived of the

REM portion of sleep, learning curves went down. Fishbein continues by identifying that the REM period participates in the storage process of learning through the actions of the neurotransmitters. Sleep studies revealed oscillations in the brain wave activity that seems to be attributed to a kind of "neuronal reprogramming" (Fishbein, 1981). He suggests that during this period, previously stored material and daily activities are reviewed and re-integrated each night and throughout the lifespan.

Dreaming, as an integral part of REM, becomes more significant to the healing process. Dreaming and dreams have been studied by many disciplines. In the 1960s, biophysics, engineering, experimental psychology, as well as psychiatric and psychoanalytic literature reported independent studies suggesting that this portion of sleep was essential for healthy functioning of the person (Fishbein, 1981). Without this portion of sleep there was less serotonin and norepinephrine available to the brain cells, and there was less sensitivity to amphetamine. Fewer neurotransmitters and amines were available for release in the brain. In dream deprived animals, catecholamine synapses do not function normally. These findings support the belief that the biochemistry of the brain and dreaming are intimately connected. Their interdependence and interaction have a restorative role, perhaps in the cortex of the brain that involves the consolidation of memory and restructuring of the neuronal pathways accounting for long- and short-term memory storage (Fishbein, 1981).

Dreams deal with emotional issues as well. In a study done by Breger, Hunter, and Lane (1971), anxiety-producing movies were shown to a group of people before sleep. Some of them were permitted a full night's rest. The remainder of the group was denied the REM or dreaming portion of their sleep. The next night the same films were shown to the same group of people. Those who were denied REM sleep were as anxious as the first time they viewed the film, while those who had the REM portion of sleep were much less anxious and ready to experience the stressful situation again. Thus, we see that something happened to prepare those with the REM sleep to deal with stress and crisis. Integration and creative problem solving may occur during the REM sleep to help individuals develop new perspectives of daily experiences to resolve old, as well as new situations (Fishbein, 1981). Reports of Avicenna and Kekulé von Stradoits presaged these findings.

Studies have also found that in new learning situations, or after stress of any kind, the period of REM sleep increases. Learning a new language is associated with increased REM sleep. Infants and children sleep as much as they do, perhaps to allow the integration of daily new experiences as well as allow the body to grow. Persons undergoing psychoanalysis for war neuroses were found to have a shortened latency for REM sleep (Fishbein, 1981). Awakened from the REM stage of sleep, persons can recount vivid dreams not reported by those awakened from other phases of sleep. In addition, the inability to restrict dreaming to the REM stage of sleep was found in persons who scored high on the schizophrenia scale of the MMPI (Fishbein, 1981).

The content of dreams ranges from the prosaic or mundane, to the exotic and inexplicable. They reflect our past experience, our conflicts, and our aspirations. They can provide us with insight and understanding of ourselves. The language of the dream is perceptual, not cognitive which accounts for the strange images and happenings in dreams. Dreams help us to repair the psychological bruises, past and present. In psychoanalysis, discussion of dreams may help the person resolve painful problems, thus leading to growth and self-understanding. When situations are too traumatic, and the person is too conflicted to reach a solution, the dream content is repeated without the resolution. When the psyche is strong enough or the individual has gained increased insight of the problem, the dream content expands indicating either a resolution of the problem or advancement toward that point. Individuals with recurring nightmares that have additional content and images indicate intense activity of the brain in resolving and integrating very complex problems compatible with the conscious. Thus, dreams are essential to healthy psychological functioning. They are the vehicle by which the past and present are interwoven to help us modify our behavior, achieve greater self-knowledge, and deal more successfully with those around us.

CONCLUSION

The sages and the poets of the past held many answers to the value of sleep that we might consider today. Sleep does indeed "weave the ravelled sleeve of care" which most of us admit to at the end of a day. Many of us, especially as we age, are aware that we may "die before we wake" and do "pray the Lord our soul to take." Studies which reveal that healing occurs during sleep both physically and psychologically, lead us to look with more attention and respect to this phenomenon. With increasing knowledge and understanding of what happens when we sleep, perhaps therapies will be developed to help those who are denied the restorative power of sleep. Those of us who deal with persons who are aged, ill, disturbed or anxious, need to incorporate into our practice those modalities proven to enhance sleep. We know now that sleep is not passive. It is a powerful tool that we can use to increase our quality of life. As research further reveals the mystery, and our understanding of the ramifications of sleep widens, many who suffer quietly will experience the healing that comes with sleep.

REFERENCES

Adam, K. (1980). Sleep as a restorative process and a theory to explain why. In McConnell, Boer, Romyn, Van de Poll, & Conor (Eds.). Adaptive capabilities of the nervous system. *Progress in Brain Research, 53,* 259-300. New York: North Holland Biomedical Press.

Adam, K., & Oswald, I. (1983). Protein synthesis, bodily renewal and the wake cycle. *Clinical Science, Medical Research Society and the Biochemical Society, 65,* 561-567.

Barkauskus, V., Allen-Stollenberg, K., Bauman, L., & Darling-Fisher, C. (1994). *Sleep assessment* (pp. 137-139). St. Louis: Mosby.

Breger, L., Hunter, I., & Lane, R. (1971). The effect of stress on dreams. *Psychological Issues, 7*(3), 27.

Chen, H., & Tang, Y. (1989). Sleep loss impairs inspiratory muscle endurance. *American Review of Respiratory Disease, 140,* 907.

Chuman, M. (1983). The neurological basis of sleep. *Heart and Lung, 12*(2) 177.

Cosnett, J. E., & Dickens, C. (1992). Observer of sleep and its disorders. *Sleep, 15*(3), 264.

Dannenfeldt, K. (1986). Sleep: Theory and practice in the late renaissance. *Journal of the History of Medicine and Allied Sciences, 41*(1), 415-441.

Fishbein, W. (1981). *Dreams and memory.* W. Fishbein (Ed.), SP Medical and Scientific Books.

Hansen, K. (1987). In M. Eliade (Ed.), *Sleep. The encyclopedia of religion* (pp. 361-364). New York: Macmillan.

Hemenway, J. (1980). Sleep and the cardiac patient. *Heart and Lung, 9*(3), 453.

Lee, K. M., & Stotts, N. (1990). Critical care endocrinology; support of the growth hormone-somatomedin system to facilitate healing. *Heart and Lung, 19*(1), 157.

Spenceley, S. (1993). Sleep inquiry: A look with fresh eyes. *Image: Journal of Nursing Scholarship, 25*(3), 249.

Swick, T. (1992). Sleep, sleep, sleep. *Mind Matters Seminars.* Houston.

Trevelyan, J. (1989). Now I lay me down to sleep. *Nursing Times, 85*(47), 34-35.

White, D., Douglas, N., Pickett, C., Zwillich, C., & Weil, J. (1983). Sleep deprivation and the control of ventilation. *American Review of Respiratory Disease, 128,* 984-986.

CHAPTER 15

The Use of Reminiscence as a Healing Therapy for Older Adults

BARBARA G. MASON, RN, RNC, EDD

God gave us memory so that we may have roses in December

James Barrie

Reminiscence is the review of past experiences. It is a natural process in which we all engage throughout life, and which becomes more frequent and more important to us as we grow older. Reminiscence is an integral part of the aging process; its increasing frequency as we age may be related to the growing awareness of one's own mortality (Beadleson-Baird & Lara, 1988).

The theoretical basis for the use of reminiscence as a healing therapy is derived from the philosophies of Robert Butler (1963) and Eric Erickson (1950). Erickson felt that the last stage of life is a time when most people seek wholeness. In order for human beings to obtain what he termed *ego-integrity* at the end of life, they need to be satisfied with the way in which they have lived their lives. Robert Butler built upon this philosophy by stating that people perform a review of their lives in an effort to make sense of the past. The recalling of past experiences and conflicts at the end of one's life is very necessary so that these revived experiences can be surveyed and reintegrated in terms of the present.

Nurses often find themselves in the unique position of assisting elderly patients or clients to achieve wholeness, whether it be through reaching for and maintaining one's highest level of wellness or through dying with dignity and meaning. Reminiscence therapy, which can be a powerful tool for the nurse, is recognized in the literature as an independent intervention with particular diagnostic and therapeutic potential for the elderly (Burnside, 1990; Ebersole & Hess, 1994; Haight & Burnside, 1992). It can build trust, increase responsiveness, and improve cooperation. It can bring someone out of their shell, make them easier to deal with, motivate them to try harder in therapy, or help them to respond to questions or instructions. As a healing therapy, reminiscence can be used as a means to resolve conflicts; to come to terms with events and feelings that one has not been able to reflect upon. It can be a supportive means for dealing with new conflicts. As Hogstel (1994) states, "It is often less threatening to talk about emotionally charged topics by reminiscing than by talking about them in the present tense" (p. 80).

Reminiscence is often used by nurses to help bring forth forgotten strengths that the elderly have possessed to cope with the many losses that they may be experiencing—loss of health, loss of family and friends, loss of home or privacy, and loss of control. Even five minutes of reminiscence can be valuable. Remembering past experiences when one was strong and capable can bring back resources to empower the elderly person to make decisions and handle problems.

As used by most nurses, however, reminiscence therapy is not the same as the life review that Butler proposed and studied. In the literature, for example, confusion regarding the life review and reminiscence allows them to be used interchangeably. According to Burnside (1990), even though the two *theories* may have commonalities, the two *therapies* are different. Burnside differentiates the two by characterizing reminiscence as supportive therapy that does not increase anxiety and positively reinforces life decisions and lifestyles. As a psychosocial intervention requiring a certain amount of clinical training, it is not psychoanalytic. It can focus on a variety of topics and include pleasant memories. Life review, on the other hand, is a therapeutic "uncovering," requiring specific psychoanalytic education and skill as the therapist works the client through the various stages of human development. There are many geropsychiatric nurses who are qualified and experienced in using this form of therapy.

With some training, reminiscence therapy can be used by most nurses. It can be used on an individual basis or in groups with one or two nurses acting as group leaders. The main attributes that nurses must have for conducting the process are caring, sensitivity, respect, and an ability to listen with empathy and without judgment; to allow the elderly person to experience their own memories whether they be pleasant, painful, or disappointing. As Huber and Miller (1989) state, "Give them the gift of listening" (p. 87).

Often the elderly person may need approval to initiate reminiscing behavior. Reminiscing is still perceived as a negative characteristic of old age by many lay people and some healthcare providers; a sign of senility

(Beadleson-Baird & Lara, 1988). The elderly themselves will complain of peers who do nothing but live in the past. In instances where the older person is hesitant about reminiscing, the nurse can effectively trigger memories by using certain words, objects, memorabilia, music, photographs, poems, and smells, such as baking bread or popping corn. Nurses who use reminiscence as a healing therapy have many techniques and tools that they employ in guiding reminiscence: techniques for sparking memories, for avoiding repetition, for keeping the conversation focused, and for dealing with emotions. An important part of reminiscing is allowing emotion and allowing silence. Many older people need quiet moments to collect their thoughts and their memories and maybe shed some tears (AARP, 1989).

Reminiscence therapy can be used in a variety of settings. It can be used in acute care settings while bathing the patient or while performing other physical nursing interventions. It can be used to calm an anxious patient prior to going to surgery or some other form of invasive medical procedure. It can be used in the emergency room to help cope with stress. Many times older patients who are acutely ill or who may be faced with a life-threatening situation will express a desire or need to recall and talk about past events (Beadleson-Baird & Lara, 1988). Acute care nurses who are knowledgeable about the healing aspects of reminiscence can be very therapeutic in these situations through their listening, exploring, and giving recognition to and acceptance of patients' positive and negative emotions. Reminiscing with patients or clients provides a type of caring that is not focused primarily on biophysiological needs.

Beadleson-Baird and Lara (1988) tell the story of a 75-year-old gentleman who was brought into an ambulatory care unit in severe pain. He was examined by the physician and became very frightened and anxious when he was told that he had a possible abdominal aneurysm. Almost spontaneously, he began talking to the nurse about the fact that he had never been this sick before, even when he had been ill in a concentration camp during World War II. The nurse listened patiently and without interruption as the elderly man recalled all of his hospital experiences; as a young boy with a broken wrist, his bicycle accident, the gunshot wounds he received during the war. He would squeeze the nurse's hand occasionally when his pain intensified. At the end of his tale, his pain was not relieved, but he appeared less frightened and more relaxed. He remarked, "It will be okay, nurse." That night the elderly man underwent abdominal surgery. Afterwards the nurse visited him in the intensive care unit. His words were, "You are my super nurse . . . you listened to my old stories when you were busy . . . I know talking about my past helped me survive this risky operation."

In the nursing home, reminiscence therapy is used in a variety of ways and for a variety of reasons. It is used to build trust and increase responsiveness. It can be used for increasing socialization, decreasing loneliness and depression, and for increasing cognitive ability. Miller (1989) found that nursing home residents seemed to need to reminisce more than the elderly out in the community. She felt that perhaps this was because they were stressed by living away from home.

Huber and Miller (1984) used group reminiscence in an extended care facility with six elderly women ages 80 to 90. All were permanent residents and all had been identified as persons who might benefit from a group experience. Three of the women had been diagnosed with Alzheimer's disease; the other three had medical diagnoses of stroke, fractured femur, and depression. Actually, four of the women were in various stages of depression. Three of the women were wheelchair dependent and all were dependent to some degree for assistance in activities of daily living. All had manifested some recent memory loss and, in spite of a caring staff, all had many empty hours each week.

The group met for one hour a day for 10 weeks. The goals that the leaders had chosen for themselves were to encourage each person to speak during each meeting, to promote relatedness and interaction among them, and to listen sincerely to each of the members. They also agreed to be active participants by sharing their own reminiscences.

The outcomes after ten weeks were not spectacular, but they were impressive. At the beginning, the participants showed no interest in one another, only in the leaders, and had to be escorted to the meeting room. The topics had to be chosen by the leaders. At the final meeting, the three who could walk were eagerly coming by themselves. One of the participants acted as a hostess, an activity that she had not done for many years, but which in her younger years she had enjoyed doing very much. The personality traits of all women stayed the same; happy or sad, negative or positive. All the women expanded their verbalization of remote memories. The last few meetings they shared humor, smiled at each other, and two participants became friends and spent considerable time together even after the group experience had ended. One very depressed participant started showing new energy by the fifth meeting. She initiated conversation, volunteered information, and helped arrange the chairs without being asked. Of the two women who were cognitively impaired, one left the group after the fourth session and would not return. The other one responded well. She told stories, occasionally interacted with another member, enjoyed humor, and several times was able to recall people and events from her childhood.

Reminiscence often is used in the discussion of dying and death. Many older people are denied the opportunity to talk about their own approaching death or the loss of someone close to them because their family and friends are too emotionally involved. Older people should be given the opportunity to talk about their total lives including death and to express sadness. When given this opportunity, the older person often experiences feelings of relief and peace. Hospice nurses often reminisce with the elderly to help them accept impending death (AARP, 1989; Burnside, 1990).

In the community, reminiscence therapy is often used at senior centers, instigated by the seniors themselves, social workers, or student nurses. It becomes a means for socialization, for elevating self-esteem by helping them feel that what they have to say is worthwhile and important. All of my students have at least one clinical experience interacting with well elderly at a nutrition site, senior citizen residence, or senior center. One of their favorite activities is to sit with a group of seniors, or perhaps just one, and begin reminiscing. They try to include those who appear to be just "people watching" or who are sitting by themselves and those who are relatively new to the center. Some do not participate by telling stories, but often they will nod or smile. The directors of the senior center have told us how much the seniors look forward to the students' visits and whenever we leave we always have many thank-you's and a chorus of "When are you coming back?"

One of the purposes of encouraging students to use reminiscence with older people is to improve or enhance their feelings and knowledge of the aging process and the elderly. The rewards of reminiscence are twofold. The student often benefits just as much, if not more, than the elder participant. The relationship that is established during reminiscence can have a very positive effect on students' perceptions of old people, the process of aging, and themselves. Many students are not aware of their biases and often are quite surprised at how much older people are just like themselves.

Burnside (1990) feels that having students reminiscence with the elderly is the single most effective way to reduce ageism in students. Students who have not had much interaction with the elderly often set out for the senior centers almost with fear and trepidation, certain that they will have a very negative experience. Most of them are pleasantly surprised at the seniors' willingness to talk to them, their trusting nature, and the wealth of their knowledge. Ross (1990) in a study of 25 students enrolled in a geriatric training program found that students' sensitivity to aging moved through several steps: (1) initial distaste or unease, (2) surprise at newly discovered values and characteristics, (3) genuine respect, (4) heightened awareness of their own aging, (5) a desire to retain new attitudes, and (6) a hope to transfer their new outlook to improved care for elderly patients.

Reminiscence as practiced by nurses is not a new intervention. It is probably practiced more widely than acknowledged. Most nurses who use reminiscence as a healing therapy find it successful. However, as Burnside (1990) points out, the success may be serendipitous as no one is quite sure why it succeeds and the practice often is not based on any theoretical foundation.

There are very few research studies by nurses on the use of reminiscence as a healing therapy. Part of this may be due to the fact that it is not easy to conduct intervention studies on the elderly, particularly the frail elderly. Burnside (1990) states that the problems researchers have include small samples, problems with the facility, attrition, varying levels of depression, unknown causes of depression, difficulties with tools, and researchers having to be therapists as well as data gatherers.

Reminiscing about earlier times provides the elderly with an important sense of continuity. As we go through life, it is our memories that help us maintain a sense of who we are and help us "pull together the elements of our existence into a coherent whole" (Kovach, 1991, p. 28).

REFERENCES

American Association of Retired Persons (AARP). (1989). *Reminiscence: Finding meaning in memories.* Washington, DC: Author.

Beadleson-Baird, M., & Lara, L. L. (1988). Reminiscing: Nursing actions for the acutely ill geriatric patient. *Issues in Mental Health Nursing, 9,* 83–94.

Burnside, I. (1990). Reminiscence: An independent nursing intervention for the elderly. *Issues in Mental Health Nursing, 11*(1), 33–48.

Butler, R. N. (1963). The life review: An interpretation of reminiscence in the aged. *Psychiatry, Journal for the Study of Interpersonal Processes, 26*(1), 65–76.

Ebersole, P., & Hess, P. (1994). *Toward healthy aging: Human needs and nursing response.* (4th ed.). St. Louis: Mosby.

Erickson, E. (1950). *Childhood and society.* New York: Norton.

Haight, B. K., & Burnside, I. (1992). Reminiscence and life review: Conducting the processes. *Journal of Gerontological Nursing, 18*(2), 39–42.

Hogstel, M. O. (1994). *Nursing care of the older adult* (3rd ed.). Albany: Delmar.

Huber, K., & Miller, P. (1984). Reminiscence with the elderly—Do it! *Geriatric Nursing, 5*(2), 84-87.

Kovach, C. R. (1991). Reminiscence behavior: An empirical exploration. *Journal of Gerontological Nursing, 17*(12), 23-28.

Miller, C. M. (1989). A past well remembered . . . *Geriatric Nursing, 10*(1), 28-29.

Ross, H. K. (1990) Lesson of life. *Geriatric Nursing, 11*(6), 174-275.

PART THREE

THE NURSE AS A PROFESSIONAL WHO ATTENDS TO HEALING

PHYLLIS BECK KRITEK, RN, PHD, FAAN

Having sampled the essence and some of the core components of healing in Parts One and Two, we move to some real life considerations embedded in our commitment to healing. This part of the book opens with a dialog on the professional nurse. In exploring healing, we discover that the healer cannot serve in this role without two givens. The first is that the healer's efficacy is linked to his or her own healing processes; to the degree that the healer seeks to heal himself or herself of woundedness, the efficacy of the healer increases. The second is that healers cannot assist others in healing without effecting their own healing processes, both in discovery of previously unacknowledged wounds and in the enhancement of the healing process the healer is personally engaged in. This no doubt is summarized well in the aphorism "healer, heal thyself!" Honoring this truism, it seemed imperative to discuss the healer before describing some of the more focused descriptions of nurses practicing their healing arts. Thus the healer is the focus of this part of the book.

Personal stories, thoughtful essays, scientific papers, and conceptual frameworks open a window on the process of healing that involves healing ourselves. Poetry provides an alternate lens. Alice Hill's poem, which she calls "A Reminder," serves notice initally by its title. Healing ourselves is always a process linked to consciousness. She aptly reminds us of the despair that wounds can evoke. Her final observation reminds us that healing is also about reframing the meaning of the wounds in our lives.

In the first paper, by Verolyn Bolander, a comprehensive and thoughtful analysis of alternative healing methods is provided. The author gives an overview of the history of alternative healing methods, shows the long relationship nursing has with these methods, and introduces some much needed clarity about the diverse terms used to describe these methods. She identifies nurses as the providers in Western medicine who, with their patients, have most often "refused to enclose the person in the human body . . ." and notes that our tradition is one of dealing with the body, mind, spirit, society, and culture of our patients. As such, we are the most equipped discipline to build a bridge between the prevailing paradigms of medicine and the range of alternative healing methods available. Noting the many terms used to describe Western medicine, such as allopathic, biomedicine, orthodox, or traditional, she also notes that the latter two seem more geography and history bound than not, since other cultures in other locations on the globe have traditional and orthodox approaches quite unlike biomedicine's approach.

To deal with the muddle of indistinct terms, and after reviewing existing taxonomies, Bolander devises a taxonomy of the alternative methods of healing categorized by two dimensions: those who practice either complementary (those who promote health) or allopathic (those who treat disease) is first, the degree of acceptance by the general public is the second, ranging from currently licensed professionals to quackery. One may question the former but it has an aura of realism about it, acknowledging the political and cultural implications of the current structures of healthcare. The latter is an honest report of the key ingredient actually driving the integration of alternative methods of healing: public choice. She teases apart the resistance of allopathic medicine practitioners to alternative healing methods, and notes that, given this resistance, nursing has an opportunity to more honestly embrace its healing mission while serving as a valuable bridge between the communities involved in allopathic medicine and those involved in complementary practices. This opportunity calls for extensive research and a conscious effort to create this bridge, one that can do much to heal the fractured community of practitioners of healing methods.

Linda Rounds presents a personal account of her journey toward active practice as a nurse practitioner (NP). She recounts her early nursing practice experiences and the untoward effects lack of decision-making power has on a hospital nurse. She provides a history of women as healers, discussing the early history of such women, including the devastating witch hunts of Europe and America that decimated this population of healers, calling them evil, dirty, dangerous, and occult. Tracing the rise of allopathic medicine in this country, she describes the establishment of a male-dominated culture where women were at once told they were either too unintelligent or too frail to become physicians, yet were grossly exploited as cheap labor, doing often backbreaking work and readily controlled and "ordered" about, particularly as student nurses. In sketching this history, she unveils the oppressed status of nursing and identifies some of the key traits of oppressed groups that manifest in our discipline: conformity, low risk-taking behaviors, fatalism, fear of autonomy and responsibility, and horizontal violence.

It is in this context that Linda describes her own decision to become a nurse practitioner and the sense of freedom it has given her to practice autonomous nursing at its best. She acknowledges that, while some nurse practitioners may actually abandon nursing, the vast majority do not, and have actually moved nursing forward to its next critical level of competence, autonomy, and commitment to enhancing the quality of patient care. She is clearly saddened by the split in nursing that emerged from the NP movement, and observes that much of the behavior directed toward those leading or participating in this movement was characteristic of oppressed groups. It is her hope that by further understanding both our oppressed group behavior and the meaning healing has for all of us, we might begin to heal this rift. She observes that such behavior is rarely to our advantage, since organized medicine so consistently works to constrain our autonomy and authority.

For Linda, the NP movement gave her the opportunity to determine appropriate care for her patients, have a sense of control over her practice, and enable her to do for her patients what she knew was best for them. Beyond this liberation, she also discovered healing, the healing of the fragmentation she felt when she lacked the opportunity to do for her patients what needed to be done. It is in this sense that her choices have given her a sense of wholeness as a nurse, a healing experience.

Christina Esperat, Geraldine Dorsey-Turner, and Patricia Davis Gilmore continue this theme in their paper, an analysis of the impact of oppression and a description of the power of choosing a transformative process for both the culturally oppressed and the healthcare practitioner. They provide an analysis of cultural oppression by the dominant culture in the United States, its current subtle nature, and the degree to which such oppression is practiced with neither awareness nor insight into consequences. Focusing on the nurse as healer, they note the incongruity of claiming the role of healer while concurrently inflicting serious emotional wounds through continuing cultural oppression in the practice of nursing. They observe how often the minority patient is first demeaned for being different, then punished for this difference.

Acknowledging the importance of empowerment and the need for the oppressed to reclaim their rights, they observe that there is a great danger that many in the dominant culture actually act on this in a paternalistic fashion, furthering the harms. They believe that approaching this issue seeking transformative power is a more constructive conceptualization, since its outcome heals both the oppressor and the oppressed. They do an excellent job of showing how oppressing others actually dehumanizes both the oppressed and the oppressor, and see transformative power as an approach that creates humanizing options for both parties.

Chris, Geri, and Pat advise that everyone can encourage transformative power; members of the dominant group can observe and seek to change institutional policies that perpetuate cultural oppression and they can consciously discover and correct their own blind spots. They clarify the fact that passivity here abets oppressive practices by sustaining them . Organizations do need to be confronted. The authors then propose building a bridge between the culturally oppressed and nurses, an oppressed group themselves, noting how reluctant nurses are to face and experience the tension and abasement of recognizing their own oppression. They observe that this is an essential first step in healing the wounds of oppression. They conclude with advice to nurses: this model, useful for cultural oppression, is a model appropriate for nurses' oppression, and the only real path available if we seek autonomy, freedom, and responsibility for ourselves.

Karen Brykczynski delves into the concept of holism to explore nursing's need for healing. Holism, she notes, is more than the sum of the parts. It implies an integration substantial enough to create something entirely new. Observing nursing's collective commitment to holism, she then explores the nature of our divisiveness. She posits that it is in part grounded in our history of building a science on the eroding foundation of logical positivism and its commitment to seeing parts only, to feigning the role of the external, objective, truth-seeking observer of others, and to its investment in dichotomization. Holistic unity is not dichotomous, but our discipline's politics demonstrate our commitment to dichotomies, with one side right and one side wrong. Holism would posit rich diversity, value in the multiplicity, collective enhancement from the union, and *balance,* the term we associate with integration and healing.

She notes that our divisiveness is worsened by its expression through the use of an adversarial stance focused on opposition and conflict. To illustrate, she offers a powerful example of one of our favorite conflicts: our scope of practice. Describing the elastic boundaries of scope of practice (it expands for night shifts in hospitals and indigent populations needing nurse practitioners), she posits that we are ill-advised to pretend these are fixed or certain since they are most often simply associated with medicine's commitment to restraint of trade and their political machinations to sustain this restraint.

Karen recommends that the idea of holism is intrinsic to healing. We might better spend our time and resources, she notes, on coming together as a discipline, on learning how to build political alliances with others and how to manage competing interests, and recommends the use of conflict resolution by accessing neutral third parties. She calls for unity among all nurses, a commitment to healing the wounds inflicted by conflict and divisiveness.

Susan Scoville Baker shows how her personal role as a healer helped her better understand that her work of healing was also healing her, vitalizing her as a healer. She clarified for herself that the increased use of her gifts as a healer had led to increased vigor and engagement in healing, and she shares her gratitude for this realization, taught to her by two adolescent patients on a unit where she does faculty practice.

Susan's personal story demonstrates a deepened understanding of the power of the role of healer when an adolescent mirrors back to her an awe at her competency and power as a practitioner: after sitting with her as she assisted a frightened teen, the girl asks her if she is a witch. The patient, having observed Susan using both her psychiatric nursing competencies and alternative healing methods, such as therapeutic touch, presence, sight, sound, and comfort, was amazed at her efficacy. Susan realized that while her work was often exhausting, it was also revitalizing, and gave her access to the healing powers of practice, feedback, and growth.

Helen Kee takes us to another unit of analysis and another level of complexity in her discussion of the leader as healer, especially during times of rapid institutional change. The leader she describes is the nurse executive facing healthcare changes at an institution where she has considerable authority and responsibility. Helen notes that healthcare institutions are intricately organized, and the disruption of rapid, often unwelcome change increases the level of uncertainty and ambiguity, heightening fear. While we nurses often propound the need to assist our patients in healing, seeking wholeness in body, mind, and spirit, we fail to realize that an institution is not only an organism in its own right, but is composed of humans, each of whom needs help in healing after intense mandated change.

Helen then provides a sobering analysis of the history of organizational theory, noting the erroneous conviction of the utility and viability of bureaucracies, and our unwillingness to let go of this model, despite its demonstrated deficiencies. She notes that the nurse leader, stressed by rapid change, may not only not serve as a healing leader, but may begin to exercise more control, become more competitive, engage in more power wielding, and argue for rationality alone as the basis for action. She believes that these behaviors wound the organization and require healing. Helen recommends useful antidotes to this tendency. She advises the nurse leader to broaden decision making to all levels, increase communication, do active listening, show compassion and empathy, and develop a trusting environment based on consistency and truth telling. She acknowledges that all members of the organization have a role to play in these healing practices, and the leader must continue to grapple with the complexities of change and mission, yet observes that the nurse executive has a unique opportunity to make the difference as the leader who is also a healer.

Priscilla Koester provides yet another window on a moving personal story that describes the death of her brother from AIDS, a young man beloved by his sister. As a nurse, she works at the task of healing from such a profound life event—the confrontation with death and a disease still confusing both to those who suffer its ravages and to those who seek to help and care. The author tells the story of all the people who helped, the love, devotion, sensitivity, and concern shown her, the lessons about healing taught to her by those who, like her also, loved her brother.

For readers who have not personally experienced the loving communities that often spring up to assist in the dying process of a person with AIDS, the story serves as a lesson in how we might better help others heal from their wounds. This story is also evocative of that insight that we too often lose sight of in nursing. Philosophy precedes theory, and theory without story is often too sterile and detached. It is story that motivates us to act, and activates our passion.

Patricia Davis Gilmore describes a familiar dilemma, and tells how she confronted and continues to confront that dilemma. While nurses are deeply valued for their caring and their empathy, they are concurrently rendered powerless by both society and the institutional policies and politics in this country. Describing a physician who blamed a nurse for an error he made that put a patient in jeopardy, she was catalyzed to ask herself more profound questions about the powerlessness of nurses and her personal options for addressing this issue.

Like many authors in Part Three, she notes the relationship between powerlessness and oppression, and the effects on nursing: our excessive conformity, our low risk-taking behaviors, our reactive stance on most issues. She observes that, to alter this, we must empower ourselves, struggle to exercise power with other providers in the control of resources, definitions of health, and ways to implement health-enhancing policies and actions. In order to reclaim our strengths, rights, and abilities, we must first heal ourselves of our enmeshment in powerlessness.

For Pat, that has included earning a law degree, interweaving the two disciplines of nursing and law in her practice, teaching, professional involvement, and personal commitments. Pat makes a useful distinction between the internal and the external influences on nursing, and notes that we tend to focus on the external, but must also attend to the internal factors, including our willingness to harm one another. She concludes that if indeed we care about the profession, we will seek the healing process of empowerment, and work to create harmoniousness in nursing through a balance of empowerment and caring. We can have both.

Harriett Riggs relates a wonderful vignette that could also be understood as a parable. She describes a brief experience with a child in a Sunday school class, where the child, seeking healing from Harriett, also gives Harriett the gift of healing herself. The child shares a series of confessions with Harriett, and in the process activates her own power to heal herself. Harriett, privileged to be part of this tender process, realizes anew that healing is often about the fragility of relationships and the resulting joy in their preservation.

The poetry I wrote for this part of the book is sequential, and provides four snapshots on the process of moving through woundedness and healing. Retrospectively, I find that I am often naive about a life reality before a wound, and experience a horror at the process of wounding. It is only through the process of healing that I discover that I can choose to learn and grow from the wounding, and that I am indeed more human for the healing.

In shamanic practices, there is a strong tradition of the "wounded healer." There is a belief that until one has been wounded and healed, one does not have the wisdom or power to become a shaman. It is through our own personal journey of wounding and healing that we begin to become useful healers, for we discover not only pain and suffering but also enrichment, humility, personal strength, and wisdom.

Virginia Rahr completes this section with a practical, yet visionary discussion of the possibilities we can actualize if healing becomes central to the process of educating the next generation of nurses, a process that can also involve healing the nurse educator and the student. She describes the reframe necessary if we intend to educate our baccalaureate students within a healing philosophy of nursing. She observes that, while all healthcare providers engage in curing, caring, and healing, for her the most essential of these is healing. For Rahr, healing involves moving beyond a focus on physical signs and symptoms and includes formal study in wholeness, comfort, patient dignity, and self-empowerment; the study of the lived experience of the patient. For these, mutual relationships are essential, and the "tasks" we perform have greater range and creativity. She gives an excellent example of a nursing intervention of this nature.

Virginia describes healing as "any intervention that assists an individual to maintain or strengthen his or her coping abilities, self-esteem, self-care, and comfort, and that promotes the individual's attainment of a 'desired wholeness.' " She believes it is not an endpoint but a "work in progress," and posits that a curriculum with this focus would require an organizational climate characterized by relationships of mutual trust and respect. It is fun for me to muse on healing as central to an educational process for our young, rather than the terror often felt over pathophysiology exams or clinical tardiness. Virginia wisely notes that creating the climate comes first, which may indeed be a striking example of our collective need for healing as nurse educators.

Part Three unveils the many ways that we healers might heal ourselves as essential to facilitating patients in their healing. It notes some ways that we are not healed, some possible pathways to healing, the power and potential of healing ourselves, and the way our patients can be excellent teachers for us if we are open to their lessons. What becomes clear in reading the various viewpoints shared in Part Three is that wonderful theories, well-intentioned scholarship, and outstanding clinical interventions will do little for our patients if we have not yet placed ourselves on a path toward our personal healing. Our woundedness need not be a weakness; indeed, it is my belief that it is the key to our strength and promise. In opting to practice what we preach, we open a rich vista of opportunities for growth and for hope.

A Reminder

by Alice S. Hill, RN, PhD

"The wound is deep"
I heard her say;
"It will leave a scar"
she said with dismay.

"My beautiful face
no longer shall be;
I know people will stare
and point at me."

Just when she was absorbed
in tears,
Along came a man who had been
disfigured for years.

I heard Him ask, "why do you
weep?"
She replied, "my face,
the wound is very deep."

In a still quiet voice, I heard Him say,
"Beauty is from within anyway."

She listened attentively, but then
exclaimed,
"We are all judged by our skin
and not from within."

"Who will take the time to know my
soul,
when my face is marred and I look
old.
My face is disfigured, I'm scarred for
life,
what man in his right mind would
want me for a wife."

Just then the man raised His head,
and with a stern look He boldly said,
"Perhaps those who judge your beauty
from without,
are not the people you should keep
about."

"My child," I know you think your
beauty is gone,
but the scar is a reminder
that the healing is done."

CHAPTER 16

The Nurse, the Client, and Alternative Healing Methods

VEROLYN BARNES BOLANDER, RN, MS, C

> *I'm good enough, I'm smart enough, and doggone it, people like me!*
> *(A very healing affirmation for Stuart Smalley)*
>
> —Al Franken

Nearly 25 years ago, before most of us had ever heard of what is today referred to as a *near-death experience,* Pam experienced one. She didn't make it far enough through the tunnel to be reassured by what lay before her—she was suddenly whisked back, to intensive care and to a respirator. An intelligent and caring nurse, Pam felt isolated and fearful as she later recounted to her doctors and nurses what she had experienced. She found that her listeners could not understand her experience, but they were willing to treat what they referred to as the anxiety over her "nightmare." The planned treatment was electroshock therapy and she found she had to fabricate "recovery from the terrors of her nightmare" in order to get out of the hospital without treatment on the psychiatric unit.

It was not until Pam read Kübler-Ross' classic book on near-death experiences that she finally understood what had happened to her. In subsequent years, Pam learned more and began to practice, teach, and write about spiritual nursing care. Without a similar "trip through the tunnel," many other nurses began doing these same things and many nursing schools began to focus on the spiritual nature in addition to biological, psychological, and sociocultural aspects of the recipients of nursing care.

And yet today, with the exception of religious approaches, without special or advanced training, relatively few nurses practicing in the United States could state more than a few specific nursing interventions for clients in spiritual distress.

To meet the expectations of its clients, the nursing profession needs more nurses who study human spirituality and spiritual nursing care. As

Benoist and Cathebras (1993) said, "people accept biological knowledge but they do not accept a purely biological conception of their own body. They conceive that there is an immaterial part in the human body; however it is not supernatural but a part of nature" (p. 857). This concept is not merely a cultural belief to which nurses of a particular culture must respond, rather, "the refusal to enclose the person in the biological body appears as a constant through human societies" (p. 857).

Attending to the spiritual nature of clients is an accepted part of nursing practice. However, attempting to influence spiritual entities that are believed to exist outside of (and to benefit or harm) human beings, such as is done with shamanism, for example, is not usually considered a part of nursing practice, at least in the United States. Nonetheless, most nurses accept the fact that some clients may be partial to shamanic practices and understand that, when this is the case, the clients' beliefs are to be respected both in and beyond the nursing care plan. This is true whether or not the nurse understands that ". . . various experiments indicate that gifted healers may benefit their clients paranormally" (McClenon, 1993, p. 120).

What is paranormal? At one time, hypnosis and other methods of working with the human mind were considered to be "paranormal." This is no longer so. For example, in addition to providing ordered analgesics, Sean routinely uses the avoidance strategies of guided imagery and teaching self-talk to distract his burn patients from their intense pain. He is not trained in hypnosis or he might be able to use hypnotherapy to good effect, as well (Patterson, 1992, p. 17).

In contrast, Gloria has been certified as a hypnotherapist and occasionally uses hypnotherapy in her clinical practice as a nurse advocate. Other nurses certified in hypnotherapy use hypnotic age regression in their work in mental health nursing. Some also use hypnotic age progression "to promote growth on multiple levels, facilitating treatment goals and deepening the working-through process" (Phillips & Frederick, 1992, p. 99).

Maria, a masters-prepared nurse, uses and teaches others to use Delores Krieger's methods of therapeutic touch to assess patients and to help them to heal. An eclectic practitioner, Maria also uses massage of various types, such as Shiatsu.

Historically, in the United States, these areas of interest have been marginalized, the rewards of study few, and the efforts to study them not well supported. In fact, as Navarro (1993) pointed out in his review of health services research in the United States, "priorities in the research agenda are defined either by the federal government or by the private foundations, whose positions rarely conflict" (p. 6), because "scholars study what the money-granting agencies decide and accept; for the most part, it is not the academic community that decides what to study" (p. 7). As he notes, "Researchers can, of course, conduct research outside the acceptable constraints, but only at a very high personal and professional cost." For example, although "a growing number of surveys of random national samples of American and European countries reveal the extensiveness of psychic experiences and occult belief" (McClenon, 1993, p. 109), "scientists who find evidence supporting belief in the paranormal are stigmatized as deviant since their *individual* claims can be evaluated as insufficient for overturning better established explanations regarding the 'laws of nature'" (p. 111).

Although it is slowly changing, the emphasis in U.S. healthcare has been on physical care. The treatment of disease and the research dollar has been spent accordingly. Kerr White (1993), one of the editors of *Health Services Research: An Anthology,* says, "The need has never been greater for deeper appreciation of the diverse interlocking determinants of health and disease . . . and nowhere is the problem more urgent than in the United States, where an automotive culture pervades medical practice by assigning high priority to 'spare part' replacement technology" (p. 603).

In the areas of alternative therapies, researchers in other countries are generally more progressive. For example, as Mowrey (1986) pointed out, the healing properties of whole herbs, with few exceptions (such as garlic), ". . . are seldom if ever investigated . . ." in the United States (p. v). He attributed this lack of research to the reluctance of pharmaceutical companies to support the enormous cost of bringing a drug to market and the fact that an herb is not classified as a drug. Citing 1986 costs, he said,

> *The FDA estimates it costs over $7 million to bring a new drug to market. Pharmaceutical companies put that figure closer to $70 million. They say they need two million users of a substance just to break even. Since natural substances cannot be patented, there is even less room for profit in them. Hence, it really doesn't matter how strong the demand for a natural substance might be. It would never be economically feasible to go through the expensive process of getting it approved for use by the FDA. No pharmaceutical company would market garlic when the money is in penicillin. (p. xi)*

Thus, the pharmaceutical companies, which could afford to complete the research, are not motivated to do it while others, who might be motivated to do it, can seldom afford the cost. Yet herbal remedies have been used for centuries and are still being used today (Achterberg, 1991;

Mowrey, 1986; Weiner & Weiner, 1994). Bookstores display numerous publications on herbs. Newspaper and magazine articles tell how to grow and use them. A number of herbs are readily available, even without consulting an herbal practitioner. Many grocery stores and health food stores sell herbal products. And the public obviously consumes them for purposes of enhancing health and curing disease as well as for enhancing the flavor of foods. Nurses, who counsel clients regarding nutrition, including the use of food additives, vitamins, and minerals, can ill afford to be ignorant of the use of herbal remedies and yet little (if any) time is given to herbals in most basic nursing programs. There are nurses like Paul, however, who are quite knowledgeable about herbs. In fact, Paul grows herbs and prepares herbal preparations as his family has done for several generations. Paul also practices aromatherapy. As part of his nursing practice, he teaches about the use of herbs, as necessary, as he does client counseling.

Pam, Sean, Gloria, Maria, and Paul are all using interventions that were not even considered to be within the realm of nursing 25 short years ago. Today, these practices have come to be accepted as interventions nurses can use. These interventions are all *alternative healing methods*. Because many of them are relatively new to modern nursing, questions naturally arise concerning their use. Are these alternative therapies legally appropriate for the nurse to use? Are they ethically appropriate? Are they accepted by their nursing colleagues? What additional education or training is needed to learn these techniques? Is a higher degree necessary or not? What certification or licensure is required, if any? Is the licensing or certification accepted nationally or only by individual states? What is the structure of what we refer to as *alternative healing?* We need definitions and classifications, particularly classifications that establish the parameters under which we may or may not legally and safely practice. We need the answers to those basic questions.

If we are going to fulfill our roles as practitioners, consultants, teachers, and researchers, we need to start with an understanding of how much the general public understands about alternative healing. What is the prevalence of alternative healing in general as well as in specific cases in which we might have interest? What are the patterns of use? What are the trends? Who are the persons who use alternative healing methods? Why are alternative methods chosen over other methods? How much does the public spend on healthcare and, of this amount, how much is directed toward alternative healing? Of the money spent on alternative healing, how much does the client spend on products versus practitioners? Are clients insured against the costs of alternative healthcare? How is the insurance reimbursement dollar apportioned to various healthcare products and practitioners?

In this chapter, I have attempted to answer some of these questions and to suggest how the nurse may practice safely, legally, and professionally in a healthcare system that increasingly uses alternative healing methods.

DEFINITIONS

When we talk about alternative healing methods, just what do we mean? Alternative to what? In the U.S., alternative care is most often written about as an alternative to Western medical care. Western medicine is the traditional, conventional medical practice that is termed *biomedicine* or *allopathy*. It is often referred to as *orthodox* medicine. Allopathic medical practitioners (medical doctors, physicians) use modern technology to treat diseases mainly by surgical intervention or by less invasive techniques such as the prescription of pharmaceuticals. Examples of allopaths include these familiar types of practitioners:

- family practitioners
- general practitioners
- internists
- psychiatrists
- surgeons
- other specialists

It should be understood that allopathic medicine is traditional medicine in North America and in most industrialized nations, but traditional medicine in other countries is the native medicine practiced there as distinguished from Western medicine, which is often practiced alongside of it. Thus, the term *traditional medicine* differs in meaning according to geography and history.

Although some alternative healthcare practitioners treat disease, many promote health or attempt to heal or assist in healing, instead. Alternative practitioners often focus on healing the mind, body, and spirit by improving the interrelationship among these three parts of the person (Zagorsky, 1993). Many if not all practitioners of alternative healing practices believe that the real power of healing comes from within the client (Engebretson & Wardell, 1993).

To understand the concept of *alternative healing methods,* it may be helpful to look at Boisset and Fitzcharles' (1994) definition of *unconventional medicine;* that is, "medical interventions not widely taught in North American medical schools or generally available in North American hospitals" (p. 148). Because Boisset and Fitzcharles refer to the practice of medicine and because they define the concept by telling what it is not, rather than what it is, it is preferable to look at Montbriand's (1993) definition of *alternative healthcare,* which is, "all health-related practices initiated or prescribed by patients, their family, or friends or an alternate healthcare [*sic*] healer" (p. 1195), as opposed to medical practices initiated or prescribed by a licensed allopathic physician or by someone who does not have the patient's best interests in mind (a quack). These two definitions seem to complement each other but both are incomplete.

Some authors use the term *alternative healing methods* to refer to *complementary treatment methods* (healthcare practices that are prescribed by, and work hand in hand with, the practices of allopathic physicians, rather than as an alternative to these allopathic practices). Other authors use the terms *alternative* and *complementary* healing methods interchangeably. I support Frost (1994) who adamantly states, "complementary approaches should be regarded as just that and not as an alternative to routine therapies" (p. 331).

The term *alternative healing methods* usually refers to the practice of therapies such as:

acupressure	homeopathy[+]
acupuncture[+]	hypnotism[++]
affirmations	iridology
aromatherapy	meditation
biofeedback[++]	naturopathy
centering	osteopathy[+]
chakra balancing	rolfing
chiropractic[+]	shiatsu
flower remedies	therapeutic touch
guided imagery	visualizations
herbalism	vitamin therapy

(Engebretson & Wardell, 1993; Vecchio, 1994; Warpeha & Harris, 1993). The methods marked by a plus sign are in the process of becoming accepted as part of mainstream medical practice in the United States, Canada, the United Kingdom, and Australia and those marked by a double plus sign are often accepted as complementary methods. These indicators will change over time.

Methods complementary to medicine usually refer to practices such as:

art therapy   pharmacology
diet therapy   physiotherapy
music therapy   psychology
nursing care   recreational therapy
occupational therapy

These are therapies that are more frequently prescribed than practiced by the majority of allopathic physicians. They are accepted as ancillary parts of mainstream medicine and are practiced by licensed healthcare workers who may work dependently (under the direction of a physician in regard to certain responsibilities) or independently (as a licensed practitioner of a profession in regard to other responsibilities). It could, of course, be argued that the practice of medicine is complementary to the practice of nursing, which is a more central profession, but that is another paper, entirely. For now, let us accept the premise that all of these professions are commonly viewed as complementary to medicine and to each other.

Just as some authors incorrectly use the terms *alternative* and *complementary healing methods* interchangeably, other authors may use either or both of these terms (or their synonyms) to refer to outright quackery. Neither of these methods should be confused with quackery. With quackery, unscrupulous persons misrepresent their knowledge and ability to treat disease and make extravagant claims about the efficacy of their treatments. Quacks are usually identified by the secrecy of their remedies and by their claims that the established medical community is persecuting them in order to prevent them from selling their cure. Examples of quacks include those who would encourage persons with disorders such as cancer or AIDS to stop orthodox treatments and, instead, use treatments such as those identified by the American Cancer Society in their discussion of questionable cancer treatments such as:

• Ozone injections into cancerous tumors on the basis on the work of Puharich, Arnan, and deVries reported in 1985 where they "postulated that ozone is effective [in curing cancer] because in neoplastic cells the 'terminal respiratory chain flow of electrons is reversed,' as it is in photosynthesis" ("Questionable methods of cancer management: Hydrogen peroxide," 1993, p. 54). According to the American Cancer Society, Puharich, Arnan, and deVries claimed that they confirmed their theory "by finding 'Chlorophyll bodies' in the cytoplasm of neoplastic tissue."

• Hoxsey external and internal herbal treatments, developed and first used by Harry Hoxsey in the 1920s. The external herbal remedy was "corrosive enough to destroy body tissue on contact," and the mixtures of herbs for internal use have never been demonstrated to be "more effective than no treatment at all." Hoxsey was convicted three times of practicing medicine without a license but he moved to other states and continued practice until finally stopped by the FDA in the 1950s. Since his death, his former nurse, Mildred Nelson, has opened a clinic in Tiajuana, Mexico, where treatments continue (Questionable methods of cancer management: 'Nutritional' Therapies).

Unfortunately, a number of allopathic practitioners have lumped together all alternative healing methods as quackery and have been so biased that they were not open to some truly therapeutic methods. One example is Panush (1993), who doesn't use the term *quackery,* but whose attitude speaks volumes about how he defines what he terms *unproven* therapies. He says,

> *My previous view of unproven therapies had been unrelentingly harsh. I was unsympathetic of gullible patients, intolerant of advocates of such approaches, and critical of failures to follow scientific methods. My presentations on this topic were heavily laden with sarcasm. I showed slides of my dog for whom we acquired certification as a nutritional consultant. (p. 201)*

He uses the term *alternative remedies* interchangeably with the term *unproven remedies,* and throughout his article, he speaks of *unproven* remedies as we would expect of someone warning against quackery. When he finally allows that some of these "unproven remedies" had perhaps not been so bad, he admits,

> *Exciting reports are now emerging that patients with arthritis have improved with participation in aerobic dance programs, water aerobics, treadmill exercise programs, stationary cycling exercise programs, and Nautilus-type training—all programs we previously eschewed for our patients. (pp. 204-205)*

With this disclosure of what he had been so reluctant to accept, compared with what he admits was his previous stance, he has come a very long way, indeed. And one wonders what he might possibly think about a truly alternative modality such as aromatherapy or therapeutic touch.

Obviously the confusion in meanings among *traditional methods, complementary methods, alternative methods,* and *quackery* is not helpful to the consumers of the literature. Also unhelpful is the number of terms used to refer to alternative healing methods, many of which are often incorrectly used interchangeably. For example, the *alternative* portion of the term *alternative healing methods* has been referred to as *alternate, unconventional, unorthodox, nontraditional, folk, holistic, nontoxic, additional, complementary, new age, tradomedical, traditional, paramedical, unproven, untested, questionable, inappropriate,* and *fringe.* The *healing methods* portion of the term *alternative healing methods* has been referred to as *healing practices, health practices, medical practices, medicine, remedies, modalities,* and *therapies.*

Considering that nurses practice nursing to assist clients in promoting and maintaining health and that physicians practice medicine to treat disease, this confusion in the language describing alternative healthcare echoes the confusion in the literature regarding who is providing the care.

Also adding to the confusion is the semipermeability of the boundaries between any two of these systems, with concomitant movement of some modalities from one system to another. Examples are many, including: (1) the movement of acupuncture from an alternative practice to growing acceptance as an allopathic practice; (2) the movement of hypnotism from an alternative practice (when first used by Mesmer) to a quack remedy or an entertainment device (after Mesmer's fall from grace) and back to a complementary practice (as it is currently used in psychiatry); and (3) the movement of certain allopathic prescription medications to the status of over-the-counter remedies, which can be used as alternative treatments.

Just how these movements occur is a matter for a number of studies. O'Neill (1994), for example, makes a fascinating case for the Australian government accepting chiropractic, osteopathy, and acupuncture into mainstream medical practice because, these "practices become intrinsically dangerous as their efficacy is accepted. Consequently, the argument is that only established practitioners are safe enough to use them" (p. 497). Note also that some remedies may be recommended by both allopaths and practitioners of alternative healing methods (Zagorsky, 1993), for example, massage, nutritional changes, and exercise.

In addition to good definitions, we need a universally accepted classification scheme for all of the methods and for all of the practitioners in these systems. Some classifications have already been suggested in the literature.

CLASSIFICATIONS OF PRACTITIONERS

Engebretson and Wardell, two nurses from the University of Texas Health Science Center, Houston, correctly stated that "currently there is no classification system that adequately describes the types of healers practicing in the United States" (p. 51). They admitted that "an attempt to classify some of the 'New Age' healers was impossible, because healers were often practicing more than one type of healing and would frequently incorporate many different methods into their practice" (Engebretson & Wardell, 1993, p. 51). They attempted a classification of healthcare modalities according to the preparation of the healer (physical manipulation, ingested or applied substances, uses of energy, and mental/spiritual).

As orthodox practitioners using these modalities (those with the most preparation and with their practice based on scientific principles), Engebretson and Wardell (1993) list "Surgery, Physical Therapy, Pharmacology, Laser Surgery, Psychiatry, and Psychology" (p. 52). As marginal practitioners using these modalities (those with some formal education and with credentials but no recognition by the U.S. medical establishment), they list "Chiropractic, Homeopathy, Vitamin Therapy, Acupuncture, Acupressure, Secular or Spiritual Counseling, and Established Support Groups, e.g., 12 step programs" (p. 52). As alternative practitioners using these modalities (those with knowledge gained through an apprenticeship type of learning and/or intuition), they list ". . . Rolfing, Feldenkrais, Naturopathic remedies, Herbs, Flower remedies, Reiki, Magnetic Polarity Healing, Therapeutic Touch, Self-Help Groups, Visualizations, and Affirmations" (p. 52). As alternative practitioners who are practicing even more on the basis of intuition, they list "Cranio-sacral alignments, Massage Therapy, Yoga, Akido, Tai Chi, Reflexology, Aromatherapy, Diet alternatives, Chakra Balancing, Radionics, Use of color, gems & Crystals, and Psychic, Spiritual, or Intuitive Healing" (p. 52).

There are at least three problems with this scheme: (1) No attempt is made to identify complementary practitioners; (2) some of the modalities seem to be misplaced; for example, registered nutritionists would probably take exception to "diet alternatives" (p. 52) being listed among modalities of the least formally educated, most-intuitive practitioners. Surely the work nutritionists do is as orthodox as the practice of pharmacology; and (3) nowhere is there a place for eclectic practitioners, such as nurses.

Even with its problems, this classification scheme is an excellent beginning and should serve as a starting point for a dialogue concerning the classification of practitioners. With a long history of working with a wide variety of practitioners of orthodox medicine, including complementary therapies, and with clients who use all manner of alternatives, nurses are very well suited to undertake the task of devising a classification scheme for practitioners.

Using the Engebretson and Wardell model as a starting point, I would suggest a model that can be used to classify practitioners on a continuum from the highest level of acceptance by the general public in the United States to the lowest level of acceptance by this same public. See Table 16.1 for a model of the relationship of orthodox practitioners, complementary practitioners, alternative practitioners, and quacks. With this model, general acceptance is evidenced, from highest to lowest levels, by: (1) completion of an orthodox curriculum in the United States and earning state licensure; (2) completion of an orthodox curriculum in another country or completion of U.S. training at less than a professional level and earning some credential and practice privileges from the state; (3) completion of a short course of training in the United States with receipt of a training certificate or completion of a longer period of training in another country, but (in either case) no specific license to practice; (4) no credentials certifying training at all but anecdotal evidence of safety and efficacy in the practice of an unlicensed activity; (5) (regardless of education, credentials, or practice privileges) questioning of methods by public agencies; and (6) (also, regardless of education, credentials, or practice privileges) censure by public agencies with denial of the right to practice. This last would be the lowest level of acceptance by the general public (prior to criminal charges being filed).

This model separates those who treat disease, such as allopaths, and complementary healthcare workers who promote health, such as nurses, because groups of practitioners in these areas do not cross the line. The marginal healthcare workers below the professional and semiprofessional healthcare workers are generally those who have received some acceptance by the more orthodox above them, but acceptance is not yet unanimous. As time passes, these marginal practitioners may cross the semipermeable line above them to join the ranks of mainstream medicine or they may cross the semi-permeable line below them to return to the ranks of the less-well accepted alternative practitioners. Again, the two groups of practitioners are separated by whether they treat disease or promote health. The line separating the two groups is impermeable.

Alternative practitioners are grouped together in the belief that they all promote health. There is a semipermeable line between them and quacks

TABLE 16.1.   Relationship of orthodox practitioners, complementary practitioners, alternative practitioners and quacks

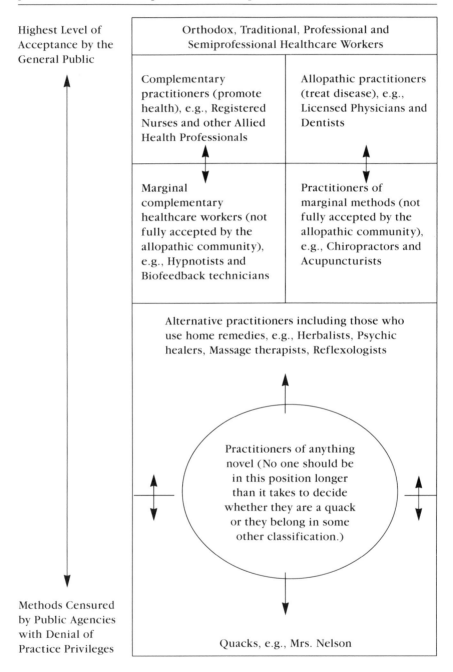

Highest Level of Acceptance by the General Public

Orthodox, Traditional, Professional and Semiprofessional Healthcare Workers

Complementary practitioners (promote health), e.g., Registered Nurses and other Allied Health Professionals

Allopathic practitioners (treat disease), e.g., Licensed Physicians and Dentists

Marginal complementary healthcare workers (not fully accepted by the allopathic community), e.g., Hypnotists and Biofeedback technicians

Practitioners of marginal methods (not fully accepted by the allopathic community), e.g., Chiropractors and Acupuncturists

Alternative practitioners including those who use home remedies, e.g., Herbalists, Psychic healers, Massage therapists, Reflexologists

Practitioners of anything novel (No one should be in this position longer than it takes to decide whether they are a quack or they belong in some other classification.)

Methods Censured by Public Agencies with Denial of Practice Privileges

Quacks, e.g., Mrs. Nelson

below them, but there is a "holding area" between the two groups where practitioners of novel methods may be placed, temporarily, until their method of healing has been evaluated. Under the correct circumstances, the alternative practitioners may move into the quack area below or into one of the two marginal areas above and the quacks may move into the alternative area. But neither can move into the holding area for novel practices. Those in the holding area can move down to the quack area or up to the alternative practitioner area. They may also move to higher levels of acceptance, but this usually takes some time.

More needs to be said about the question of who is marginal and who is not. It depends on circumstances. In the United States, for example, some alternative care practitioners, if they are allowed to practice at all, require licensing by individual states; for example, practitioners of homeopathy, chiropractic, and acupuncture. In some states, homeopaths are licensed medical doctors, but in others they are not. Some practitioners of Western medicine have adopted homeopathic medicine, chiropractic techniques, and acupuncture and use these modalities as part of their medical practice. In such cases, these alternative techniques have crossed over the line and practitioners are still considered to be practicing orthodox medicine.

In other states, these practitioners are licensed as professionals in their own right, but like physiotherapists or occupational therapists, they serve in complementary roles to the physicians who practice Western medicine. Others who are licensed practice independently and outside of the traditional medical practice as alternative practitioners.

In still other states, they are not licensed and may or may not practice at all, depending on the state laws. Because chiropractors and acupuncturists, among others, are not yet accepted as professionals in their own right in all states, they seem to fit best as examples in this marginal area of the model.

With the proper training, all healing methods used by alternative practitioners should be available for use by the practitioners above them in the model. It seems reasonable that the adoption and use of these methods by practitioners (who are more acceptable to the public) is one way to help to make the methods more acceptable and is a way to help assure their safety. I do not advocate use of these methods without adequate research, but I question whether adequate research will be done without trained investigators to do it. Because orthodox medicine has not had a strong record of being open to alternative healing methods, this area of research is ideal for nurse researchers. Let us go on to look at these alternative healing methods, then.

CLASSIFICATIONS OF ALTERNATIVE HEALING METHODS

The classification of alternative healing methods is well along the way. Montbriand and Laing (1991) did some initial work in which they listened to patients in a Canadian hospital and found that alternative healing methods used by these patients could be divided into physical, mental, and spiritual methods. They noted that:

> *Physical alternative practices were tangible in nature. They were substances causing physiological change in the body such as vitamins or herbal products, physical manipulations such as massage, or physical objects such as talismans. Spiritual alternative care evoked a cosmic source to cure the illness or help the patient to cope. The cosmic source was often God or a saint. Psychological alternative care included all healthcare practices using the mind as the director of care, for example, self-initiated distraction, attitude change, or visualization therapies. (p. 327)*

Except for some attention to the physiological, these authors did not separate body, mind, and spirit of the client in that they did not attempt to classify each type of modality according to a specific hoped-for physical, spiritual, or mental effect. They looked mostly at the desired end of healing and classified remedies by their action, instead. With little change, we could say that each remedy can be classified according to whether it is expected to work to heal the total person: (1) by its direct chemical or physical action on or in the client's body; (2) through the direction of the client's mind, with or without touching or use of tangible objects, such as a swinging watch to induce a hypnotic trance; or (3) through a cosmic or spiritual force, which may or may not involve touching the client or using a tangible object, such as a talisman. And I would add (4) by a combination of two or more of the preceding three methods.

Because use of a talisman is actually reliance upon some cosmic or supernatural force to protect or to heal the individual, I have moved the example of the use of a talisman from the physical and into the spiritual realm of healing. But I would still include the use of physical devices, such as heating pads, as physical methods important to those of us raised in the United States and Canada. In fact, Montbriand (1993) found that, most of his informants were "attracted to the physical types of alternate therapies, either alone or in combination with psychological or spiritual choices" (p. 1197).

With the biological, the psychological, and the spiritual covered here, it is tempting to try to force in a classification of social or cultural. As nurses, we are attuned to the biopsychosocial and cultural nature of our clients. There *are* entire alternative healing systems that are culturally based. However, although the outcome of a healing practice can be strongly influenced by the cultural context in which it is practiced, it should be remembered that specific cultural systems use methods that can be broken down into one or more of the three main classes mentioned—physical, psychological, and spiritual. To try to use cultural healing practices as a separate class of healing methods would be to add confusion to the classification system. For example, a traditional healer from Africa might provide herbs to take away pain (a physical method), might use incantations to scare away evil spirits (a spiritual method), and might "treat the total personality of the client to allay . . . fears, anxieties, stress and strain" (Osujih, 1993, p. 192) (a psychological method). Thus, to say that healing practices within specific cultures are *cultural methods* would not be helpful in a classification scheme. It may be useful, however, to consider the cultural context within which healing practices occur.

If nurses could agree upon this classification, or upon any other, it would improve our ability to research alternative health methods. We could complete studies that would allow direct comparisons among groups of subjects who have been treated by alternative practitioners. As it is, many investigators allow their subjects to define what they see as alternative care and to answer surveys on this basis (Fawcett, Sidney, Hanson, & Riley-Lawless, 1994; Montbriand & Laing, 1991). The results vary considerably in quality as do the generalizability of the results.

Costs

Because of a lack of universally agreed upon definitions and classifications, it is very difficult to know exactly what is spent on alternative health methods. When people suffer chronically from the pains of rheumatoid arthritis, for example, they will most often seek help from their family physician and perhaps from a rheumatologist, both of whom may order prescription and nonprescription drugs, thermal applications, devices such as splints, and visits to such complementary practitioners as physiotherapists or nutritionists. Clients may also visit one or more alternative therapists, such as an acupuncturist, herbalist, or homeopath who may prescribe other remedies. These same clients may also purchase over-the-counter medications and medical devices recommended by friends or by advertisements. Or they may try one of the newer arthritis home remedies to come to the attention of orthodox medicine: white raisins soaked in gin (in fact use of this remedy is highly likely as anecdotal evidence is very positive regarding the efficacy of the active ingredient in the juniper berries that go into the gin).

Some of the expenses of those plagued with rheumatic pain may be covered by insurance while other expenses are out-of-pocket. Considering all of those who are insured, it may be difficult to know what part of the total premiums covers the care for this specific disorder, and of that part, what part covers alternative care for the same disorder. Some policies cover alternative treatments such as chiropractic treatments to some extent (with or without deductibles) and other policies do not.

Of the out-of-pocket expenses, what part goes for the alternative care of this disorder? What part of the cost of the bottle of over-the-counter analgesic can be assigned as a cost of alternative healing of the client's inflamed joints and what part of the alternative healing to her daughter's two-day headache or her son's sore throat (when the analgesic was ordered by a physician for the sore throat but not for the headache)? Estimating the costs of alternative care is not a simple matter.

By way of example, investigators in one Canadian study attempted to look at the costs of alternative care for a small group of unselected, consecutive rheumatology patients attending a rheumatology clinic. They found that the expenditures reported by patients in the past 12 months for alternative practitioners averaged $500 per person, and expenditures for over-the-counter products including herbs, vitamins, minerals, and topical remedies averaged $100. The investigators were careful to point out that their definition of over-the-counter products excluded single daily multiple vitamin pills and calcium supplements because these are frequently prescribed by physicians (Boisset & Fitzcharles, 1994). How many other investigators were careful enough to make such exclusions? According to the investigators in this study, the frequent use of over-the-counter products among their patients was in accordance with the literature. But just how much confidence did they have in this?

With the many problems entailed in establishing expenditures, it is easy to understand just how uncertain any estimate might be, but we do have some figures to give us a rough idea of the costs of alternative healthcare. Eisenberg et al. (1993) reported a study in which "expenditures associated with use of unconventional therapy in 1990 amounted to approximately $13.7 billion, three quarters of which ($10.3 billion) was paid out of pocket" (p. 246). They added, "this figure is comparable to the $12.8 billion spent out of pocket annually for all hospitalizations in the United States" (p. 246). In the United States in 1991, Wallis estimated that alternative healthcare was already a $27 billion per year industry (1991). In the United Kingdom, Pfeil (1994) reported that alternative therapy currently produces "a turnover of about £450 million per year" (p. 218). This equals approximately $688.5 million per year at the current exchange rate. It is evident that alternative healthcare, however it is defined, is big business.

PREVALENCE AND PATTERNS OF USE

Northcott and Bachynsky (1993) point out that 20 percent of Canadians used some form of alternative healthcare in the first six months of 1990 and half of these visited a chiropractor. Some populations use all healthcare, including alternative care, more than others. One group of high users is rheumatology patients. Boisset and Fitzcharles "observed a 66 percent prevalence of current use of alternative medicine in an unselected consecutive group of rheumatology patients attending a rheumatology clinic" (p. 150) in Canada. Of the 66 percent who used alternative methods "54 percent used over-the-counter products, 39 percent spiritual aids (including prayer, relaxation, meditation), and 13 percent each had visited alternative practitioners or used dietary intervention" (p. 148). In a study of those attending a rheumatology clinic in Australia, 40 percent had attended one or more alternative practitioners at some stage of their rheumatology illness (Vecchio, 1994, p. 145). This was a much lower rate than should have been expected when compared with the rate in the Canadian study because the Canadian study only asked about *current* use. When compared with the rest of the literature, lifetime use should have been in the 82 percent to 94 percent range (Boisset & Fitzcharles, 1994).

Another group of high users of healthcare is cancer patients. Montbriand and Laing (1991) found that, of the 75 hospitalized Canadian cancer patients they studied, 67 (89%) were using a physical, spiritual, or psychological alternative healthcare method—58 used a physical method, 23 used a spiritual method, and 18 used a psychological method. Eighteen of the 67 used two types of alternative methods. Seven used all three. Of those who chose a physical alternative method, the most popular methods were megavitamins or herbal products.

In 1990, in the United States, a national telephone sampling of adults found that, excluding exercise and prayer, 34 percent of the persons responding used "at least one unconventional therapy in the past year, and a third of these saw providers for unconventional therapy" (Eisenberg et al., 1993, p. 246). The investigators limited the therapies to be studied to exercise, prayer, and 16 other commonly used alternative methods. The largest percentages of users of unconventional therapies used were exercise (26%), prayer (25%), relaxation techniques (13%), chiropractic (10%), and massage (7%). Of those who saw a provider of alternative healthcare, most went to a provider of acupuncture (91%), with the next largest percentages going to providers who offered chiropractic (70%), hypnosis (52%), and massage (41%).

U.S. patterns of use can be compared to those found in England where data from two community surveys show prevalence rates of 27 percent to 29 percent for men and 33 percent for women and where an opinion survey showed rates of 34 percent for men and 46 percent for women. Results of the opinion survey showed that "Physical treatments, particularly of the manipulative type, were the most commonly used, followed by homeopathy and acupuncture" (Murray & Shepherd, 1993).

In the United States, how does the use of alternative health methods compare with the use of allopathic physicians? According to Eisenberg et al. (1993), among the U.S. population in 1990, 425 million visits were made to providers of alternative therapies and this "number exceeds the number of visits to all U.S. primary care physicians (388 million)" (p. 246).

As Boisset and Fitzcharles (1994) say, "It has been well established that many patients use both conventional and unconventional medicine concomitantly, and . . . numerous studies have reported a very low physician awareness of such use" (p. 151). In the United States, 72 percent of the users of alternative therapies have elected not to inform their physicians of this fact (Eisenberg et al., 1993). But just who are these "secret" users of alternative methods?

CHARACTERISTICS OF THE CONSUMERS

Alternative health methods are being used by people from all walks of life, but in the United States, the users are generally nonblack, middle to upper middle class, well-educated women, aged 25 to 49 years (Eisenberg et al., 1993; Engebretson & Wardell, 1993; Zagorsky, 1993).

The class status of users of alternative health methods in the United States differs from that of users in Canada. Without taking into account the use of chiropractors, Northcott and Bachynsky (1993) found that Canadian "Utilization patterns for alternative healthcare therapies . . .

suggest that females, younger adults, the not currently married, the better educated, renters, and persons who are less well-off financially are more likely to use alternative healthcare" (p. 434). Boisset and Fitzcharles (1994) disagree with Northcott and Bachynsky, stating, "Patients in the upper middle income group and French speaking patients used more bought products, but no other differences were observed . . . [in] . . . level of education, income or cultural background" (p. 148).

In England, women were more likely to have used alternative health methods. In Europe, studies show that women are more likely to use home-opathy and herbalism and men are more likely to use massage and osteopa-thy (Murray & Shepherd, 1993).

Directly comparing the patterns of use by persons with specific health-care problems is not easy because of differences in reporting of disease conditions.

- In Canada, "a high prevalence of use of unconventional methods has been noted in patients suffering from chronic disorders, including acquired immunodeficiency syndrome, cancer, chronic back pain, irritable bowel disease and arthritis" (Boisset & Fitzcharles, 1994, p. 148).
- In the United Kingdom, users of alternative methods have been noted to be persons suffering from "chronic pain, allergies, musculo-skeletal, psychosomatic, and functional conditions" (Murray & Shepherd, 1993, p. 983).
- In the United States, in 1990, the 10 medical conditions most fre-quently reported in persons who used alternative health methods were: back problems (36%), anxiety (28%), headache (27%), sprains or strains (22%), insomnia (20%), depression (20%), arthritis (18%), digestive problems (13%), high blood pressure (11%), and allergies (9%) (Eisenberg et al., 1993).

Why did all of these people turn to alternative healing methods? Why have alternative healing methods become so popular?

THE GROWTH OF ALTERNATIVE HEALING METHODS

Prior to the 19th century, Western medicine was not very successful in treating the major scourges befalling humankind. Cholera epidemics, yel-low fever epidemics, smallpox, and other plagues fell upon the population with regularity. Children died of "teething" as well as whooping cough, diphtheria, and the croup. With few exceptions, "regular medicine" had little to offer in the way of effective cures. Those who used the services of the physician or the barber could look forward to being purged or bled as likely as not. But sweeping changes were to come about that would improve the health of all in the United States and elevate the physician to the status we give to those who hold knowledge and skills that are beyond attainment by the masses.

The 19th century saw great movements in preventive medicine with sanitary commissions to clean up the water and sewerage systems in major cities, with increasing attention to standards for the production of milk and foods, and with the enactment of laws to protect the health of our citizens. There were movements in which the general public got involved in improving the health of the citizenry through exercise, diet, and temperate living. The average life expectancy crept steadily upward.

By the 20th century, the infection rate had dropped due to the availability of vaccines and the science of hygiene. Women no longer strapped themselves into corsets so tightly that fainting resulted before the stays were released at bedtime. The use of local and general anesthetics allowed humane dentistry and surgery and the practice of sterile technique greatly increased survival from these procedures. As the century progressed, the science of surgery advanced, as did the world of medicine. Sulfa drugs became available and then antibiotics. People began to survive that which had previously decimated entire populations.

By mid-century, truly effective antipsychotic drugs became available for the first time. So few people went off to T.B. sanitoria that these hospitals began to close down. Polio was conquered and the iron lung became a relic of the past. Group therapies began to be used to help the mentally ill in larger numbers than ever before possible and mental hospitals began to close their now-empty units. Technology seemed to be there to solve any health problem. And if there wasn't an answer to your health problem today, why, there'd be one tomorrow. There was always hope.

In the 1960s and 1970s, we believed that whatever was wrong science could fix it. And now, some 25 years later, a good percentage of our population seeks medical care from alternative sources. Alternative healing methods have gained increasing popularity over the past 25 years, not only in the United States, but elsewhere in the industrialized world.

What turned so many of us away from the mainstream of medicine and toward alternative healing methods? There is no one answer. Pfeil (1994) says emphasis on science during the 1950s and 1960s "resulted in a decline in the caring aspects of medicine. This made technology appear cold and inhuman and turned medicine into a purely physical, restorative profession. . . . Hence the desire to explore alternative approaches to healthcare arose" (p. 217). But surely all of medicine did not suddenly become so cold and uncaring that this alone accounted for the trend.

Wallis (1991) says that "The growth of alternative medicine . . . reflects a gnawing dissatisfaction with conventional . . . medicine" (p. 68). Murray and Shepherd (1993) believe that "Negative attitudes toward modern medicine arose from perceptions of excessive technological intervention and iatrogenic disorders arising from long term drug treatment" (p. 983). They found that, among the users of alternative health methods they studied, "many orthodox treatments were believed to entail greater risk of harm since they required either surgery or potentially toxic drug treatment" (p. 986).

As Wallis (1991) said in a Time magazine article:

Conventional medicine has always put its emphasis on crisis intervention, and that is where it is most successful. It is what you want when they haul you in from a car wreck, or your Achilles tendon has snapped on the tennis court, or you've got a tumor in your lung. Standard medicine is about doing battle with a disease, bringing up the big guns of surgery and drugs to search out and destroy the miniature monsters that make people sick: bacteria, viruses, cancer cells, auto-antibodies and other biological evils. If your baby daughter has a 105 degree fever, she needs big-gun medical attention, not brown rice and meditation. (p. 69)

But if your baby daughter is just fussy and suffers from teething, you don't want the "big guns." One of the perceptions of Western medicine, today, is that there seems to be little that allopathic physicians can offer for the chronic problems and for day-to-day health maintenance that is as successful as the potent medicine used in many acute cases. Many people turn to alternative healing methods, instead. Montbriand noted that his respondents chose alternative healing methods for four reasons:

- Influence of a social group endorsing an alternate practice.
- Anger directed at the medical system for bungling or delaying diagnosis.
- Fear of the disease, the treatment, or possible death.
- Desire for control.

Along with these forces, the last three of which could tend to drive one away from allopaths, there must also be some forces driving one toward alternative methods; forces greater than mere social endorsement. Murray and Shepherd (1993) say that some commentators believe that the alternative healthcare movement "signifies a fundamental change in values, a reaction against a materialistic age, a desire to return to a more 'natural' lifestyle, and a belief that a state of total health is achievable through personal preventive actions" (p. 983).

If alternative healing methods cannot raise our hopes for a cure, they still can raise our hopes of feeling better, somehow, and if alternative practitioners listen to us and make us feel we are in control, they are meeting a need that will keep us coming back. In fact, these sentiments are echoed in one study of patients with multiple sclerosis who sought help from an alternative health practitioner (AHP). Their responses to the question, "What have been the high points in your experiences with AHPs?" were: improvement in well-being (38%), supportive relationship (19%), the availability of alternative treatment options (19%), and holistic philosophy of the AHP (12%) (Fawcett, Sidney, Hanson, & Riley-Lawless, 1994).

But we have not given up on allopathic practitioners. As Murray and Shepherd (1993) say of their study of persons who use alternative healing methods, "None of the respondents had rejected orthodox medicine, indeed most were frequent attenders. Alternative treatments were used for minor ailments and first aid purposes and as prophylaxis for recurrent problems . . ." (p. 986), and "unfamiliar or 'serious' acute conditions (involving severe pain or fever) were always brought for medical attention before any decisions were taken on the use of alternative treatments" (p. 986). This is a common finding. Indeed, in the study by Eisenberg et al. (1993), 83 percent of the 1539 respondents reported one or more "principal medical conditions" for which 58 percent saw a medical doctor but not an alternative care provider, 7 percent saw a medical doctor and an alternative care provider, and 3 percent saw an alternative care provider but not a medical doctor. A whopping 33 percent saw neither.

THE ROLE OF THE NURSE

The area of alternative healing methods is one that begs to be explored. The experience gained by the professional nurse during years of holding a position between orthodox medicine and clients who make use of alternative healing methods is experience that can be used to great advantage in the process of exploration. This experience, added to the research skills of nurse investigators, makes nurses remarkably suited to study this area.

But research is not all that is necessary. Nursing students need to be educated to the growing use of alternative healing methods, to the trends behind this growth, and to related nursing obligations. In the United States, where 34 percent of the population has used alternative healing methods, we devote precious little of our total nursing curriculum to this material. And, where 72 percent of the people who use alternative healing methods do not tell their physician about it, it behooves the nurse to become expert at ferreting out this information and adjusting the nursing care plan based upon it.

In service to the community, nurses can be expert resources concerning alternative healing methods. It is up to us to publish helpful information and to otherwise become teachers for the communities which we serve.

REFERENCES

Achterberg, J. (1991). *Woman as healer.* Boston: Shambhala.

Benoist, J., & Cathebras, P. (1993). The body: From an immateriality to another. *Social Science and Medicine, 36*(7), 857–865.

Boisset, M., & Fitzcharles, M-A. (1994). Alternative medicine use by rheumatology patients in a universal health care setting. *The Journal of Rheumatology, 21*(1), 148–152.

Eisenberg, D. M., Kessler, R. C., Foster, C., Norlock, F. E., Caulkins, D. R., & Delbanco, T. L. (1993). Unconventional medicine in the United States. *The New England Journal of Medicine, 328*(4), 246–252.

Engebretson, J., & Wardell, D. (1993). A contemporary view of alternative healing modalities. *Nurse Practitioner, 19*(9), 51–55.

Fawcett, J., Sidney, J. S., Hanson, M. J. S., & Riley-Lawless, K. L. (1994). Use of alternative health therapies by people with multiple sclerosis: An exploratory study. *Holistic Nursing Practice, 8*(2), 36–42.

Franken, A. (1992). *I'm good enough, I'm smart enough, and doggone it, people like me!: Daily affirmations by Stuart Smalley.* New York: Dell.

Frost, J. (1994). Complementary treatments for eczema in children. *Professional Nurse, 9*(5), 330–332.

McClenon, J. (1993). The experimental foundations of shamanic healing. *Journal of Medicine and Philosophy, 18*(2), 107–127.

Montbriand, M. J. (1993). Freedom of choice: An issue concerning alternate therapies chosen by patients with cancer. *Oncology Nursing Forum, 20*(8), 1195–1201.

Montbriand, M. J., & Laing, G. P. (1991). Alternative health care as a control strategy. *Journal of Advanced Nursing, 16*(3), 325–332.

Mowrey, D. B. (1986). *The scientific validation of herbal medicine.* New Canaan, CN: Keats Publishing, Inc.

Murray, J., & Shepherd, S. (1993). Alternative or additional medicine? An exploratory study in general practice. *Social Science and Medicine, 37*(8), 983–988.

Navarro, V. (1993). Health services research: What is it? *International Journal of Health Services, 23*(1), 1–13.

Northcott, H. C., & Bachynsky, J. A. (1993). Research note: Concurrent utilization of chiropractic, prescription medicines, nonprescription medicines and alternative health care. *Social Science and Medicine, 37*(3), 431–435.

O'Neill, A. (1994). Danger and safety in medicines. *Social Science and Medicine, 38*(4), 497–507.

Osujih, M. (1993). Exploration of the frontiers of tradomedical practices: Basis for development of alternative medical healthcare services in developing countries. *Journal of the Royal Society of Health, 113*(4), 190–194.

Panush, R. S. (1993). Reflections on unproven remedies. *Rheumatic Disease Clinics of North America, 19*(1), 201–206.

Patterson, D. R. (1992). Practical applications of psychological techniques in controlling burn pain. *Journal of Burn Care & Rehabilitation, 13*(1), 13–18.

Pfeil, M. (1994). Role of nurses in promoting complementary therapies. *British Journal of Nursing, 3*(5), 217–219.

Phillips, M., & Frederick, C. (1992). The use of hypnotic age progressions as prognostic, ego-strengthening, and integrating techniques. *American Journal of Clinical Hypnosis, 35*(2), 99–108.

Questionable methods of cancer management: Hydrogen peroxide and other "hyperoxygenation" therapies. (1993). *CA-A Cancer Journal for Clinicians, 43*(1), 47–56.

Questionable methods of cancer management: 'Nutritional' Therapies. (1993). *CA-A Cancer Journal for Clinicians, 43*(5), 309–319.

Vecchio, P. C. (1994). Attitudes to alternative medicine by rheumatology outpatient attenders. *The Journal of Rheumatology, 21*(1), 145–147.

Wallis, C. (1991, November). Why new age medicine is catching on. *Time,* pp. 68–73.

Warpeha, A., & Harris, J. (1993). Combining traditional and nontraditional approaches to nutrition counseling. *Journal of the American Dietetic Association, 93*(7), 797–800.

Weiner, M. A., & Weiner, J. A. (1994). *Herbs that heal: Prescription for herbal healing.* Mill Valley, CA: Quantum Books.

White, K. L. (1993). Comments on Navarro's review of Health Services Research: An Anthology. *International Journal of Health Services, 23*(3), 603–605.

Zagorsky, E. S. (1993). Caring for families who follow alternative health care practices. *Pediatric Nursing, 19*(1) 71–75.

CHAPTER 17

The Nurse Practitioner: A Healing Role for the Nurse

LINDA R. ROUNDS, RN, FNP, PHD

As a new graduate RN, I worked on a busy surgical unit. I was the evening charge nurse and the only RN on the unit. The two other nurses were LPNs. I remember passing meds and checking IVs, always trying to find the time to be with patients. It was hard to do except through casual conversation or a touch of the hand as I made rounds or rehung IVs. On the rare occasions when I wasn't the charge nurse or when I found a little extra time at the end of the shift, I took the opportunity to give backrubs to patients. I still remember two women—one had had general surgery, a gall bladder removed, and the other a hysterectomy. The first just couldn't get comfortable or sleep, despite pain medication. I spent 10 minutes giving her a backrub and talking. At the end of that time, she relaxed and fell asleep. The other woman was in a great deal of pain and also had urinary retention. Again, the physical touch and presence of a concerned person helped her relax enough to sleep.

These are not accounts of how wonderful I was; they are recollections of how therapeutic and healing nursing is when one has the opportunity to practice all aspects of nursing. These were the moments I sought, but was often denied in the hospital setting. It was busy, understaffed, and seldom valued nursing beyond the tasks that could be performed and documented. Nurses kept patients medicated, hydrated, safe, free of infection, or clean. All valuable and necessary, yet they don't encompass the totality or the potential of nursing.

Seldom are nurses given the autonomy to decide what is most important or most needed by patients. Rather, nurses follow orders. Nursing has failed to gain the autonomy of practice experienced by other professions. Nor have nurses always been willing to accept autonomy and the concomitant accountability that characterizes more male-dominated groups, such as medicine.

EARLY HEALERS, THE ROOTS OF NURSING

The roots of nursing are powerfully intertwined with the culture and experience of the women healers of European history. Authors (Achterberg, 1991; Ehrenreich & English, 1973, 1978) have recounted for us the experience of these women. With the exception of ancient cultures which worshipped the Earth Mother or Earth Goddess, women have seldom been permitted to be fully autonomous healers. The degree to which society has been willing to permit women to function as healers has varied through the ages. Evidence exists from Stone Age artifacts that women were revered as both healers and priestesses. During the European Middle Ages, women healers were often the only source of healthcare for women and the poor.

However, with the evolution of medicine as a profession and the early development of science, women healers were systematically banned from practice. Men dominated the practice of medicine. Women were not entirely discounted as healers, but since they were not allowed to seek education or licensure in medicine, which was reserved for upper-class men, they were not accepted as legitimate healers. Women healers and midwives of the Middle Ages ministered to the poor who had no doctors or hospitals.

The climax of the fear and subjugation of women as healers took the form of the witch trials which spanned the 14th to the 17th centuries in Europe. The witches were accused of three crimes: possessing female sexuality, being organized, and helping or healing (Ehrenreich & English, 1973). The wise woman, as the witch was called by her patients, was accused of practicing magic, not medicine, though her prescriptions were often the same or more effective than those of the trained physicians. The witch relied on trial and error, intuition, cause and effect, and her senses rather than dogma and doctrine. Estimates of the number of witches who were burned or hung range from 30,000 to millions. Eighty-five percent of those who were killed were women.

Women healers never recovered completely from the devastation of the witch hunts and trials. The witch trials placed the male physician on the side of God and Law, "while it placed [the female healer] on the side of darkness, evil, and magic" (Ehrenreich & English, 1978, p. 35). As early as the 13th century, medicine first entered the universities in Europe. With little exception, women were not permitted study at the university and thus were easily banned from the professional practice of medicine.

During the development of scientific thought and the expansion of European civilization, the position of women continued to unfold. It was viewed as necessary to dominate nature if civilization were to advance. Woman was seen as the embodiment of nature and thus also had to be dominated. "The emerging scientists conscripted what they believed to be feminine wisdom, and developed a methodology that lauded the masculine attributes of reason and objectivity" (Achterberg, 1991, p. 111). Women's roles in healing and society were redefined, emphasizing domestic duties. Objections to women as healers shifted from a religious argument to the lack of mental capacities and other similar deficiencies. The only legal healers remaining were the midwives. They, too, were later attacked by the medical profession and nearly eliminated in the first half of 20th-century America. This struggle continues to this day.

CONTEMPORARY NURSING

Contemporary nursing in the United States and Europe developed as an essentially female profession. With this came the notion of woman's work and so-called inferior feminine characteristics. Women were not suited to higher education, according to some male "experts," because of their inferior intellect, emotional instability, and physical weakness, especially associated with menstruation. Further, "woman's greatest charms—her modesty and delicacy—[had to] be protected at all costs" (Achterberg, 1991, p. 149). Thus, women were discouraged from entering medicine to protect them from the horrors of dissection and surgery and the mysteries of the human body. However, physicians encouraged women to become nurses. Nurses were trained, not educated, and could "leave the home, work at backbreaking tasks, and be exposed to the 'indecencies' of hospital life" (Achterberg, 1991, p. 149).

Early in the development of formal nursing, the medical profession acknowledged the contribution of well-trained nurses to the promotion of health and well-being for patients in both public and private settings. Medicine also supported the idea that a primary attribute for becoming a nurse was female gender (Showalter as cited in Dickson, 1993). Not content with the supervision of nurses by other women, the medical profession also took responsibility for the education of nurses, and the AMA suggested that the instruction of nurses fall under the supervision of county medical societies throughout the United States (Dickson, 1993).

There was little financial support for establishing nursing schools in traditional institutions of learning. Hospitals quickly discovered the advantage of free labor from student nurses, also noting the decreased mortality rates when students were used (Achterberg, 1991). Originally, schools of nursing based on the Nightingale model had been established as autonomous programs. However, when any financial difficulties ensued, this was used as an excuse for hospitals, run primarily by physicians, to take control of the school and the education of nurses (Torres, 1981).

As nursing developed in the United States, the goal of professional recognition emerged. The model emulated was that of medicine, a profession dominated by white males. With the notion of professionalism came the ideal of scientific study as the basis for professional development. Other essentials included service and higher education. In the rush to be professional and scientific, which meant also accepting medicine as the dominant culture, nurses and women relinquished the practice of healing. Physicians assumed the role of professional healers and human experiences become medical problems demanding a scientific solution (Dickson, 1993).

The modern nurse often views her position as liberated from the power of physicians: no longer needing to stand and relinquish a seat when a physician enters the room; understanding and controlling the technologies needed to care for patients; writing nursing diagnoses and nursing orders, and initiating nursing interventions; or seeking education in a university. Nursing leaders exhort nurses to assert professional control over education and practice and to determine the profession's destiny. Roberts (1983) and Torres (1981) described the evolution of nurses and the profession of nursing today as the evolution of an oppressed group.

OPPRESSION MODEL

Freire (1990) outlined a theoretical construct that describes the situation of oppressed groups. Oppressors take many forms, but generally identify the norms and values of a society or group and assert these values as the "right" ones. Oppressors also have the power to enforce the values of a society or group. The "behavior of the oppressed is a prescribed behavior, following as it does the guidelines of the oppressor" (p. 31). Freedom from oppression is often feared by the oppressed as it would require them to rid themselves of the image of the oppressor and replace it with autonomy and responsibility.

Characteristics of Oppressed Groups

Some of the characteristics of an oppressed group include the belief that the views of the more powerful oppressor represent reality, attempts to look and act like the oppressor in order to gain more power and control, self-hatred and poor self-esteem, a preference for conformity, fatalistic attitudes expressed often as docility, and emotional dependence. Often oppressed groups practice horizontal violence, striking out at their own comrades or colleagues.

The perceived inability to revolt against the oppressor and the view that the oppressor exists within some colleagues, results in a form of intragroup violence practiced by the oppressed. Some oppressed individuals who are eager to be powerful attempt to become like the oppressor and to assimilate that culture. Individuals who are successful at assimilation are termed marginal as they are not members of the dominant group and are on the fringes of their own group (Lewin as cited in Roberts, 1983). This often results in self-hatred and low self-esteem. Nursing exhibits many of these characteristics.

As Torres (1981) describes, the oppressor perceives that it is in the best interest of all that the power and privileges of the dominant group be maintained. In order to do this, devices are constructed that sustain the status quo. "These devices include limiting the quality and extent of education . . . , keeping the oppressed group divided among themselves, and granting periodic acts of false generosity . . . [such as] token rewards for continued loyalty [or] elevating a member of the oppressed group to a high status position" (p. 4).

Liberation from Oppression

Liberation from oppression is not by chance. According to Freire (1990), it must be sought, but only after the causes of the oppression can be identified. The liberation and its associated freedom will threaten not only the oppressor, but also oppressed colleagues who are fearful of even greater repression. Oppressed individuals and groups must view "oppression not as a closed world from which there is no exit, but as a limiting situation which they can transform" (p. 34).

The oppressed group is not only confronted with their own fears as a barrier to liberation, but also must face their perceptions which create a barrier as well. The oppressed have internalized an image of the oppressor as powerful and right and accepted the oppressor's interpretation of reality. They "have no consciousness of themselves as persons or members of an oppressed class" (Freire, 1990, p. 30). In an attempt to gain the power and advantages of the oppressor, a member of the oppressed group often rises to a position above colleagues and becomes like the oppressor. However, the oppression has not changed, and the individual who has gained power actually becomes tougher and more difficult than the oppressor. A reluctance to take risks also impedes the oppressed in any attempt at liberation. To overcome these barriers, the oppressed must first recognize their position and its oppression and then reject the myths and beliefs that have formed the core of the oppression. "Freedom therefore involves rejecting the negative images of one's own culture and replacing them with pride and a sense of ability to function autonomously" (Roberts, 1983, p. 25).

Nurses as an Oppressed Group

Roberts (1983) eloquently describes the oppression of modern nursing. Despite an ancient history of healing by women and nursing which took place in the home and community, the nursing profession today has failed to attain professional freedom. As early as the Middle Ages, women healers were dominated by the male culture of medicine as they were banned from practice and burned at the stake. The systematic oppression of modern nursing in the United States began in schools of nursing and hospitals. Nurses lack autonomy. Despite the attempts to develop and emphasize the nursing aspects of patient care, nurses in general must still rely on physicians to decide on and order essential elements of patient care. It is extremely difficult to offer holistic healthcare when the determination of what is acceptable comes from several sources.

Nursing and the public at large have accepted medicine's view of healthcare as reality. Few dispute the belief that medicine is the primary form of healthcare from which all others emanate. How many times has a capable nurse been asked why she didn't become a physician or have doctorally prepared nurses been asked why didn't they get an M.D.? How many nurses struggle to define nursing? How many lay people can answer the question "What is a nurse?" In academia, the bodily systems model of medicine is commonly accepted as a means for discussing not only medical care, but nursing care as well. Nursing has begun to identify its own culture through the development of nursing theory and laying claim to aspects of healthcare that are nursing. "As nurses are discovering their cultural identity, the disparity with that of physicians becomes more clear"

(Roberts, 1983, p. 26). However, in an attempt to achieve power and status, nursing adopted the image of the professional established by male-dominated scientific professions. Dickson (1993) describes how faculty found themselves teaching the values of caring, healing, and nurturing against the backdrop of science which reduced human responses to quantifiable variables. The dominant scientific model of research was accepted by most nurse researchers. Such situations actually left the nurse in the position of being marginal in efforts to be transformed into the dominant culture.

The acceptance of science as defined by the dominant male culture has left nursing in a rather closed system (Chinn, 1989) which limits the knowledge generated, disseminated, and taught (Dickson, 1993). Consequences include the lack of recognition given to qualitative research, a traditional science-based system of promotion and tenure, and little respect for nontraditional or complementary healing methods.

Nurses traditionally have accepted their position as being secondary to that of the physician, only recently trying to rid themselves of the image of the submissive hand maiden. Much of the media still portrays nurses in this image. Nurses still must work very hard to be heard in public forums and political arenas and few nurses or others acknowledge nurses as the colleagues of physicians. Such secondary status has led to a long-standing history of poor self-esteem by nurses as a professional group.

Oppressed groups show a preference for conformity. Nurses share this characteristic. There is seldom a willingness to break with tradition. Often this is prompted by fear of the consequences. How will administration react? What will the physician say? Nurses as a whole do not stand out as nonconformists or risk-takers.

Fatalistic attitudes, which in the oppression model lead to docility, are not uncommon among nurses. The acceptance of a lack of power within the healthcare system and the unwillingness to join professional organizations reflect a fatalistic approach. This results in docility as a profession and as a political force. Often this is assumed to be a feminine trait and so it is accepted as ingrained in the profession because of its primarily female composition. However, Freire (1990) describes this as an historical and sociological result of oppression rather than a natural characteristic of a group. Such fatalistic attitudes persist until the oppressor is recognized and the consciousness of the oppressed can be discovered.

According to Freire (1990), emotional dependence results when the oppressed are "under" the oppressor and dependent on him. The oppressor is in the position of having something, usually at the expense of the oppressed. The tradition of nursing is clearly "under" medicine. Seldom in modern nursing have groups escaped from the control of medicine and independently practiced nursing. With the exception of groups such as the nurse midwives, public health nurses of the early 20th century, and more recently enterprising nurse practitioners, nursing has been dependent on medicine for much of its practice. Medicine flourished as the preeminent provider of healthcare, but could not have done so without nursing to provide the daily care and treatment of patients.

One of the most frustrating and most frequently discussed characteristics of nursing is the continual internal struggle to agree and unify. Often striking out at each other, nurses have criticized each other for having attained higher education, independent forms of practice, and positions of authority. Nurses have failed to agree and continue to argue about entry into practice, necessary education for advanced practice, and representation by professional organizations. All of this is consistent with horizontal violence, the struggle against each other rather than the more risky revolt against the oppressor.

There have been exceptions to the above by individuals and subgroups in nursing. However, nurses generally have poor self-esteem as a professional group, often accept the roles and the duties given to them without question, conform to rules and standards created by others, and frequently strike out vehemently against their fellow nurses. This model may be difficult for many nurses to acknowledge and accept as the characteristics have become a part of the nursing culture. As Cleland (1971) notes "dominance is most complete when it is not even recognized" (p. 1543).

THE NURSE PRACTITIONER MOVEMENT

The nurse practitioner movement began in 1965 in an attempt to expand the scope of nursing practice (Ford, 1979). Nurse practitioners were quickly criticized for joining the enemy, abandoning nursing, and becoming junior doctors. Nurse practitioner programs initially were not accepted in graduate nursing programs as the content was believed to be medicine and not associated with nursing. Nursing faculty successfully resisted the placement of nurse practitioner programs at the master's level for many years. The resistance resulted in a proliferation of certificate programs or, if and when accepted into graduate nursing programs, little support for the faculty or the curriculum. Even after thirty years, some of these same criticisms persist.

Nurse Practitioner Education

The educational preparation for a nurse practitioner does include elements of practice that are within the legal description of medicine. Like
earlier expansions in nursing practice, this an example of an evolving and
dynamic scope of practice. For instance early in the 20th century, nurses
were not permitted to take blood pressures. Thirty years ago, nurses did
not perform comprehensive physical examinations. Today both of these
are considered standard nursing practice. Nursing's scope of practice is
actually the broadest form of healthcare with medicine providing only a
portion of the care which patients need (Diers & Molde, 1983). Nurse
practitioners, equipped to provide both nursing and medicine, offer a
unique blend and broader scope of healthcare. Physicians can offer only
medicine.

Nurse Practitioner Practice

The practice of nurse practitioners ranges from close relationships with
physicians in clinics and private practices, to schools and nursing homes
to independent practice by nurse practitioners. The central theme of this
practice is health. Health is achieved through health promotion, health
teaching, management of illness, counseling, and referrals. *Nursing's Social Policy Statement* (1995, p. 6) defines nursing in part as the "diagnosis and treatment of human responses to actual or potential health
problems." It is further elaborated to include "attention to the full range
of human experiences and responses . . .; integration of objective data
with . . . subjective experience; application of scientific knowledge to . . .
diagnosis and treatment; and, provision of a caring relationship that facilitates health and healing" (American Nurses Association, 1995). Within
the document, advanced nursing practice is described as "specialization,
expansion, and advancement in practice" (p. 14). Expansion in particular
refers to the acquisition of new knowledge and skills that legitimize role
autonomy. This may include areas of practice that traditionally overlap
the boundaries of medical practice.

Both the definition of nursing and the description of advanced practice
are congruent with the practice of nurse practitioners. Nurse practitioners routinely diagnose and treat actual or potential health problems. These
problems range from the actual responses of fever, cough, depression, or
acute abdominal pain to the potential responses associated with the risks
of smoking, inadequate nutrition, or the prevention of communicable

diseases through immunization. Routinely, nurse practitioners integrate subjective and objective data as well as diagnose and treat health problems. Nurse practitioner practice has, since its inception, pushed the boundaries of traditional nursing practice, in some cases regaining the lost practices of the ancient healers or the original public health nurses.

Nurse practitioners have always had a relationship with medicine. The first program was developed jointly by a nurse, Dr. Loretta Ford, and a physician, Dr. Henry Silver. In individual practice, collaboration has always existed. However, at the level of professional organizations, medicine has not supported the development of the nurse practitioner role as independent of medicine nor encouraged significant collaboration between the two disciplines (DeAngelis, 1994; Fagin, 1992). At the level of individual practitioners, however, the roles have been seen as complementary and supportive. Organized medicine has more commonly seen the role of the nurse practitioner as a threat, both economically and culturally.

Much like the female physicians of 19th-century America (Achterberg, 1991), medicine has accepted the nurse practitioner in special circumstances where need is great and physicians are lacking, such as practice with rural and urban underserved populations. However, when nurse practitioners have sought prescriptive authority and third-party reimbursement to establish independent practice and challenged the cultural boundaries of medicine, the negative response has been swift and decisive. Nurse practitioners have quickly been attacked for practicing medicine without a license.

OPPRESSION MODEL APPLIED TO NURSE PRACTITIONERS

Looking at the nurse practitioner within the framework of the oppression model, nurse practitioners have gained a degree of autonomy that is only matched by the nurse midwives and the nurse anesthetists. In some states, nurse practitioners are free to practice independently and are accountable for their practice only to themselves and the board of nursing. Some nurses would say that the nurse practitioner has sold out to the oppressor, medicine. Rather than maintaining the purity of nursing, nurse practitioners have been accused of assimilating and practicing medicine thus becoming mini doctors or physician extenders. Such behavior would be considered cultural assimilation, leaving the nurse practitioner a marginal role, neither a nurse nor a physician.

Certainly, there are nurse practitioners who have aligned themselves with medicine and lost their identity as nurses. These individuals often have become critical of nursing, failing to see the nursing aspects of the nurse practitioner role. This does not reflect the nature of nurse practitioners or nurse practitioner practice in general. For some, the close identification with medicine may have evolved from a poorly defined concept of nursing or from a failure to make the role transition from nurse to nurse practitioner. Regardless, it is critical that nursing and nurse practitioners understand the essential practice of nurse practitioners rather than dwell on the exceptions.

Characteristics of Nurse Practitioner Education and Practice

The original intent of the nurse practitioner role was to expand the scope of nursing practice. In so doing, aspects of medical care were included in the practice of nursing so that nurse practitioners could provide holistic, comprehensive care with a focus on health. To do this, nurse practitioners went to the only credible source for learning those aspects of medical care, the physician. Physicians taught much of the medical content in early programs and are still involved, but to a much lesser degree. However, the control of the curriculum and the interpretation of the role of medicine within the nurse practitioner's scope of practice is under the direction of nursing faculty. Nurse practitioner education has evolved to a point where the standards of the curriculum are based on a nursing model of education and practice (Boodley et al., 1995). It is not that nurse practitioners have tried to look and act like the oppressor for the sake of power and control. Rather, nurse practitioners recognized and understood the culture of nursing and expanded the culture to incorporate aspects of healthcare previously considered medicine.

Liberation of Nurse Practitioners

In contrast to joining the oppressor, nurse practitioners as a professional group have enjoyed liberation from oppression. It was not a chance occurrence. The purpose of the role and the education were well planned by Ford and Silver in the 1960s. The development of this new role was deliberate and intent on expanding the boundaries of nursing.

As outlined in the oppression model, liberation is threatening to both the oppressor and oppressed colleagues. The nurse practitioner as a form of liberation was threatening to both nursing and medicine, and remains so, particularly to organized medicine. Both the program and its founders were criticized by faculty, deans, and organized nursing (Fondiller, 1995). This resulted in a delay in the placement of nurse practitioner programs at the master's level as well as a reluctance to acknowledge nurse practitioners as genuine members of the nursing profession. Until the very recent shift in healthcare to a primary care focus, some nurse colleagues have continued to deny the equality of nurse practitioners in education and practice.

Nurse practitioners were also able to identify some of the causes of oppression in nursing. Nurse practitioners understood that nursing was not inferior and had a significant contribution to make to the health and well-being of individuals and families. Nurse practitioners are and always have been risk takers (Ford, 1979; Lewis & Brykczynski, 1994), a characteristic necessary to challenge oppression.

The ability and willingness tò incorporate medicine into the nursing role and provide holistic care allowed nurses to make a significant contribution to healthcare. This resulted in a positive self-image and a healthy self-esteem. Loretta Ford recalled a comment regarding the first nurse practitioners, by Esther Lucille Brown, who said, "This is nursing at its finest" (Fondiller, 1995, p. 10). Dorothy DeMaio (1979) in a review of the expanded role of the nurse practitioner stated, "Their practice, with emphasis on casefinding and health teaching, counseling, and maintenance, has always seemed to me to be *nursing* practice, in the truest sense of the definition" (p. 272).

Koerner and Bunkers (1994) suggest that a healing consciousness requires cooperation and unity. Nurse practitioners have demonstrated cooperation and unity on many occasions. The nurse practitioner movement has instilled its members with pride and a sense of unity. Though intragroup disagreement still exists among nurse practitioner organizations, it is much more common to move forward for the sake of the whole rather than sacrifice a goal completely. The horizontal violence which has characterized nursing is much less evident among nurse practitioners.

Some nurse practitioners have joined the oppressor, embracing medicine and discounting nursing and nursing colleagues. Their marginal position leaves them in professional limbo, not really fitting in with any professional group. This is a rather precarious position, and one that is neither free nor liberated.

The struggle for liberation continues as nurse practitioners seek fully autonomous practice. The efforts to gain prescriptive authority, hospital privileges, and third-party reimbursement for all nurse practitioners continue. Repeated attacks by organized medicine demand cohesive organizations and unity and cooperation among the specialties of advanced practice. To fully escape the oppression that nursing has experienced, nurse practitioners must demonstrate what Mason, Backer, and Georges (1991) describe as power-sharing in addition to practicing mutual respect and equality with peers. This leads to shared influence and empowerment. The ability of nurse practitioners to overcome oppression and seek autonomy and equality is healing. For more traditional nursing, it is a lesson in the possibilities.

On the level of the individual, there is also liberation and a healing which occurs with the experience of becoming a nurse practitioner. Often this is a difficult transition. Freire (1990) describes liberation as a painful childbirth. For nurses becoming nurse practitioners, this is an apt description.

The role transition and role crisis which occurs among nurse practitioner students and graduates (Anderson, Leonard, & Yates, 1974) is upsetting and unsettling. It calls into question the individual's values as a nurse. Students are forced to confront their definition of nursing as their scope of practice expands. Some cannot accept that medical aspects of care have become the practice of nursing. Others abandon the essentials of nursing practice. However, the majority grapple with the conflicts and overcome the inner confusion and the oppression. The rewards are autonomy, a heightened self-image, and the freedom to decide what is appropriate and necessary for patients.

CONCLUSIONS

Nurse practitioners are not totally liberated from the oppression of medicine, but the experience of becoming a nurse practitioner is a significant step toward such freedom. The knowledge that freedom is possible and that one is a legitimate member of the struggle for liberation is a healing journey.

For me personally, and I believe for other nurse practitioners, the freedom to determine appropriate care—whether it is as fundamental as a backrub or as complex as managing a diabetic drug regimen—is a liberating and healing experience. The frustration I felt as a new graduate RN was replaced by pride and a sense of control over my practice when I became a nurse practitioner.

Achterberg (1991) reasons that healing involves "some independent effort to help others become 'whole'" (p. 173). In the case of the nurse practitioner, the transformation from nurse to nurse practitioner fostered by faculty, clinical preceptors, and professional colleagues helps the individual nurse to become whole. It is both a liberating and healing experience.

REFERENCES

Achterberg, J. (1991). *Woman as healer.* Boston: Shambala.

American Nurses Association. (1995). *Nursing's social policy statement.* Washington: Author.

Anderson, E., Leonard, B., & Yates, J. (1974). Epigenesis of the nurse practitioner role. *American Journal of Nursing, 74,* 1812–1816.

Boodley, C., Harper, D., Hanson, C., Jackson, P., Russel, D., Taylor, D., & Zimmer, P. (1995). *Advanced nursing practice: Curriculum guidelines and program standards for nurse practitioner education.* Washington: National Organization of Nurse Practitioner Faculties.

Chinn, P. (1989). The editors respond. *Image, 21,* 249.

Cleland, V. (1971). Sex discrimination: Nursing's most pervasive problem. *American Journal of Nursing, 71,* 1542–1547.

DeAngelis, C. (1994). Nurse practitioner redux. *Journal of the American Medical Association, 271,* 868–871.

DeMaio, D. (1979). The born-again nurse. *American Journal of Nursing, 79,* 272–273.

Dickson, G. (1993). The unintended consequences of a male professional ideology for the development of nursing education. *Advances in Nursing Science, 15*(3), 67–83.

Diers, D., & Molde, S. (1983). Nurses in primary care: The new gatekeepers? *American Journal of Nursing, 83,* 742–745.

Ehrenreich, B., & English, D. (1973). *Witches, midwives and nurses: A history of women healers.* Old Westbury, NY: The Feminist Press.

Ehrenreich, B., & English, D. (1978). *For her own good: 150 years of the experts' advice to women.* Garden City, NY: Anchor Press/Doubleday.

Fagin, C. (1992). Collaboration between nurses & physicians: No longer a choice. *Nursing & Health Care, 13,* 354–363.

Fondiller, S. (1995). Loretta C. Ford: A modern olympian. *Nursing & Health Care: Perspectives on community, 16,* 6–11.

Ford, L. (1979). A nurse for all settings: The nurse practitioner. *Nursing Outlook, 27,* 516–521.

Freire, P. (1990). *Pedagogy of the oppressed.* New York: Continuum.

Koerner, J., & Bunkers, S. (1994). The healing web: An expansion of consciousness. *Journal of Holistic Nursing, 12*(1), 51–63.

Lewis, P., & Brykczynski, K. (1994). Practical knowledge and competencies of the healing role of the nurse practitioner. *Journal of the American Academy of Nurse Practitioners, 6,* 207–213.

Mason, D., Backer, B., & Georges, C. A. (1991). Toward a feminist model of the political empowerment of nurses. *Image, 23,* 72–77.

Roberts, S. J. (1983). Oppressed group behavior: Implications for nursing. *Advances in Nursing Science, 5*(4), 21–30.

Torres, G. (1981). The nursing education administrator: Accountable, vulnerable, and oppressed. *Advances in Nursing Science, 3*(3), 1–16.

CHAPTER 18

Transformative Power: Healing the Wounds of Cultural Oppression

M. CHRISTINA R. ESPERAT, RN, PHD

PATRICIA DAVIS GILMORE, RN, MSN, JD

GERALDINE DORSEY-TURNER, RN, MS, PNA, CS

American society has come a long way since the turmoil of the fifties and sixties, when the civil rights movement reached a pitch and gave way to changes aimed at redressing the ills of racial discrimination that had plagued this nation for more than a century. Since then, political and legal actions have done much to rectify the impact of racism and improve the plight of minorities. Nonetheless, while many gross inequalities have been addressed, the limits of political and legal actions are obvious, especially in regard to the more subtle forms of cultural oppression that continue to plague people who are seen as different by the socially dominant culture.

In this chapter, we will explore the idea of cultural oppression as a ubiquitous element of American society, where subtle and less than apparent effects continue to inflict upon its victims wounds more insidious and debilitating than blatant discrimination. We have elected to use the term "cultural" as more comprehensive in scope, but recognize racial oppression is a major manifestation of cultural oppression in the United States. We will also discuss how oppression continues to be institutionalized in ways that legal and political actions are unable to redress. Cultural oppression, for example, exerts effects that are particularly enervating in healthcare, where the healthcare provider often enables healing, but knowingly or unknowingly fails to alter the relationship of oppressor to oppressed. In response, we offer the concept of transformation as an alternative means of empowerment, which promotes healing for the oppressed and the oppressor. The nurse, both as an oppressor and as an oppressed participant in healthcare, can certainly become an important part of that transformative healing.

THE WOUNDS OF CULTURAL OPPRESSION

Years after reaping the fruits of the civil rights movement, a self-deception reigns among a significant number of Americans that cultural discrimination no longer exists. This self-deception can lull people into believing that those who still claim to be oppressed by cultural discrimination are nonetheless better off in many ways than those who are not or who do not claim to be oppressed. The current distaste for "affirmative action" and the increasing calls against "reverse discrimination" bear witness to this unnerving development. While it is true that the more severe and gross forms of cultural oppression are no longer tolerated generally, and institutionalized support for discriminatory practices are proscribed, there are an infinite variety of ways that the oppression of people who are different, or who claim difference, continues to flourish. Because they are subtle and sometimes embedded in a paternalism aimed at ameliorating blatant discriminatory practices, such attitudes and behavior are much more difficult to confront.

The issue of class rather than race as an explanation for the misery of culturally oppressed groups in this country has also been debated in many circles. Indeed, studies have evidenced that controlling for the variable of race, class can explain the plight of people at the lowest rungs of the American social ladder. Dalton (1995) contends that this issue is often propounded by well-meaning academicians made uncomfortable by the race issue. The argument suffers fundamentally in that it assumes that class and race are independent of each other, and can be teased out easily (p. 123). Rather than struggle with academic distinctions between concepts that are closely intertwined in many complex ways, it would seem to be more pragmatic and accurate to conceptualize cultural oppression more broadly, encompassing not only economics and class, but race and cultural mores as well.

Dealing with the issue of race will continue to be a very painful process, especially when it reflects back upon an individual's position and circumstance. And while those who believe, even with the best intentions, that class can explain the ills of cultural oppression, caution is essential. For in our society at least, one of the major determinants of class is the racial pecking order itself.

The effects of cultural oppression are more than evident in the lives of those at the receiving end. Taylor (1992) points to the psychological harm that results from racist attitudes and discriminatory behavior as particularly injurious. Within healthcare, such harm is evidenced in the disparities in health status among minorities, intertwined with powerlessness—a structural problem woven into social institutions that continues to perpetuate oppressive cultures (Braithwaite, 1992). People who are powerless do not have control over their destinies, an idea which has also been developed as a working hypothesis for the study of people's susceptibility to disease (Wallerstein, 1993).

Jones and Mitchell (1987) contend, for example, that despite advances in medical care, gross disparities still exist between blacks and whites on every measure of illness and health. This is true of most other minority groups as well. Adequate healthcare would modify these disparities. Institutional racism cannot be forgotten as a possible explanation for the inequalities in healthcare in American society, and an important reason why minorities underutilize health services. Covert racism does persist in many health institutions, apparent in the manner in which poor people of color are treated, and sanctioned by the adoption, administration, and implementation of policies specific to them.

Institutional views toward the treatment of the poor overlap extensively with attitudes toward minorities (Jones & Mitchell, 1987). Sociocultural barriers such as long waits for care, onerous processes for establishing eligibility, demeaning attitude of providers, dearth of bilingual providers, and lack of institutional sensitivity to individual values and beliefs are factors that promote non-utilization of health services by powerless individuals. To add insult to injury, these individuals are reproached for the opprobrious behavior of being "stupid and ungrateful" for the services made available to them at taxpayer's expense.

The wounds inflicted by a sense of powerlessness are deep and lasting. Behaviors emanating from generalized distrust, alienation, and hopelessness tend to separate a disenfranchised individual from those who purport to help. Examples of this abound in healthcare. Consider a situation wherein a Medicaid child belonging to an ethnic minority group is brought into the hospital for a workup of failure to thrive. The family is under a state surveillance for possible child abuse or neglect. The mother is uncooperative and belligerent, not only with the floor nurses, but also with the staff of the various services to which the family has been referred. Healthcare workers, including nurses, express their frustrations at the family, and label them "noncompliant." The helping relationship that needs to be established is never really initiated because the family, which has been always socially marginal, has been further marginalized in the healthcare system with the imposition of the label.

Censure is often directed at people without health insurance who enter the healthcare system "with an attitude," implying that if they can't pay for their healthcare, if "the taxpayers have to pick up their tab," they better act subservient and be eternally grateful. "Blaming the victim" is a phenomenon that we often observe in healthcare.

In time, the victims of oppression begin to internalize the labels pinned on them by their oppressors, and their outward behaviors mirror that internalized self-deprecation in ways that serve to cement the oppressors' opinions about them. Paulo Friere (1970), a noted Brazilian philosopher/educator, describes the process: "So often do they hear that they are good for nothing, know nothing, and are incapable of learning anything—that they are sick, lazy, and unproductive—that in the end they become convinced of their own unfitness" (p. 49). Thus it is that the victims of cultural oppression are accessory to their own denigration and dehumanization.

TRANSFORMATION—THE PATH TO HEALING

The dehumanization inflicted on the oppressed reflects upon the oppressor as well. Freire (1970) posits that dehumanization "is a distortion of the vocation of becoming more fully human" (p. 28), and that being human is constantly being thwarted by injustice, exploitation, oppression, and violence by the oppressors. He further states that oppressors cannot inflict wounds that dehumanize other individuals without inflicting those wounds on themselves as well. In an unbalanced power relationship, such as that which exists between dominant and subordinate cultures, it would seem that the dominant party has the ability to influence that imbalance. Seemingly, one would expect that the oppressor merely has to relinquish some of the power held over the oppressed in order to bring into balance the power equation. However, the idea of an oppressor relinquishing power voluntarily seems to be a contradiction in terms.

Empowerment is a term that has crept into the healthcare lexicon and is a convenient catchword that means anything from feminist liberation to community activism. Rappaport (1987) uses the term to refer to a process of "becoming able or *allowed* to do some unspecified thing because there is a condition of dominion or authority with regard to that specific thing" (p. 129). The use of this term as defined is inappropriate when one thinks of healing the wounds of cultural oppression. In attempting to break the shackles of cultural oppression, one must be particularly wary of the lure of pseudo-empowerment through manipulation and paternalism. It is easy to be lulled into thinking that the oppressed have been empowered when in fact what has happened is that they have internalized the values of the oppressor.

The idea of *transformative power* is a more appropriate concept in explaining how the wounds of cultural oppression can be healed. Gaining transformative power is an active process on the part of the culturally oppressed, wherein the oppressed *obtain for themselves* the ability to control their own destiny, to make decisions about their lives and circumstances, and to work with others to establish an environment where freedom and liberty in all the important aspects of life can flourish and prosper. In other words, gaining transformative power enables the culturally oppressed to *construct their own reality, on their own terms.* Freire (1970) believes that the only way that oppression can be overcome is through the active efforts of the oppressed—no one else can liberate a victim from oppression. However, in the process of liberating oneself, by "taking away the oppressor's power to dominate and suppress, the humanity lost in the exercise of oppression is restored to that oppressor" (p. 42).

This process of transcending dehumanization from cultural oppression involves increased consciousness of the oppression (Collins, 1977). The role of this consciousness in the process of self-liberation is very important; it is, in fact, an ontological necessity for the transformative process. It is only through this process that the oppressed can "take possession of the reality" (p. 65) of their oppression, and act on it to be liberated. The Rev. Martin Luther King referred to this as creating a tension that will propel the movement by oppressed people to rise above prejudice and racism. A precondition for the work of transformation is that the victims of oppression must be made uncomfortable enough about their situation to do something about it themselves.

The value of transformation in the process of self-liberation by oppressed people is two-fold. First, it requires that the victims take action for themselves, not have their transformation bestowed upon them. In so doing, it ensures that the outcomes in rectifying the imbalances in the power equation between the oppressed and the oppressor will be real. Secondly, when the dehumanization of cultural oppression is transcended, it allows the burgeoning of the humanity of both the oppressed and his oppressor. There cannot be a more effective healing process than the restoration of the humanity of both victim and oppressor. This may seem to be an oversimplification of the process. Indeed, it is difficult to imagine that the oppressor will willingly give up dominance over the oppressed just to have humanity restored. The reality for some is that this process may never take place, and what may come out of successful efforts of the oppressed to be liberated is an uneasy truce with the oppressor, supported by a layer of simmering resentments and hatred that never is far from the surface. However, transformative healing calls for change in all those involved. This change must involve not only cognitive and affective ways of responding, but just as importantly, conative patterns as well.

TRANSFORMATION IN HEALTHCARE

Transformational healing of the wounds of cultural oppression is necessarily a component of healthcare. Nurses, particularly those from minority groups, have a responsibility of being sensitive to the need for this type of healing. Nurses from the dominant culture must also be cognizant of the need for transformational healing, for the changes in the demographics of our society portend more, not less, people of color in the healthcare system.

How can the acquisition of transformative power for the culturally oppressed be realized in the healthcare arena? At one level, the idea that systematic supports of culturally oppressive practices are still ubiquitous in many of our healthcare institutions must be recognized and confronted. When healthcare workers are able to treat, with impunity, people who are different in ways that dehumanize them, when gross insensitivity to cultural values and norms get in the way of understanding vulnerable people's realities and prevents effective interaction for healthcare delivery, when institutional policies fail to break down sociocultural barriers to people's access and utilization of healthcare services, then the environment is inimical to the transformative process for the victimized people. Institutional passivity in the face of blatant oppressive practices is just as destructive as overt promulgation of those practices. Change in institutionalized norms and patterns cannot take place without concerted effort. Therefore, not only does inactivity fail to prevent or avoid cultural oppression, but more importantly, it maintains it as a part of the system (Kavanagh & Kennedy, 1992).

Institutional norms and values are engendered from the top. Unless concerted and committed actions are taken from the top in eradicating a culturally oppressive healthcare environment, the conditions for transformative healing will not converge. That convergence can be facilitated by educating oppressors at that top layer concerning the devastating effects of their oppression on the clients that they purport to serve. An individual who is already disadvantaged by ill health and the vicissitudes of fringe existence faces overwhelming hurdles in the effort to transcend the oppressive state. An environment that does nothing to promote recognition of the immorality of cultural oppression actually promotes cultural oppression. Conversely, an environment that actively suppresses the conditions that promote cultural oppression, actively promotes transformative healing. Thus, it is incumbent upon minority nurses as part of that oppressed group to take on the responsibility of educating those in power. This education would facilitate the transformational process through institutionalized norms for culturally sensitive practice for the vulnerable people they serve.

At the individual level, a person may not intentionally act to dehumanize another, but it is not unusual for persons who have always been part of the dominant and powerful group to have blind spots that prevent them from recognizing that some of their attitudes and behaviors toward people who are viewed as subordinate by the dominant culture are in fact dehumanizing. Those who are not personally prejudiced or racist can be oblivious to the fact that by failing to prevent the discriminatory treatment of others, they are contributing to the cultural oppression of people who are different (Kavanagh & Kennedy, 1992). Thus it is incumbent upon those who hold the edge in an unbalanced power relationship, whether by virtue of professional position or membership in the dominant/majority group, or both, to be aware of the vulnerability of individuals who have suffered cultural oppression. Furthermore, healthcare professionals working with disadvantaged people must realize that their effectiveness hinges on the ability of those individuals to transcend their oppressive state. Only then can the transformative process be possible. In an effort to promote healthy behavior in minority persons, the healthcare professional must recognize that health behaviors are culture bound, and that primary healthcare must emerge from a recognition and famiiiarity with the target culture so that health interventions are culturally sensitive and linguistically appropriate (Airhihenbuwa, 1992).

One of the mistakes that persons in helping professions make in their attempts to provide services to minority groups is to address beliefs and norms within the context of their own dominant culture, rather than within that of the persons to be served. A dominant culture nurse may find the parenting style of a single African-American mother on public assistance particularly troublesome. Viewed from her white, middle class upbringing, the strongly authoritative approach that the mother uses on her child may seem severely harsh and punitive, and a report to children's protective services may seem to the nurse to be a necessary option in the management of the child. There may be a survival instinct underlying that seemingly authoritative parenting style that attempts to prepare the child for the tough conditions of oppression. Unless the child is in imminent physical or psychological danger as a result of the mother's treatment, it would serve everyone well if the nurse takes the time to reflect on the situation further before taking action.

It is a mistake to assume that the substance and meanings of beliefs and norms are the same within subgroups of a specific culture, just because they are similar in form (Airhihenbuwa, 1992). As a function of their degree of "assimilation" within the dominant culture, subgroups in American society may have differing values and practices from their identified cultural origins. To impute images and behaviors on persons based on their membership within a larger group without verification through interaction and communication is as dehumanizing as denying their right to be different at all. Belonging to a group does not mean that individual values, beliefs, practices and norms cannot deviate from those presumed to be held by the group.

The Nurse Participant in Transformational Healing

Nurses have historically suffered dual oppression in their status within the healthcare system. The oppression of being physicians' handmaidens had long been an impediment to the recognition of nurses as colleagues and leaders, and to taking their rightful place as the largest group providing healthcare to the public. The oppression of being second class citizens in the male-dominated healthcare system has meant a constant struggle for recognition as full participants within this system. Thus, the burden of cultural oppression is an experience not unknown to nurses.

It might be expected then that dominant culture nurses would be most sensitive to the plight of minority groups and the dehumanization of oppression, and that this sensitivity would allow them to naturally take on the cause and advocacy for them. However, this is not necessarily so. Freire (1970) indicates that in the struggle of the oppressed to liberate themselves and their oppressors, they do not initially strive for liberation, but instead become oppressors, or "sub-oppressors." Striving to become more empowered, they envision themselves in the same position as their oppressors, ones with the power and the ability to make change happen. Thus nurses who have internalized this vision of empowerment can be said to have a "fear of freedom." Freedom would require them to eject the "oppressor" image and strive to replace it with autonomy and responsibility.

Those nurses who "fear freedom" have become resigned to their roles as oppressed and are unwilling or incapable of running the risks associated with the struggle for autonomy and responsibility. These nurses are conformists, not listening to the appeals of others, nor even to the appeals of their own consciences; they simply follow the guidelines set up by others in determining how they should or should not practice in the context of nursing. Thus, the "healer" caring for patients cannot truly promote healing, because of his or her own limitations. Nurses with the zest for transformation, who feel the need to become free from oppression by the healthcare system at large, who want to push forward the concept of "patient advocacy" and healing, not only of self but others, have embraced the concept of "freedom." They have internalized the concept of autonomy and responsibility, and are willing to struggle to achieve freedom in their nursing practice. These are the nurses who can participate in transformational healing, not only for themselves, but also for the people that they purport to serve.

What do nurses need to do in order to participate actively in transformational healing? First and foremost, nurses need to feel the tension and the abasement of being oppressed. Unless the nurse feels the discomfiture and the feeling of degradation that being oppressed engenders, then the energy needed to participate in the transformation process will not emerge. Strong identification with the plight of the oppressed helps to build the commitment to pick up the cause on their behalf. Nurses also need to become fully aware that they have been, and are, oppressors of others as well. Recognizing that one has it in oneself to dehumanize others makes one much more sensitive to the situation in which that tendency realizes itself. Finally, nurses need to remember that just as they, as an oppressed group, have to liberate themselves, so too, do the victims of oppression have to battle for themselves. The environment that nurtures the possibility of liberation can be created and facilitated; the liberation process cannot be undertaken by someone other than the one that needs to be liberated.

One of the most important concepts that nurses who work with persons from minority groups must internalize is the concept of individual realities. It is fairly easy to mouth the rhetoric of "walking in someone else's shoes," but does that have any meaning when one is experiencing the frustration of trying to convince an elderly Asian-American addicted to opium to use his social security checks to buy his antihypertensive medications rather than to pay for maintaining his addiction? Or the anger at the single mother who uses welfare checks to go to bars to have a good time rather than spend the money on buying nutritional food for her children? We may have good reason to rail against those individuals, but that exercise does nothing to help us to be more effective in working with them. We have to come as close as we can to realizing their realities—then can we understand what opium means to him, and what having a good time means to her.

In an era and society where cultural diversity is increasingly becoming the norm, the healthcare system will not be able to withstand the pressures to address the specific issues that such a diversity brings with it. Cultural oppression still exists, and will probably continue to exist as long as there are differences and power imbalances in human relationships. Although we claim our society to be a democracy, it is an incomplete democracy, with all the blemishes of its imperfection. The sooner we accept that, the sooner can we strive to create the conditions where the people we wish to help can overcome those imperfections for themselves.

REFERENCES

Airhihenbuwa, C. (1992). Health promotion and disease prevention strategies for African-Americans: a conceptual model. In R. Braithwaite & S. Taylor (Eds.), *Health issues in the black community.* San Francisco: Jossey-Bass.

Braithwaite, R. (1992). Coalition partnerships for health promotion and empowerment. In R. Braithwaite & S. Taylor (Eds.), *Health issues in the black community.* San Francisco: Jossey-Bass.

Collins, D. (1977). *Paulo Friere: His life, works and thoughts.* New York: Paulist Press.

Dalton, H. (1995). *Racial healing: Confronting the fear between Blacks and Whites.* New York: Doubleday

Friere, P. (1970). *Pedagogy of the oppressed.* New York: Herder and Herder.

Jones, W., & Mitchell, R. (1987). *Health care issues in Black America: Policies, problems, and prospects.* New York: Greenwood Press.

Kavanagh, K., & Kennedy, P. (1992). *Promoting cultural diversity: Strategies for health care professionals.* Newbury Park, CA: Sage.

Rappaport, J. (1987). Terms of empowerment/exemplars of prevention: Toward a theory for community psychology. *American Journal of Community Psychology, 15*(2), 121-143.

Taylor, S. (1992). The mental health status of black Americans: An overview. In R. Braithwaite & S. Taylor (Eds.), *Health issues in the black community.* San Francisco: Jossey-Bass.

Wallerstein, N. (1993). Empowerment and health: The theory and practice of community change. *Community Development Journal, 28*(3), 218-227.

CHAPTER 19

Holism: A Foundation for Healing Wounds of Divisiveness Among Nurses

KAREN A. BRYKCZYNSKI, RN, RNCS, FNP, DNSC

Over the past twenty-five or so years, while studying, practicing, teaching, or researching nursing, I have been struck by the impression that although there is much diversity in educational preparations, specialities, and positions, nurses are much more the same than we are different. I am deeply disturbed by my observations and experiences of hostility of nurses toward nurses—a phenomenon referred to as horizontal violence when seen within the framwork of oppressed group behavior (Friere, 1970; Hedin, 1986; Roberts, 1983). The tension between individualism and community (Bellah, Madsen, Sullivan, Swidler, & Tipton, 1985; Taylor, 1992) along with our tendency to dichotomize and classify according to rigid criteria certainly contribute to this behavior. Furthermore, the separatism and polarization that result from extreme individualism and pervasive dichotomization are diametrically opposed to the fundamental tenets of holism on which nursing rests. I believe that revisiting the fundamental significance of holism to nursing practice can promote healing among nurses.

HISTORICAL ASPECTS

The term holism was coined by General Jan Smuts in the early 1900s. According to the philosophic theory of holism, wholes occurring in nature are not reducible to the sum of their parts. Smuts (1926) maintained that a thorough understanding of wholes and consistent application of this understanding to humans could solve the mind-body problem. Smuts claimed that the major significance of holism is a complete transformation of

234

causality as follows: "When an external cause acts on a whole, the resultant effect is not merely traceable to the cause, but has become transformed in the process" (p. 119). The fact that in spite of espousing belief in persons as holistic beings, nurses and nursing continue to adhere to the world view of mechanistic atomism in which causal determinism is fundamental calls for reflection.

Nursing has been constrained in the full development of holism because of the influence of positivism. Profound changes were produced in physics and philosophy of science with the broad acceptance of the quantum nature of matter. Concepts of the discontinuity of matter and the uncertainty principle led to re-examination of long-held ideas about the continuity of matter, objectivity, and causal determinism (Wolf, 1981). What followed was a new awareness of the interdependence and interaction of knowing (epistemology) and being (ontology) commonly referred to as the mind-body problem. The fact that the momentum for the transition of nursing from a job to a career intensified at a time when the positivist conception of science was prevalent in nursing education was a significant factor influencing nursing's development (Watson, 1981; Webster, Jacox, & Baldwin, 1981).

Positivism has served nursing well particularly in the research arena. The value of nursing research has been recognized nationally with the establishment of a Center for Nursing Research at the National Institutes of Health. However, a major problem with implementation of the positivist philosophy is that reality is far more complex than its rigid tenets provide for. Webster and his collaborators explain that the 17th-century worldview basic assumptions underlying the Received View of Logical Positivism, such as belief in the fundamental independence of parts (atomism), followed the tendency to view simple dichotomies and mutually exclusive and jointly exhaustive categories as sufficient and appropriate (Webster et al., 1981). Dichotomies and polarities provide a way to order the continuities in the world around us (Hefner, Rebecca, & Oleshasky, 1975). They result in an emphasis on differences.

The tendency in nursing to conceptualize issues using dichotomous classifications such as content versus process, objective versus subjective, nursing diagnosis versus medical diagnosis, change versus stability, qualitative versus quantitative, theory versus practice, baccalaureate versus nonbaccalaureate, and clinical specialist versus nurse practitioner, to name a few, may be understood as an application of the principle of parsimony to simplify the complexity of nursing phenomena. There is a tendency to search for certainties and absolutes to guide our actions and to construct dichotomies in an effort to comprehend the nature of nursing and eliminate ambiguity. There is something fundamentally uncomfortable about ambiguity and indeterminism, particularly from a positivistic philosophical perspective.

BEYOND DICHOTOMIES

Maslow (1968), a prominent proponent of holism, has asserted that it is crucial to abandon "our 3000-year-old-habit of dichotomizing, splitting, and separating in the style of Aristotelian logic" (p. 174). In arguing for holistic rather than atomistic thinking, he points out that dichotomization impedes integration. In describing the integration characteristic of higher level functioning, he explains that "dichotomies, polarities, and conflicts are fused, transcended, and resolved . . . What I had thought to be straight-line continua, whose extremes were polar to each other and as far apart as possible, turned out to be rather like circles or spirals, in which the polar extremes came together into a fused unity" (p. 91). Transcendence of the polar opposites does not signify singularity so much as an integral holistic diversity.

The major difficulty with dichotomies is that they fail to provide for any connection or interaction between the polar extremes. Yet there is an interrelationship or connection. Take for example the simple commonplace extremes of day and night and white and black. They seem so totally opposite and distinct. Now consider the terms dawn, dusk, and gray and the picture becomes much less determinate with many possible gradations. Whitehead (1925) resolves this difficulty with dichotomies through the observation that the problem derives from interpreting abstract notions as if they were concrete entities. This is what he terms the "fallacy of misplaced concreteness" (p. 51).

This concept can perhaps be better understood by reference to the formalization tendency of positivist science. According to the original version of the received view of the nature of science, if one could reduce science to the language of mathematical logic, then one would have certainty (Suppe, 1977). As a result of the formalization assumption, theories were either true or false. Consequently, theories were considered real or factual. This is what Whitehead implies by the "fallacy of misplaced concreteness"—that theory was interpreted concretely. In other words, the map or theory (abstraction) was taken to truly represent, to *be* the territory or reality (concrete entity).

According to Whitehead's process philosophy, there are no separate, mutually exclusive parts (1925, 1933). There are no clear demarcations, and this is as it should be since everything is interacting and developing or becoming. Our longstanding difficulty in clearly distinguishing the body from the mind is evidenced by research in biofeedback; the placebo effect; recent awareness of human auras from Kerlian photography and therapeutic touch; as well as the recognition of the phenomenon of personal space. If one accepts the concept of the creative advance of the universe, there are no fundamental changeless certainties or static entities (Whitehead, 1925). Ambiguity must not merely be tolerated, it must be understood as fundamental!

PRACTICAL APPLICATIONS

There are many currently available research approaches for expanding and complementing the positivist worldview such as critical theory, discourse analysis, Heideggerian hermeneutics, and action research. In concert with the holistic perspective advanced here, these approaches should be considered in addition to the predominant positivist methods as complementary rather than alternative, *and* rather than *either/or*. A situational approach based on interpretive phenomenology can be particularly useful for moving the insight gained through the process philosophical perspective on to practical application. The goal in interpretive phenomenology is to get beyond dichotomous classifications of mind and body (subjectivity and objectivity) characteristic of mechanistic atomism by assuming that through common background knowledge, language, habits, skills, practices, situations, meanings, and being embodied, we can understand others not as private subjects, but as embodied participants and members of a shared human community (Benner, 1994).

Interpretive phenomenology provides one of many alternative perspectives to the rational, economic, technical, exchange-oriented view so pervasive in society today. As shared meanings are brought to awareness and open discourse through phenomenological research, advanced practice nurses can learn to appreciate qualitative similarities and distinctions in advanced practice roles and to celebrate the unity within the diversity that exists in present day clinical nursing. We need to adopt peer supportive rather than peer critical behaviors in nursing as Mauksch (1981) advocated. In fact, the most important single directive is for nurses to learn to nurse other nurses! We need to incorporate holism as a concept in our relationships with other nurses not just in our relationships with our patients, their families, and communities.

Just saying that we need to be peer supportive and use holistic concepts in our relationships will not make it so. There are serious differences of opinion and outright conflict among nurses over the issues surrounding clinical nurse specialists and nurse practitioners. Part of the problem is the adversarial stance taken, that is, the nurse practitioner and the clinical nurse specialist are pitted against one another by defining the situation as nurse practitioner versus clinical nurse specialist. A polarized perspective such as this sets us up for opposition and conflict.

An alternative evolutionary viewpoint, as in the process organism perspective, sees a gradual transition with the distinctly different advanced practice roles of the nurse practitioner and the clinical nurse specialist becoming more alike than different over time. We can choose to take a proactive stance and move to combine the strengths of both roles to fashion future-oriented advanced practice roles. This would require abandoning false opposition and outdated beliefs that nurse practitioners are no longer nurses, but have become junior doctors (a position promulgated by Martha Rogers (1975), which has been steadfastly maintained by many nurses in academia) by virtue of combining aspects of medical knowledge with nursing knowledge.

The alternative evolutionary viewpoint has been aptly expressed by Ingeborg Mauksch (1981), as follows:

> *Historically, nurses have taken over tasks originally done only by physicians, such as taking temperatures and blood pressures, and so it is now with physical assessment. Yet, these tasks have never been the main component of nursing care. The primary functions of nursing fall into two other realms: first, the emphasis on health maintenance and health and self care education and second the care of the ill and the dying. (p. 4)*

Indeed, to continue to oppose the inclusion of responsibility for medical diagnoses and prescription of diagnostic tests, procedures, medications, and other treatments as legitimate and necessary components of curricula for advanced practice nurses and essential knowledge for competent advanced nursing practice is to deny the realities of the practice world.

It is well-known among nurses that the scope of nursing practice grows geometrically during the late night and early morning hours even in major hospitals and shrinks proportionately during normal working hours. Similarly expanded scopes of nursing practice are observed in rural areas and low income minority sections of large cities. This is a very complex issue that needs to be addressed carefully. Double standards such as these have been widespread in our illness care system. Underlying the notion of a double standard, is the false belief that physician-provided care is superior to the same care provided by a nurse. Research comparing care provided by nurse practitioners and physicians has shown that nurse practitioners provide care of equal and in some cases better quality than physicians (Safreit, 1992). In essence, Safreit, Associate Dean of Yale Law School, observed that this is more a restraint of trade issue than an issue of quality of care.

Physicians have succeeded thus far in maintaining a monopoly over patient care in preferred locations during normal working hours by cleverly representing the situation as one of public safety and quality of care. Now that evidence is accumulating that nurse practitioners, nurse midwives, nurse anesthetists, and physicians' assistants can provide 70 percent to 90 percent of primary healthcare in a more cost effective manner with sometimes better patient outcomes, it is becoming more difficult for physicians to maintain control. They have begun attacking us at our weakest point—the lack of consistency in standards of quality in academic preparation across programs.

Advanced practice nurses of all types (nurse practitioners, clinical nurse specialists, nurse midwives, and nurse anesthetists) need the educational and experiential background as well as the authority to assume responsibility and accountability for holistic patient care. The complementary nature of nursing practice in relation to medical practice needs to be emphasized in establishing collaborative relationships. Political alliances need to be strengthened among advanced practice nurses and physicians' assistants, psychologists, and others to move toward greater balance of power and authority.

Commonalities between nurse practitioners and all other nurses have been demonstrated through descriptions of the domains and competencies of nurse practitioners (Brykczynski, 1989). Similarities between the practice of nurse practitioners and clinical nurse specialists have also been demonstrated (Fenton & Brykczynski, 1993). To claim that there are irreconcilable philosophical differences is to define the problem as unsolvable.

Achievement of an integrated perspective, however, can be expected to be difficult. It is no accident that nursing's dominant research perspective is characterized by separatism, dichotomization, linearity, and hierarchy that reflect its underlying positivist philosophical foundation. Our American culture rests on a long history and traditional foundation of individualism. The tensions between the attitudes, values, beliefs, practices, and goals of individual versus collective interests become more predominant as our society becomes more diverse. Perhaps instead of seeking to resolve all our conflicts or forging ahead by simply ignoring them, we can learn to manage competing interests. For example, our nurse practitioner faculty sought consultation for successfully implementing our integrated curriculum for primary healthcare. This experience serves as an example for curriculum planning in the face of competing specialty interests.

Our curriculum planning was at an impasse because of incommensurability among the various nurse practitioner specialty groups (pediatric, obstetrical/gynecological, family, and adult/geriatric). Our consultant facilitated an all-day faculty workshop where feelings, concerns, and issues were expressed. After everyone had the opportunity to share their thoughts and feelings, we engaged in brainstorming and came up with the strategy of all specialty faculty putting essential content on index cards and collecting them on a table in a neutral area. The designated course coordinator volunteered to collate the content areas; then group meetings were held to organize the content. We overcame divisiveness, yet maintained our uniqueness, and created a program that integrates common areas while keeping selected specific specialty content areas separate thereby maximizing resources and minimizing double teaching. A similar process could be implemented to integrate core components of our new acute care nurse practitioner program with our primary care nurse practitioner program.

CONCLUSION

Increased awareness of the common core of nursing knowledge and skill can serve to unify and integrate many of the false dichotomies that have developed among nurses. All nurses are responsible for making clinical judgments and acting on those judgments to create situations where patients can heal themselves or die peacefully. This holistic perspective of the unity of all nurses, can serve as a unifying force to promote healing of our wounds inflicted by conflict and divisiveness.

REFERENCES

Bellah, R. N., Madsen, R., Sullivan, W. M., Swidler, A., & Tipton, S. M. (1985). *Habits of the heart. Individualism and commitment in American life.* Berkeley: University of California Press.

Benner, P. E. (1984). *From novice to expert. Excellence and power in clinical nursing practice.* Menlo Park, CA: Addison-Wesley.

Benner, P. E. (Ed.). (1994). *Interpretive phenomenology.* Thousand Oaks, CA: Sage.

Brykczynski, K. A. (1989). An interpretive study describing the clinical judgment of nurse practitioners. *Scholarly Inquiry for Nursing Practice: An International Journal, 3*(2), 75–104.

Fenton, M. V., & Brykczynski, K. A. (1993). Qualitative distinctions and similarities in the practice of clinical nurse specialists and nurse practitioners. *Journal of Professional Nursing, 9*(6), 313–326.

Friere, P. (1970). *Pedagogy of the oppressed.* (M.B. Ramos, Trans.). New York: Continuum Press. (Original work published 1968).

Hedin, B. A. (1986). A case study of oppressed group behavior in nurses. *Image: Journal of Nursing Scholarship, 18*(2), 53–57.

Hefner, R., Rebecca, M., & Oleshansky, B. (1975). Development of sex role transcendence. *Human Development, 18,* 143–158.

Maslow, A. H. (1968). *Toward a psychology of being.* (2nd ed.). New York: Van Nostrand.

Mauksch, I. G. (1975). Nursing is coming of age . . . through the practitioner movement. Pro. *American Journal of Nursing, 75,* 1834–1843.

Mauksch, I. G. (Ed.). (1981). *Primary care. A contemporary nursing perspective.* New York: Grune & Stratton.

Roberts, S. J. (1983). Oppressed group behavior: Implications for nursing. *Advances in Nursing Science, 5*(7), 21–30.

Rogers, M. E. (1975). Nursing is coming of age . . . through the practitioner movement. Con. *American Journal of Nursing, 75,* 1834–1843.

Safriet, B. (1992). Health care dollars and regulatory sense: The role of advanced practice nursing. *Yale Journal of Regulation, 9*(417), 418–488.

Smuts, J. C. (1926). *Holism and evolution.* New York: Macmillan.

Suppe, F. (1977). (Ed.). *The structure of scientific theories* (2nd ed.). Champaign, IL: University of Illinois Press.

Taylor, C. (1992). *Multiculturalism and the politics of recognition.* Princeton: Princeton University Press.

Watson, J. (1981). Nursing's scientific quest. *Nursing Outlook, 29,* 413–416.

Webster, G., Jacox, A., & Baldwin, B. (1981). Nursing theory and the ghost of the received view. In M. Grace & N. McCluskey (Eds.), *Contemporary issues in nursing.* Boston: Blackwell Scientific.

Whitehead, A. N. (1925). *Science and the modern world.* New York: The Free Press.

Whitehead, A. N. (1933). *Adventures of ideas.* New York: The Free Press.

Wolf, F. A. (1981). *Taking the quantum leap.* San Francisco: Harper & Row.

CHAPTER 20

"Are You a Witch?"
A Clinical Story

SUSAN SCOVILLE BAKER, PHD, RN, CS

Strange things have a way of happening to you when you work in adolescent psychiatric nursing. After a while, it just becomes part of the landscape. It also seems that, since adolescents who are admitted are more acutely ill and stay for shorter periods of time, the opportunities for therapeutic intervention are few and far between. At times it is difficult to explain the necessity for advanced practice nursing in an area in which nursing often seems reduced to medication administration, order transcription, and behavior management. Once in a while, however, a situation arises in which all your training and a good measure of inspiration can have remarkable results.

For several years, one evening a week, I had a faculty practice as a clinical nurse specialist for the inpatient child and adolescent psychiatric units at the University Hospital. As part of the staff and the unit, I often accepted a patient care assignment, usually selecting particularly difficult or problematic patients, to give the regular staff a break or even occasionally a new idea about patient management. So it happened that I was approached by one of "my" patients for assistance with a peer who was experiencing what everyone referred to as one of her "spells."

The 15-year-old girl (let's call her "Tina") was seated in the dining area with several other teens, staring into space, weeping, and shaking. Her body was otherwise stiff. I sat with her for a while, then escorted her to her room. She said repeatedly, "I want to die, I want to kill myself right now. Then I will be happy. I have to kill myself." She continued to stare and shake. I sat with her saying, "Tina, you are safe. I am with you," and so on, to move her attention away from the internal voice telling her to kill herself. Another patient (let's call her "Amy") came into the room and sat with us also. Amy held Tina's hand and also stated repeatedly who she was and where we all were, and that we would keep her safe. After a while, Amy went back to her own room and returned with a stone, an alabaster egg, and a ring. She placed the egg in Tina's hand, and held it closed, putting the ring on her own finger, and holding the stone to her own neck. Tina continued to stare and shake.

I asked Tina what she was seeing. "A woman," she responded, describing her as beautiful, with long blonde hair. I was holding Tina's other hand, softly working the stiffness out of it with slow soft massage, at the same time trying to help her take control over the self-destructive image in her mind, by telling the image to go away. Tina said she couldn't tell her that, and that the woman was laughing at her. The next 30 minutes involved intensive work, using a critical combination of active touch (a light kneading-type massage of her hand), and a transmission of strength and will through that touch and repeated soft verbal assurance of safety and support along with gentle verbal instruction. At last Tina was able to follow the instructions to turn and walk away from the image, even though she remained unable to tell the image to go away. She began to blink her eyes and move her arms and legs from their frozen positions. Soon she was able to respond appropriately to our questions and comments.

In a short time, Tina was able to return to the dining area and join the group activity in progress. I heard Amy talking to one of the staff in the hallway while I was in the office nearby reporting and documenting the incident. When I finished charting and went back to the hall, the staff member said, "She thinks you're a witch." I asked what that meant, and the girl marvelled, "Do you have special healing powers?" I said, "Well, really I just think it is nursing, but I do practice therapeutic touch and massage and such things." "I knew it," she said, in awe. "I never could have gotten her out of that myself. I wasn't strong enough. But you have a lot of power."

There is a body of feminist literature about witchcraft, wisdom, and healing. Cultural anthropology also is replete with exemplars of the mysterious cosmic healing powers of native healers, many of them women, who can help channel another person's healing potential. This phenomenon, it seems to me, is psychiatric nursing at its best—and maybe it helps explain the difficulty we in the field have historically found in expressing exactly what it is that we "do." We often even take it for granted, seemingly needing to apologize for the very personality qualities which drew us into the field of psychiatric nursing in the first place and which make us uniquely effective in our patient interventions.

I think we perceive this healing power most clearly when someone else identifies it, or when the usual, recognizable forms of communication are nonfunctional. For me, it is especially evident in work with psychotic, catatonic, or severely brain-damaged persons. Then the use of sensory healing techniques involving touch, sight, sound and a general effect I have to call "presence" become all-important. This quality I call "presence," is almost an hypnotic effect of a person's way of being. It is a carefully planned combination of posture, expression, dress, voice tone, body language, and way of moving, and must be individualized to the particular situation.

I remember working with one young woman, whose severe cognitive impairment was expressed in violent, uncontrollable outbursts of frustration when she perceived that other teens were making fun of her limitations (the result of severe childhood physical abuse by family members who had tried to kill her). After one particularly violent outburst, other staff wanted to seclude or restrain her, but I asked to try some alternative strategies first. I spoke softly as I entered the patient's room. She was thrashing on the bed, wailing, and smashing her fists and feet against the wall. In a soft, even tone, I told her I was there and that I wanted to come close to her, that I wanted to be with her and share her pain, that I would not hurt her in any way. Already her thrashing became less violent. Then I told her quietly that I would like to touch her shoulder. She did not move away or strike or protest. Slowly I approached, close enough to touch her and too close for her to land a very strong kick or punch. When I put my hand on her shoulder, her wailing resolved into shudders and sobs and, as I continued to speak softly and massage her neck and shoulders, she began to talk of her unspeakable pain. I could feel and share her despair and rage at being ridiculed for the physical deformities created by her mother's efforts to destroy her.

I've been thinking about these incidents and others like them, how they both exhaust and revitalize me, and particularly about the patient I've called Amy, who assisted me in my intervention and attributed its effectiveness to witchcraft. She impressed me with her sensitivity to the tremendous amount of energy required for these healing interventions. I have also given considerable thought to her identification of the objects she had brought into the room as her "stores" where she has stored up psychic energy for times when she needed it. Certainly these healing interventions are tremendously taxing, and are only effective when the nurse has the energy and the focus necessary. In order for these qualities to be replenished, time and attention need to be given to activities and interests which serve to revitalize the healer. Another interesting aspect of these healing powers is that the more you use them, the more vigorous they become.

Unfortunately, all too often the demands of psychiatric nursing in the 1990s, particularly in the inpatient setting, revolve around documentation requirements and cost-cutting strategies. Nurses must counter the tendency of administrators to consider them interchangeable components by expressing their importance as unique individuals with special healing potential that requires opportunity for practice, feedback, and growth.

CHAPTER 21

The Healing Role of the Nurse Leader in Response to Organizational Change

HELEN K. KEE, PHD, RN

Leaders have been known as visionaries, persuaders, strategic planners, and motivators. But they are not typically called healers. This chapter will identify behavioral and functional activities which are the healing aspect of the leader's role, particularly in times of organizational change.

NATURE OF LEADERSHIP

Leadership is the process of persuasion or example by which an individual (or team) induces a group to pursue objectives held by the leader or shared by the leader and his or her followers (Gardner, 1990).

Peters and Austin (1985) describe leadership in more vivid terms— visionary, cheerleading, enthusiasm, love, use of symbols, coaching, creating heroes. They indicate leadership must be present at all levels in the organization. It is a million little things done with obsession, consistency, and care, and superimposed upon trust and beliefs.

Though leaders exist outside of organizations, most persons who assume leadership roles attempt to accomplish their goals within large intricately organized systems. Depending on the state or health of the organization and the external forces that influence it, the leader may experience profoundly stressful times. This is especially so in today's turbulent, ever-changing economically driven healthcare environment. The basic characteristics and roles of leaders are unchanging; however the environment that surrounds the leader has changed from a world that was controlled (or so they thought) to a world of uncertainty and ambiguity (Lucas, 1985).

246

Construct of Healing

The word "heal" is derived from "hal" an English word meaning to make whole. Healing has been defined as the integration of all of humankind in body, mind, and spirit. Primitive people knew intuitively that healing was to make whole (Keegan, 1994).

Healing can occur physically, psychologically, socially, and spiritually. Individual people need to be healed, but, so also do institutions and societies. To make whole—to heal suggests an end, complete, or finished state. But that is not so! Healing is an ongoing process that requires energy and motivation and may, indeed, be one's primary motivation for certain acts and behaviors.

An example of an environment that needed healing was the Barrack Hospital at Scutari, where Florence Nightingale in 1854 found herself with 39 other nurses surrounded by four miles of beds with approximately 4,000 patients enmeshed in filth and disease. Florence improved the sanitary conditions, scrubbed and cleaned the walls and floors, opened windows, and aired the space. Mortality decreased from 60 percent to only 1 percent through her efforts at creating a healing environment (Shealy, 1985).

We as members of specific environments may take advantage of opportunities for our own healing. Greenleaf (1977) in his book *Servant Leadership* cites this example: twelve ministers and theologians of all faiths and twelve psychiatrists of all faiths had convened for a two day, off-the-record seminar on the theme of healing. The chairman, a psychiatrist, opened the seminar with this question: "We are all healers, whether we are ministers or doctors. Why are we in this business? What is our motivation?" There followed only 10 minutes of intense discussion and they were all agreed, doctors and ministers, Catholics, Jews, and Protestants. "For our own healing," they said.

When I worked in a psychiatric institute in Los Angeles many years ago, it was not unusual to hear nursing or medical staff comment (with tongue in cheek) on the belief that the caregivers entered the psychiatric workforce because they, too, needed to be treated—healed.

Organizational Structure

Most of the leadership and much of the healing occurs in healthcare organizations, thus, it behooves us to understand the history of the development of these entities. Organizations in our society were built with the belief held that there was a natural order of events in the world, and that the world and these events could be controlled (Kuhn, 1962). Weber's 1864-1920 (1947) philosophy of organizational structure supported this belief. His organizational characteristics included a hierarchy of authority, division of labor, specialization rules and regulations, impersonality, and rational allocation of various functions. The premise of the Weberian model of organizational structure is that efficiency is better attained through rational control. This structure has come to be viewed as an "iron case": rigid, inflexible, inhuman, and inefficient. Failings that develop within this structure include:

1. An excessive chain of command causing decision making to be slow and tortuous
2. Proliferation of subcultures
3. Maintenance of a turf syndrome that leads to rivalry and conflict development
4. An organization that functions because of informal groups and informal networks as well as informal politics controlled by power brokers (Kotter, Schlessinger, & Sathe, 1979).

Because there are elements in the world that cannot be controlled—that are ambiguous and uncertain—those leadership theories of the past that were predicated on world order with emphasis on control, competition, power wielding, and rationality, are no longer useful. Belasco and Stayer (1993) discuss their old leadership paradigm functioning like a "herd of buffalo." Their leadership role was to plan, organize, command, coordinate, and control. They expected and received supreme loyalty without any initiative or motivation from the people who were just "waiting around to be told what to do." This lack of desire and interest to have people act independently caused changes to be made too slowly and the organization to suffer in the market place. Their new leadership paradigm was to develop the organizations structure and function like a "flock of geese." The employees became a group of responsible, interdependent workers with changing leadership according to projects, and with each employee (goose) accomplishing the objectives of the organization through his or her own efforts as leader or follower.

Despite the growing recognition that organizations must change and adapt to changing societal needs, the organizations continue to retain a legacy of rigidity in their central structure.

Changes Affecting Leadership

Both nationally and internationally, major changes are occurring because of several historic happenings. Some of these are: the dominance of the Japanese market, the electronic revolution, the collapse of communism, the decline of industry, the increase of service economies, and the decline of the birth rate with a concomitant increase in the aging population (Albrecht, 1994).

In healthcare in the United States, major changes in the way government agencies reimburse providers of healthcare has caused a restructuring of healthcare business practices. Healthcare costs have risen exponentially with an advancing belief that we are not getting our money's worth. The prevailing view is that the healthcare institution is no longer an economically neutral institution. These costs are often associated with overbedding, overuse of high technology, a noncompetitive market place, and a high use of entitlements for employees.

Historically, organizations, including those concerned with healthcare, were very stable, slow changing, and predictable. The healthcare industry was unwise in normal business practices, believing there was no need to be skillful in this area, uneconomical, and noncompetitive. However, people knew who they were, what they stood for, and knew the meaning of their lives in the organization where they worked. Now people are being asked to rethink basic values, adapt to new business ways, reinvent processes and let go of the past—downsizing, rightsizing, boundaryless corporations and managed care are all new words that must be incorporated into leadership roles and activities. A pervasive uncertainty about the future of organizations also causes people to question long standing values and priorities in their work world and in society-at-large. The new reality can be frightening and unsettling and human beings cannot function indefinitely in a world that does not have some kind of order and predictability (Albrecht, 1994). Our predictable world has changed to one with a central priority—quality patient care in a cost effective environment! True! There is much wastage, duplication, and overuse, but what are the criteria for the definition of cost effectiveness and who makes those decisions?

Healthcare organizations have historically been institutions of stability and balanced equilibrium with the leadership expected to maintain that equilibrium as well as to maintain the integrity that provided for economic neutrality, noncompetitiveness, recognition as a pillar of society, and a good place to work. Now, there is disequilibrium, a competitive market place, a costly industry exposed to the public eye. Our image is changing! Is healthcare a business with a bottom line to worry about or is it a nonprofit structure that only follows accepted business principles? There is no question the healthcare industry has been wounded. It needs to be healed!

Looking at it another way, perhaps the staid institution of yesteryear no longer meets the needs of today's changing society. Hospitals as a service industry are a good example of technology *not* increasing productivity. Over the century, hospitals have moved from being entirely labor-intensive with little capital investment to supremely capital intensive facilities highly invested in bodyscanners, analyzers and other modern technology. This environment has created the need for more specialized personnel, thus, increasing the total number of people in these institutions. The result: an economic monstrosity causing healthcare costs to soar (Drucker, 1992).

THE HEALING ROLE OF THE LEADER

This changing world has caused turmoil and profound stress for the people working in these institutions. More than ever the leaders in these organizations must work to provide a healing environment during this paradigm shift. An example of a healing approach is illustrated thus. A recently appointed head of a large, important but difficult to administer public institution realized that he was not happy with the way things were going. His approach to the problem was a bit unusual. For three months he stopped reading newspapers and listening to news broadcasts; he relied wholly upon those he met in the course of his work to tell him what was going on. In three months, his administrative problems were solved. By active and intentional listening, a skill we do not use sufficiently, this person learned what he needed to resolve the issues (Greenleaf, 1977).

In addition to listening which is the most important communication skill, the leader must show compassion and empathy and a genuine caring attitude toward the people in the institution. Murphy (1994) discusses a Native American concept "Cangleska Wakan" as the theoretical basis for organizational healing. Cangleska Wakan is described as "the sacred medicine circle, or hoop—a vision of unity arising from complexity. The concept suggests that there is equality among all and that the traditional linear structure does not support organizational healing.

Further, the concept indicates that all group members contribute to the whole. Mobilizing "the whole" toward healing is a process that requires that the leader (a) lead through "strategic humility," characterized by becoming one with the issues, needs, and pressures affecting the group, and to promote a "profound understanding," laying the path for effective change; (b) build heroic partnerships, that are fundamental alliances binding group factions together, creating a stronger entity than the individual parts; and (c) walk in a "sacred" manner, which embodies the "intangible power" or potential for change and improvement.

The changes occurring in healthcare organizations have had a profound effect on employees in terms of productivity, uncertainty, insecurity, and fear of job loss. These conditions of change require "healing." Greenleaf (1977) and Albrecht (1994) have provided insights into the major characteristics of the bureaucratic organizational model. The hierarchy of authority defines the level of control and rationality for each organization while the division of labor breaks institutions down into manageable units with specialized functions in each unit. Both of these characteristics underpin a very controlling and segregated environment. This environment does not lend itself to teamwork, recognition of a common mission and the acceptance that decision making should occur at the lower working levels. The result is a strengthening of the informal culture which prevails in organizations with tight controls because the formality of the organization does not meet the needs of employees in their day-to-day work.

The three characteristics and the rationale for moving from the current bureaucratic model to a more participative model of decision making is shown next. These changes assist in the process of environmental healing.

The role of the leader is to develop a healing environment where goals are clarified and responsibilities are clearly articulated. It is helpful if the leader is seen as a healer to the staff. The characteristics of a

Past-Present	**Rationale**	**Future**
Rigid hierarchy, command authority	Changes in society reflect increase in communication, i.e., media	Encourage creativity of employees
	Change from industrial to information age	Strengthen lower level authority and decision making

Past-Present	Rationale	Future
	Better educated employees, knowledge specialists	Share governance, listen to employees
	Desire for greater autonomy in decision making	Allow expertness of staff to come out in project leadership roles
	Blurring of roles	
Division of labor	Healthcare changes require reinforcement of common mission	Reinstate single goal mentality
	All departments must move in same direction	Develop teams, help people to value results from working together
Informal organizational culture	Numerous cultures in one organization wanting to be heard	Must buy into organizational culture
	Strong societal values, aging, geographic movement	Pay attention to characteristics of the employee group
	Increase in demand for control	Recognize value by organizational culture in decision making

healing leader include the ability to define the mission (vision) set direction, describe reality, and provide resources so that the work of the institution can be accomplished. The leader must move from the command authority mentality that focuses on organizational structure toward a much more diversified thinking process. This can be done by broadening decision making to all levels of employees, particularly that of the lower level management group; increasing communication, especially the skill of listening; and using compassion and empathy when resolving issues with employees. Finally, a healing leader, particularly, in times of uncertainty and change, develops a trusting environment based on consistency and truth telling.

A FINAL CAVEAT

I have stressed the characteristics and roles of the leader as healer. It may be wise, however, to conclude with a cautionary note. Healing an organization as it progresses through the impact of major change is a difficult process. The leader as healer has a significant role in this process, but so also do the other employees in the organization. The leader's role is not infinite; there is a finite end to the leader's role and responsibility. In addition, activities designed to heal an organization cannot be effective if they in any way are in conflict with the leader's ultimate responsibility to uphold and fulfill the mission and objectives of the organization. The leader cannot abrogate these responsibilities, even though, arguably, an overly stressed employee is not a productive employee.

Finally, a healing workplace is often described as one where the staff are empowered to control their own environment. Stated without qualifiers, it becomes an euphemism. Staff do indeed control some of their activities, but do so within the framework of the mission and objectives of the organization. Thus, while employees may decide what hours they wish to work (empowerment), organizational policies and managers determine the number of staff needed per shift, the types of staff persons needed, and the manner in which labor laws will be enforced.

Despite these cautions, the final reality is that both the leaders and the followers have responsibility for the healing function in the organization. Everyone has a role to play in their own healing and in assisting the healing of their fellow workers.

REFERENCES

Albrecht, K. (1994). *The north bound train* (pp. 22–29). New York: American Management Association.

Belasco, J. A., & Stayer, R. C. (1993). *Flight of the buffalo: Soaring to excellence, learning to let employees lead* (pp. 16–18). New York: Warner Books.

Drucker, P. F. (1992). *Managing the future* (pp. 119–123). New York: Penguin.

Gardner, J. W. (1990). *On leadership.* New York: Macmillan.

Greenleaf, R. K. (1977). *Servant leadership* (pp. 7–48). Mahwah, NJ: Paulist Press.

Keegan, L. (1994). *The nurse as healer* (p. 4). New York: Delmar Publications.

Kotter, J. P., Schlesinger, L., & Sathe, V. J. (1979). *Organization: Text, cases and readings on the management of organizational design and change.* Homewood, IL: Richard D. Irwin.

Kuhn, T. S. (1962). *The structure of scientific revolutions.* Chicago: University of Chicago Press.

Lucas, C. (1985). Out at the edge: Notes on a paradigm shift. *Journal of Counseling and Development, 64*(3), 165-172.

Murphy, E. C. (1994). *Forging the heroic organization* (p. 7). Englewood Cliffs, NJ: Prentice Hall.

Peters, T., & Austin, N. (1985). *A passion for excellence* (pp. 5-60). New York: Random House.

Shealy, M. C. (1985). Florence Nightingale 1820-1910, An evolutionary mind in the context of holism. *Journal of Holistic Nursing, 3*(1), 4-6.

Weber, M. (Birthdate 1864-1920). (1947). *The theory of social and economic organization,* A. M. Henderson & Talcott Parsons. (Trans.) New York: Oxford University Press.

CHAPTER 22

Healing: The Loss of a Brother

PRISCILLA W. KOESTER, RN, RNCS, PHD

It was the year of AZT, but Alan was dying. Dying because he just wanted to love and be loved. Stories from his friends as they came to visit me, the newcomer that they had only heard about. Patty, my childhood name, was what they called me, the sister they had never met. I sat in the old Victorian house he now called Greengate, a long plane ride from my home.

It was only a few days since the phone message from his old roommate, Jim. Jim wasn't there when I called back, so I tried my brother's number. Relief, when he answered, but he sounded strange, tired maybe? "I'm trying to get a new drug, but it's not yet released. My friend next door is a pharmacist, and he said he'd help me get it." My mind raced backward to the patient I cared for last week, and the new drug was "AZT?" "Yes," he said, "that's it." An icy cold finger ran down my spine. "Oh, Alan, you have AIDS." Silence, then a soft "yes." "Do you want to come here? We have a specialty hospital." No, he would rather stay with his friends, but I could come see him. He spoke slowly, as though in a dream.

On the plane I had time to remember. Old memories, sunlit streets, and World War II. We ran with the pack. Bobby and Billy and Brad. Hide and Seek or Cowboys and Indians. Shirttails flying with mother's words, "I'll sew lace on that shirttail." Was that why? No, it was not being able to hit a baseball. That's it. It was his eyes. One was lazy, and he wore funny glasses with special black tape patches to strengthen it. That was it. And he ran a little funny; the other boys teased him. Sometimes I beat them up.

When mother returned to teaching kindergarten, we spent afternoons after school arguing. Who would wash the dishes before she came home? Who had to scrub potatoes tonight? One day we constructed a large fantasy about the potato water and its travels to the ocean. But mostly we argued and fought hard, and I was bigger and usually won. Maybe that was it.

High school pictures of Lynn and Alan. She was the minister's daughter. "I'll wait for him. Always," she assured me one evening, but that didn't happen. He went to Europe to study. It didn't bother him he was the first of the family to leave. Eagerly, if haltingly, he learned German while living in a boardinghouse where meat was a luxury. What did those years have to do with this, this disease he has?

He told me he had talked to a psychiatrist once who said he didn't need to tell anyone what it was about. Then he didn't tell me. Was it about being . . . , or was it something else? Sitting in the hospital room, I remembered the conversation. That was after he had been rejected by the draft. They said it was his eyes: his vision was 20/400, but he told us it was an error because they re-tested him right after he took out his contacts. Blinking, was that how they found out? Or was it true, that his eyes kept him from the service?

The cycling of the hypothermia machine brought me back to reality. He was shivering on the cooling blanket. My education tells me that's not good, and I want to turn it off. I hear myself calling the nurse and one nurse is talking to another. The blanket is turned off, and he is dressed again in a white gown. Poor Alan. We bathe him. Helpless, only the little blue and white pills every four hours. Sometimes they are in a cup on the table when I come in at 1. Is this the 2 o'clock dose early or the 10 o'clock dose not yet taken? Do they make a difference anyway? He is incoherent. They are not supposed to leave pills at the bedside, the nurse in me cries. Anyway they don't work unless you take them on time.

The pulmonary specialist comes in, stopping to gown, glove, and mask. Should I be . . . ? I feel suddenly naked in my street clothes, then angry because he knows so little about transmission of this disease, then forgiving because this is their first patient with this disease.

His roommate, John, and I say goodbye to the young, old man in the bed. I give a sisterly kiss and pat, but John hugs him hard. I see there really is a bond. It is true. Too many things unraveling at once—a busy friend trying to paint the Victorian house to get it ready for sale, realtors trying to sell the gaggle of apartment houses partly redone, friends asking if it's true he has AIDS, and his wishes to respect by not telling Dad and our brother. One friend comes to tell me that he went with him for the HIV test a year ago, and he was with him when he found out he was positive. "I watched him give up drinking and then smoking. And he started eating better than he ever had." I match the dates with my father's story of his college reunion when Alan came to accompany him in the parade of graduates from 50 years ago. "He read a book the whole time," Dad complained. "It's like he wasn't there." That was the week he had found out he was positive.

The two weeks went by. My job was on hold, but my wedding anniversary pulled me home to some sanity. It was still happening, but now in another city. Telephone calls to realtors, to doctors, but especially to the nurses, friendly voices of colleagues, who themselves were caring for their first AIDS patient. He wasn't that; he was my brother. The skinny blond with bad eyes who loved music, who hunted for old banisters for his houses and had a cellar full of gingerbread trim, who helped me when I had questions about real estate. One day the call came: "you've got to come back, he's sinking fast."

It was hot in the little front bedroom of his old house with the table someone said was on loan. The fan whirred. Sleep, maybe the house will sell tomorrow, or one of the apartment houses. Call Dad, get him at the airport. Don't tell. "He has a brain infection, Dad." That, at least, was true. Maybe it was the steak tartar one friend said he loved. Call our brother: I can't lie to him, and I tell and say he must come.

Protective numbing sets in. Just take care of things. See the banker. Oh, his life insurance policy is made out to his old roommate, Jim? Well, at least the investors won't get it. Talk to Harold, the old man who had lunched with Alan every week, and who would handle his affairs after . . . . The nurse in me knows the outcome although the friends are all hoping for a miracle. AZT, is it working? They're giving him blood today, and TPN, all these special things. Click, click, the machine counts out the TPN. Has he gained any weight?

After telling me that he had signed off on the insurance policy, Jim is avoiding me. The friends are busy—selling houses, going to school, appraising art, doing what people do when someone else is there for their friend. So I spend hours waiting to show the house to potential buyers, telling out-of-town family that we are doing all we can, but it doesn't look good. A long silent cousin calls, "I hear that Alan Lee is sick." "Yes." By then I can't keep the secret, "but don't tell my Dad, he'll never understand." My uncle, the doctor, assures me, "He won't hear it from me."

We arrived at the hospital one summer evening and decided to take him outside for the first time in two months. His friend is strong and lifts him to the chair. TPN swinging from an I.V. pole and his limp body propped up in an orthopedic chair with pillows, we made our way through many doors to the starlit park in front of the hospital. Who are we doing this for—him or us? He breathed the warm evening air, and thanked us.

Once his friends brought his dog in a basket, bathed and brushed to protect him from other infections. Later they sent a picture of his Yorkie commandeering Alan's realty desk. I called funeral homes between faculty meetings and arranged for cremation. Loose ends, a will to be rewritten by his lawyer friend, a brother to be consoled. The lawyer calls, "I'm sorry, there's nothing I can do. He's too ill to sign it."

What has prepared me for this? I had called Alan when my son was hospitalized. "You sound sleepy," but he was already asleep. He roused, but we couldn't talk. "So I'll call you later." I wanted him to tell *me* that everything was okay, but *he* wasn't okay. That was years ago, before I knew.

There was a family reunion organized by my brother a year ago, but Alan hadn't come because he had a sore throat that wouldn't heal. After an afternoon on the lake, while my sister-in-law and I drove back to their house, she asked "Do you think Alan is gay?" "I never really thought about it, but does it matter?" Now I remember those words and yes, it does matter.

My friends call. It isn't over. One friend calls and as she begins to hang up, I tell her "Don't go, I need to talk to someone." She stays on the line and we recall good times, even though she never knew my brother.

The Sunday afternoon telephone call that he was going brought people to our house. My German friend Elisabeth cleaned everything, so we could leave it nice for our teenagers. Another friend helped my husband put new brakes on the car we would drive north. Our two dogs followed me around and watched with their large brown eyes whenever I sat. Long after midnight the call came from the night nurse. And then Jim, "He's gone, he looks so peaceful." "I'm so sorry," I tell him. "He was a good brother," my husband reminded me.

Black suits, black ties, young men. The church was filled with them. Navy silk, navy suit, Alan would have liked that. Strange not to have Dad, but he was too worn to travel. The words were spoken by his good friends, who knew him, rather than the minister at the old church with stained glass windows which shared a parking lot with one of Alan's houses. Alan had installed a large fan in the ceiling of the church balcony after a parking lot conversation with the minister; that was their connection. Outside beside the huge stone columns, my brother grasped me, weeping so I had to hold his usually sturdy frame. "We'll pull through this," I told him." "You're always so strong," he tells me.

I don't feel strong as I let my husband drive us across three states to take the ashes to Dad's and then back three hours to the family cemetery for burial. The large yellow wreath sits lonely in the October sun. "We just thought there should be a little color," my aunt tells me, and there another minister who never knew him speaks of healing.

Home again, and the Monday–Tuesday–Wednesday–Thursday–Fridayness of my life numbs me. Speak to a class about AIDS? Sure. In room 103 I tell them about the child I nursed during the summer. That was so unfair, that a healing blood transfusion would contain HIV. And it was cruel for this disease to rob me of my brother, but I don't say so.

Thanksgiving and Dad came to visit, alone, without Alan. Last Thanksgiving Alan and I had taken Dad to buy a suit for Christmas. He wears it this year and is so proud, and I realize how frail he has become in a few months. We talk long hours about things that matter. He is worried about our daughter's work in a science laboratory because she might get AIDS. He doesn't know why Alan died, but he doesn't ask, and I don't tell him. Telling won't bring Alan back.

Alan's friend Bill calls to say that he has made arrangements for a tree to be planted in the local park in memory of Alan. "It has to be the biggest and strongest oak of all." Funds are raised and we go to the dedication the next summer. It is Festival Weekend, and many of his friends come in jeans and workclothes as they put the finishing touches on their yards. A trio of white birches is dedicated at the entrance of the park where all can see, birches like the ones in his old front yard. In the absence of the friend expected to speak, I am asked to say a few words. I hear myself telling of the kindness of friends I had not met before Alan's illness and the love they showed my brother in his adopted city, especially while he was ill. I tell of the generosity of people who housed me, loaned me cars, picked me up at the airport, and finally made these trees and the plaque possible. I recall the few ashes we left the previous fall in a small wooden box to be placed under the plaque. We share stories in the twilight.

Letting go of a brother is much harder than saying goodbye to a parent. He had no right to leave us. I depended on him, he was always there. There isn't anyone now who knows the story and will laugh when I mention potato water. Yet every year on Alan's birthday, my younger brother calls and we visit. And year by year, we are healing.

Epilogue

I wrote this story in a rush of inspiration one morning. It was time to tell the story. Revisiting the summer of '87 was like unlocking an unused room. Healing is embedded in the events preceding the horror of the loss of my brother. My nursing background prepared me for this event. My nursing students had cared for patients with AIDS for several years. But it was my assignment as a contract nurse to a person with AIDS, and the arrival of AZT in her home the previous week that made me aware of the new drug. So I knew the medicine my brother was waiting to get, and I knew why.

In the light of nine years when AZT is offered to HIV-positive patients (and often refused), it is hard to recall the excitement in those of us working with AIDS patients when AZT was released to the public. As the first drug to affect the human immunodeficiency virus directly, AZT was expected to change the course of AIDS. This story took place just two months after the Food and Drug Administration (FDA) approval when the medication was in such short supply that only very seriously ill AIDS patients could receive it. It was released to patients only upon approval of an application to the FDA. This was the process that the pharmacist neighbor stood ready to assist. Nine years later and with more experience with HIV and AIDS, we now have many other therapies, some medical and others self-designed. Some of these my brother explored such as not drinking or smoking and improving his diet. I have tried to keep the focus on the relationship I had with my brother and with the growing awareness of the seriousness of his illness. He had refused medical care for many months for various sore throats and increasingly obvious neurological problems. For example, one friend watched him spend fifteen minutes trying to close the car door. As a nurse, I wondered if earlier medical care would have made a difference given that there was no treatment for HIV or AIDS. Perhaps some of the opportunistic infections could have been successfully treated and made him more comfortable in his last year. Above all, Alan wanted privacy, so he hesitated to tell his friend, the doctor, about his illness. And thus, I found him hospitalized in the late stages of AIDS.

The nurses were kind and much more willing to discuss his progress with me on the long distance phone than I would have been in a similar position. They spent time with me and really supported my healing process before his death. It was a new night nurse who made the last call, and she could not have been more gentle. Alan would have approved. He was a gentle person, who had a hard time refusing anybody anything. He loved old things, old people, and symphonies.

The memories of many years of sharing our lives prepared me, and have helped in the healing process. We have had no contact with the childhood friends, but the fact that our present friends knew Alan and cared about him when he was ill has helped put his ashes to rest.

You think you will have your brothers and sisters all around you when you are growing older. It isn't that way. We make new families; some are our own, some are constructed of friends who become close as family, and we write new stories that become old. But fewer people know the old, old stories.

CHAPTER 23

Empowerment: A Factor in Healing

PATRICIA DAVIS GILMORE, RN, MSN, JD

Traditionally, nursing is characterized as one dimensional, as focusing on its affective domain of caring and empathy toward others. This traditional characterization of nursing, however, is a two-edged sword. It brings forth an immediate and powerful image of a health provider whose caring and empathy meets the needs of others. Yet, the reverse is also characteristic of nursing, as it has been seen: that nurses are powerless in the overall healthcare domain. Over time, the unstated philosophy that we nurses seem to have developed is that "if we take care of others, then someone will take care of us." This has not occurred. No one, no organization, nor other professions will give us what we need to empower ourselves. We must do it for ourselves and for our profession. Therefore, the purposes of this chapter are to: (1) briefly describe the impact that traditional characterization of nursing has had on nurses, (2) address the role that empowerment has in healing nurses, and (3) discuss how nurses can be empowered while retaining the positive characterization of nursing.

THE IMPACT THAT TRADITIONAL CHARACTERIZATION HAS HAD ON NURSES

A "good" nurse who overtly displays the traditional characteristics of nursing, caring, and empathy, is given high praise from both clients and coworkers. Further encouragement is provided by employers who have been known to reward "good" nurses with raises and promotions based on these attributes. One survey (Koska, 1989) revealed that hospital CEOs ranked nursing care as one of the three most significant factors in 97.3 percent of all responses. This "good nurse" feature has reinforced these behaviors over time. The nurse adopts the caring role (often described as altruism) when she does things for patients, or when she protects them from harm or from unnecessary worry (Malin & Teasdale, 1991). The caring that nurses tend to expect for themselves in their job situations is closely related to this same principle of altruism which implies that someone or something else has the responsibility of caring for the nurse. We have continuously expected and accepted this paternalistic-type relationship between employer and employee.

Paternalism implies that one person is perceived to be dependent or helpless in order to receive benevolence from another. When we perceive that in our caring for others, we are not being cared for, we will: (1) try harder, giving more of self; (2) become less caring and possibly bitter in the process; (3) stay on the present job and do the minimum of the job requirements; and/or (4) seek nursing employment somewhere else. Nurses change their positions or stay where they are because of the perception of powerlessness, a condition of being weak or unable to produce any effect (Webster, 1983).

The Disempowered Nurse

Powerlessness brings forth an image of nurses as conformists; that is, we adapt to each situation or crisis as it presents itself. More often than not, we act after the fact, rather than anticipating an outcome and preparing a strategy either for its prevention or for command over it. The characteristic of conformity can initially be blamed on childhood experiences, but later developmental influences, such as the nursing training system that rewards conformity and discourages creativity, can be equally disempowering (Chavasse, 1992). As conformists, when faced with making decisions, we tend to choose the ones associated with the least risk or challenge. Hence, in some instances, we are powerless because we choose not to be powerful. Further, our powerlessness is generally enforced through the systems in which we work. We are told and encouraged to care for the client, and, for the great majority of us, this involves only the caring dimension of nursing.

Caring is described as a process (Wolf, Giardino, Osborne, & Ambrose, 1994) with five dimensions: (1) Respectful deference to the other that incorporates a courteous regard for the other; (2) assurance of human presence that reflects an investment in the other's needs and security; (3) positive connectedness that indicates an optimistic and constant readiness on the part of the nurse to help the other; (4) professional knowledge and skill that indicates nurse caring as proficient, informed, and skillful;

and (5) attentive to other's experience that incorporates an appreciation of and engrossment in the other's perspective and experience.

Though the Wolf model is considered multidimensional, caring remains only one, albeit important facet of nursing. If we are to empower ourselves and the nursing profession, we must be willing to struggle to share the control over issues with other healthcare entities. These issues include, but are not limited to, the control over resources, the definitions of what health is, and how to implement health-enhancing policies and actions (Skelton, 1994).

One-dimensional nursing which has worked for nurses in the past will not carry us through the present, nor into the future. We can no longer afford to emphasize only one facet of our profession. Being a "good nurse," who cares and empathizes with others, is no longer good enough. This traditional characterization of nursing continues to earn us a pat on the head, but it also continues to render us powerless.

HEALING THE HEALER

How can we overcome powerlessness of nursing? The answer begins with the concepts of healing and empowerment. Healing has been defined as "causing an undesirable condition to be overcome" (Webster's New Collegiate Dictionary, 1983). The healing process is not passive; it is an action-driven endeavor. To begin healing, we must first do a thorough, unbiased self-scrutiny. After doing this, we should be able to identify the undesirable condition in our nursing practice, if one exists. We must then develop a strategy or strategies to overcome the undesirable condition. Implementation of the strategy or strategies is a vital part of the healing process, for without it, no healing will take place. During the implementation phase, continuous assessment and re-assessment should occur. The desired outcome is the alleviation or lessening of the undesirable condition.

The term *empowerment* implies solutions rather than problems; overcoming rather than succumbing; building up rather than tearing down. As Kieffer (1984) so aptly stated, "empowerment addresses people's strengths, rights and abilities rather than deficits and needs" (p. 34). A proposed redefinition (Gibson, 1991) of empowerment is that it is "a social process of recognizing, promoting and enhancing people's abilities to meet their own needs, solve their own problems and mobilize the necessary resources in order to feel in control of their own lives" (p. 359). This is done within our own context; thus we are liberated to empower those whom we serve (Chavasse, 1992, p. 2). To begin the process of healing, we must first become empowered by addressing our own strengths, rights, and abilities. Studying nurses who are considered empowered is helpful because it gives a barometer of measurement for empowerment.

Attributes of Empowered Nurses

I have studied nurses whom I considered empowered and found that these nurses had many attributes that helped to explain their various states of empowerment. These nurses also shared several common attributes: active professional nursing involvement and collaboration with their colleagues that extended to members of other professions; demonstrated networking skills; recognized competence in their area of specialty; perceived autonomy; and an aura of high self-esteem. The positive characteristics of nursing remained. Their shared perception was that they determined whether they were empowered or not. Acting on this premise, they actively sought paths that have led to successful careers in nursing.

Self-Scrutiny

Several years ago, in my own efforts to overcome powerlessness, I inventoried the attributes I already possessed as a nurse educator with an advanced degree in maternal-child nursing. Involvement in my professional nursing networking skills, collaboration with other healthcare professionals (which did not always extend to other professions), recognized competency in pediatric nursing, some autonomy, and a reasonable measure of self-esteem all contributed at least to a semblance of empowerment.

As a nurse educator, I had also contributed to the increased number of nurses practicing in the local area. As I talked with practicing nurses, however, I discovered that my teaching alone was insufficient to make a difference in the state of nursing. Any influence that I could possibly have was only extended to new graduate nurses. Furthermore, these nurses, once in practice over a period of time, had developed some of the same one-dimensional characterizations of nurses who had been in practice over a number of years. They were considered "good nurses" albeit with little or no autonomy within their employment environment. They talked of being stifled by the confines of the job, and thus began to develop other characteristic behaviors. They were eventually trying harder, giving more of self, becoming less caring and possibly bitter in the process, staying on at their present job by doing the minimum, or seeking nursing employment elsewhere. Such observations again led me to reflect upon myself. I had helped in contributing to the increased number of nurses locally, but I had not made a difference in the state of nursing.

Although I felt some degree of autonomy, I also felt that my contribution to nursing was not what it should be at this point in my career. At the same time, I became certified in Advanced Cardiac Life Support (ACLS) and Emergency Room nursing through a course known as the Trauma Nurse Core Course (TNCC). Thereafter, I obtained a position in a local hospital emergency room, first as a staff nurse and later as the ER education coordinator. Though this time was exciting and afforded me another side of clinical nursing that I had not previously possessed, there remained a missing intangible element in my career. Being "good" at what I was doing and caring for clients in the emergency room was still not enough.

The Identification of the Undesired Condition

One day, during a particularly pungent emergency situation, the missing element in my career became exceedingly clear to me. A patient had been flown in by helicopter to the hospital. After being taken to the trauma room, he fell from a gurney onto a tiled concrete floor. This incident occurred after the patient had been examined by a physician who had left the side rail down. The physician later accused the nurse, who had not been with the physician during the examination, of not putting the side rail up. This nurse's job was in jeopardy because she had not attended to the physician's duty of safety toward this patient.

While the nurse is safeguarding the physician's practice, who safeguards the nurse's practice? I could not readily answer that question. However, I had finally identified the missing intangible element of my assessment and re-evaluation of my career. The process of healing had begun for me with this identification. I realized that though caring and empathy are important to the practice of nursing, they are not enough to sustain a career in nursing. I needed to know more about the influences on nursing, both internally and externally. I felt somewhat knowledgeable about the internal influences. However, I was not certain of the external influences on nursing.

The Beginning of Self-Healing: Implementation

I determined that obtaining a legal degree and combining that knowledge with my nursing would help me to identify the external influences and to clarify the internal influences on nursing practice. I made immediate plans to attend law school. I started law school within nine months of my plans. I maintained my state nursing association professional membership during this period to keep abreast of nursing developments. I clerked with a law firm that handled medical malpractice lawsuits. I attended medical legal seminars when the opportunities arose. Further, I became a student member of The American Association of Nurse Attorneys (TAANA).

After law school graduation and upon attaining my law license, I resumed and increased my participation in nursing organizations. I was elected to the Council on Practice through my state nursing association. I kept abreast of recommended changes and amendments to the state nursing practice act. I collaborated with other professional colleagues, both in and out of nursing. I became an active member of TAANA on the national and local levels.

I continue to attend legal and nursing seminars when the opportunities present themselves. I have presented at numerous seminars on legal issues and implications in nursing practice to practicing nurses, in a variety of settings, as well as to nursing faculty and nursing students. I teach courses on ethical/legal issues or present topics in specific nursing areas to various classes, both on campus and off campus. In addition, my law practice is largely focused on nurse-related issues. I counsel nurses prior to and after peer review hearings, and I also represent nurses before the state board of nurse examiners for allegations of nursing practice violations.

Accomplishment: Empowerment

Empowerment (Kramer & Schmalenberg, 1993) is feeling that one is enabled to act. In the process of obtaining a legal degree, I became aware that social, political, economic, and demographic conditions were part of the overall structure and functional interrelations, not only of nursing, but of the entire healthcare system. Knowledge of these issues contributed toward my healing and empowerment. I have integrated them into my dual practice areas—nursing education and law—to benefit my students, my clients, and myself. As Chally (1992) notes, the teacher and students (and other nurses) come together and subsequently empower each other toward the actualization of a shared vision of knowledge. Empowerment and the positive characteristics of nursing are not incompatible. Several authors (Chally, Kramer, and Malin) have had little difficulty in characterizing empowerment through teaching/learning with caring, nurturing, growth, support, and a recognition of the humanity of both teacher and students (nurse and patients). This is important because when we explore an additional facet of the empowerment process, we must talk about the struggle to share control over issues in the healthcare system. Caring for ourselves, our profession, and our clients thus extends into the regulatory arena because it affects nursing practice. Our understanding of regulatory processes provides us with the knowledge necessary to affect the future of nursing and to protect nursing practice (Oxhorn & Rosen, 1992) which invariably affects our clients.

As nurses become more empowered, we become more actualized in a shared vision. During the healing process, nurses learn to practice the profession in many dimensions. We learn and acknowledge that empowerment is not antagonistic to caring, but is harmonious with it. The two concepts contribute greatly to the healing process of nurses.

REFERENCES

Chally, P. (1992). Empowerment through teaching. *Journal of Nursing Education, 31*(3), 117-120.

Chavasse, J. (1992). New dimensions of empowerment in nursing and challenges. *Journal of Advanced Nursing, 17,* 1-2.

Gibson, C. (1991). A concept analysis of empowerment. *Journal of Advanced Nursing, 16,* 354-361.

Kieffer, C. (1984). Citizen empowerment: Prevention in human services. *Prevention in Human Services, 3,* 9-36.

Koska, M. (1989). Quality—thy name is nursing care, CEOs say. *Hospitals, 32.*

Kramer, M., & Schmalenberg, C. (1993). Learning from success: Autonomy and empowerment. *Nursing Management, 24,* 58-64.

Malin, N., & Teasdale, K. (1991). Caring versus empowerment: Considerations for nursing practice. *Journal of Advanced Nursing, 16,* 657-662.

Oxhorn, V., & Rosen, S. (1992). Legislation: Understanding the regulatory arena. *AORN Journal, 55*(2), 623-629.

Skelton, R. (1994). Nursing and empowerment: Concepts and strategies. *Journal of Advanced Nursing, 19,* 415-423.

Wolf, Z. R., Giardino, E. R., Osborne, P. A., & Ambrose, S. (1994). Dimensions of nurse caring. *Image: Journal of Nursing Scholarship, 26*(2), 107-111.

Chapter 24

Healing Through the Eyes of a Child

HARRIETT L. RIGGS, PHD, RN, CPNP

Healing comes in various forms and in the strangest places, sometimes at the most unexpected time and place. I once found it in a situation outside of the usual hospital setting when a child's healing also healed me.

One Sunday I was substituting for one of the regular teachers in a kindergarten Sunday school class. The class, that day, dealt with children of Bible days, especially during the days when Jesus was a child. The children saw pictures of houses, trees, schools, and clothes, all typical of the day. A story was then read to the children about a typical day in the life of a five-year-old during the time when Jesus was a boy.

The children were then given crayons and paper and asked to draw a picture of the children during the days of Jesus. The children busily began their art work. All trees were apple trees and the houses resembled houses of the twentieth century. Each child was drawing the familiar. At first, each teacher attempted to correct the children, "No, no, not an apple tree but an olive tree." "The houses had flat roofs." "They didn't have TVs or bicycles."

Since I was the "new teacher on the block," I kept quiet, sat at the table, and watched the children in their undertakings. One pretty little girl, dressed in her Sunday-best, came up to me to show me her picture. Initially, I too wanted to comment on the red apples in the tree, but thought the better of it. The child in the picture was hiding behind a tree with only a portion of his body showing. It was also evident that the initial drawing was of a boy with a happy face, but the smile had been changed to a frown, almost a cry face. Something told me to be quiet.

The little girl whispered in my ear in a muffled voice, "Jesus's daddy doesn't like him." My first inclination was to respond quickly, "Of course not. Jesus's daddy loved him very much." But again, something told me to remain unruffled. The child left my side and returned to her drawing. In a few minutes, she again appeared and whispered in my ear, "Do you want to know why Jesus's daddy doesn't like him?" By now my curiosity surged. I quietly replied, "Yes, I would like to know why his daddy doesn't like him." But she turned away again, returned briefly to her work. Soon I heard a whisper for my ear alone, "He said a bad word."

Now I began to understand. The child was relating her own hurtful experience. As I sat quietly, pondering over what the child had told me and my role in the situation, she again appeared and whispered in my ear, "Do you want to know what he said?" "If you want to tell me," I replied.

The girl now returned to play with the other children and participate in the group activities. I was busy assisting the other teachers, when she pulled me aside and quietly whispered, "He said damn."

Sunday school was over and parents began to arrive for their children. Suddenly, my little friend looked up, gave a big grin, turned toward a man approaching her, said "Daddy" and happily ran into the outstretched arms of a smiling, warm father. She then turned around, smiled at me, handed me her picture of Jesus as a boy, and walked off, hand-in-hand with a loving father.

As the years have passed, I have often reflected on that Sunday morning. Her simple, childish picture is preserved among the treasures from my professional career as a reminder of the fragility of relationships and the resulting joy in their preservation.

CHAPTER 25

Four Poems along a Path of Healing

PHYLLIS BECK KRITEK, RN, PHD, FAAN

natural

she was the moment point
of the curve in the lightest breeze
she was the blue light burning
at the base of a candle flame,
that which never dances;
she was the cradling hollow of a lake wave
where ducks and things, fully present,
could for just an instant
become invisible; she was a rock:
she seemed totally natural.
And so we learned her,
enveloping our lives as she did
with elemental energy,
and, fearing an exam, unannounced
at some later date,
we memorized her
by heart.

vigil

Barefoot and disheveled in fine crystalline snow,
a small girl stubborns on the walkway,
staring down the house with boarded windows,
bolted doors and fright.

Filmy light knives cut fog paths through the night,
the hapless boarding fails,
and gelatinous music moans beneath
the half hung door.

Sounds of war are glistening in this house,
beating like maniac bands
on old odd pots and pans.

Spirit waifs float from attic vents, the chimney;
thick blood bubbles from cellar window wells,
deep crimson.

This is a warrior dance,
and the cold silent girl
watches alone.

clay

If dazed pottery could move
it would creep on clay belly
as i, from this capricious kiln;

if glazed pottery could see
it would blink bewilderment
as i, at the firing process;

chemically altered by heat,
some fool's aesthetic statement,
some clown's functional tool;

finished, yet ripening for weeks
into the nature of pottery:
holding things well.

Departure Monologue

Be clear. And as
you take your leave
of all these passions
(fantasized and real),
be clear that you are
just as surely now
alone as any certain
star that sets its
fire in the sky to
be, become, burn out,
with only arms of
silent night for lover,
silent hope. Be clear.

CHAPTER 26

The Potential Effect of a Healing Philosophy on the Educational Environment of Undergraduate Nursing Students

VIRGINIA RAHR, RN, MSN, EDD

What are the ramifications and potential effects of a "healing philosophy" on the education of undergraduate nursing students? What differences might occur in their learning environments? How might their practice of nursing be affected? What changes in faculty roles might be needed? In this chapter I will explore some of the potential effects that a healing philosophy might have on an undergraduate nursing program.

HEALING, CARE, AND CURE

Healing is a familiar term to health professionals, and yet the definitions and connotations ascribed to healing vary greatly. Some health professionals view healing primarily as a physical process, as in the healing of a surgical wound or fractured bone. Other practitioners view healing in a broader sense, but a truly holistic view, encompassing all aspects of the human being, is often considered an ideal that is seldom a realistic possibility in actual healthcare.

The word "healing" is derived from "heal," an old English word meaning "whole." "Wholeness" reflects the definition that we have chosen for healing. "Healing . . . refers to the interactive process that emerges when patients within a specified health context seek the expertise of the professional nurse to facilitate progression toward a desired "wholeness" (Kritek, 1994, p. 2). The phrase "desired wholeness" is important because it clarifies that there is a "mutuality of purpose" in the nurse-patient/client interaction. The faculty have predicated the doctoral program of study on the conviction that ". . . a state of 'wholeness' is a human good, and that assisting others toward this good is an activity of worth" (p. 2).

Quinn (1989) describes wholeness as encompassing much more than the body's physical structure and function. She emphasizes that harmony of the body, mind, and spirit are essential to healing and wholeness. While it seems that this concept should be common knowledge, all too frequently it is not put into practice. The current emphasis on efficiency and cost containment is likely to further jeopardize the less tangible "mind and spirit" aspects of healthcare, unless we keep firmly grounded in a philosophy of wholeness.

Watson (1993a) cautions that "the caring and healing arts as critical dimensions of nursing have been getting lost in the science model" (p. 19). Watson is not advocating that we reject the science and technology that is now so vital to healthcare, but that a better balance be restored. With a similar view, Smerke (1990), speaking in reference to critical care nursing, emphasizes that advancing technology must be linked with a strong model of human caring and also advocates a better balance between the "curing" forces of technology and healing.

With our conviction that an individual's progress toward wholeness is a worthy pursuit, it becomes very clear that nursing assessments and interventions must include all dimensions of human need: physical, psychological, emotional, social, and spiritual. However, a number of questions presented themselves in my reflections on the potential impact of a pervasive healing philosophy: How are "healing" and "caring" related? Are they congruent and complementary, or are there salient differences in the two concepts? And what about "curing?" Is the traditional dichotomy between "care" and "cure" (with nursing's focus on care and medicine's on cure) a useful or divisive distinction?

Care and healing seem to be entirely congruent, although healing may be viewed as the goal and caring as an essential attribute of the one who is facilitating the healing process. According to Watson, (1993b) "it is the voice of care that attends to wholeness, relation, integrity, comfort, meaning, dignity, self-care, alleviation of vulnerability, mind-body-spirit healing" (p. 10). The traditional view of "cure" is the eradication of a known pathology and is most often seen as the purview of physicians. However, some definitions view cure in a broader sense.

Mosby (1994) defines cure as "restoration to health of a person afflicted with a disease or other disorder; the favorable outcome of the treatment of a disease or other disorder" and as "a course of therapy, a medication, a therapeutic measure, or another remedy used in treatment of a medical problem" (p. 422).

These definitions indicate that healing and cure can be congruent; however, our definition of healing does not require a restoration of physical health. Individuals who are terminally ill may achieve their "desired wholeness" and therefore experience profound healing even though their physical disease was not cured.

Leftwich (1993) contends that there need be no controversy among healthcare providers regarding whose role it is to care, cure, or heal. He emphasizes that care, cure, and healing are not mutually exclusive foci of practice. Nurses and other healthcare providers may engage in all three, although the predominant focus may change from patient to patient or in different contexts of practice. This means that nurses are free to cure as well as to care and to heal and physicians are at liberty to care and to heal as well as to cure.

For purposes of the present discussion, let us accept healthcare as described by Bishop and Scudder (1990) (as cited in Leftwich, 1993), as "essentially a caring relationship concerned with the curing of illness when possible and supporting and assisting those who must live with or die from terminal illness. If cure is not possible, healthcare is concerned with supporting, comforting, and aiding those who must live with or die from illness" (pp. 14-15). Leftwich contends that "since nursing engages in care and healing, and care and healing are integral to cure, it can be concluded that cure is a function of nursing" (p. 15).

The point of this discussion about care, cure, and healing is that I believe that ascribing one or another of these essential components of healthcare to a designated healthcare provider, but not to all healthcare providers, may be detrimental to patient care. However, with the inclusion of healing, care and cure in the nurse's role, critics might argue that the healing focus of nursing can be diluted or lost. Indeed, this could happen and undoubtedly has in many instances. Awareness of the varied but complementary roles that nursing can take may actually free the nurse to engage in healing care. Freeing nurses and other healthcare providers from having a sense of failure when the physical body of the patient cannot be cured might liberate energy for creative approaches for healing. Healing can and should be the predominant feature in all types of healthcare.

Why, then, is so much of our healthcare fragmented and why does it not result in wholeness, comfort, dignity, and self-empowerment for so many of our patients? This problem is complex, and perhaps no one has the complete answer. However, I believe that we can make inroads to providing healing (wholeness) for our patients if we teach new practitioners, by actions more than by words, the importance of healing in our practice.

The differences that we would see in healthcare if healing truly was a major construct in our care is that our patients would never feel a loss of hope or dignity. They would feel respected and listened to, and they would perceive themselves in partnership with their healthcare providers. Patients would feel as free to voice psychological, emotional, and spiritual concerns as they do physical signs and symptoms.

Healing is needed most for those patients whose illness, disability, or suffering is not amenable to "cure" (in the traditional sense) by medical science or technology. These include individuals who are chronically or terminally ill, and those who are perceiving a loss of significant meaning in their lives. Healing is also a dire need for vulnerable families, groups, and communities who have few material resources or opportunities and limited education. Creating a healing effect in a community would indeed be a challenge, but not an insurmountable one.

INFLUENCE OF HEALING PHILOSOPHY ON TEACHING AND LEARNING

Very early in our undergraduate nursing students' professional studies they are introduced to pathophysiological concepts. These concepts focus primarily on physiological changes resulting from a disease or other pathology. This knowledge and understanding is very important to the students' application of nursing care principles. However, understanding pathology does not necessarily foster an understanding and appreciation of the illness experience of the individual. Benner and Wrubel (1989) differentiate disease from illness by stating that disease "refers to a taxonomy which designates the manifestation of aberration at the cellular, tissue, or organ level rather than the lived experience of illness" (p. 8). Illness refers to the personal experiences and perceptions of an individual, and these can be known only through a mutual relationship with that individual.

Teaching about illness and the "lived experience" is, in many ways, more difficult than teaching the concepts related to pathology and disease. An example will illustrate this difference. A 91-year-old woman, widowed for about ten years, lives alone in her small, comfortable home. She has several medical diagnoses: hypertension, diverticulosis, prolapse of the bladder, cerebrovascular insufficiency, hearing loss, arthritis. However, her daily experiences focus on her relationships with people and her faith in God. She complies with her medical treatment plan, which includes taking several medications and increasing fiber in her diet. She wears a hearing aid so that she can hear and communicate better. Recently, she has started drinking a "Chinese tea" that a neighbor recommended. She says that it has made her stronger and has helped her bladder problems.

During a monthly home visit by a nurse, Mrs. L.'s first words were, "Oh, I am so glad you're here. My television is not getting my channel and I am just lost without it. I don't know what to do. Can you help me?" Mrs. L.'s face was distraught and her hand movements showed great nervousness.

An unusual request for a nurse's assistance? With a bit of further investigation (assessment), the nurse discovered that Mrs. L. daily watches a special Catholic television channel. Participating in Mass and other prayers via television are the most important parts of Mrs. L.'s day. A call to the local cable company revealed that Mrs. L.'s payment for the special channel had not been received and therefore the channel had been disconnected. Mrs. L. had forgotten to mail the payment. Indeed, it was still in the mailbox on the kitchen table. After another quick call to the cable company by the nurse, Mrs. L. was assured that the channel would be reconnected that same day. Mrs. L. smiled through her tears and told the nurse that she felt restored. She said, "I can handle all my little troubles now . . . they all seem so much smaller. Thank you for helping me."

The nurse did not intervene directly with a disease process here, but she did wonders for the patient's lived experience. She assisted the patient in restoring one of her most important personal supports and in restoring a bit of wholeness or healing to her daily life. We could think about the effects of stress on an elderly person's physiological and psychosocial functioning if we needed to in order to justify this somewhat unusual nursing intervention. We could also envision a breakdown in the ability of an elderly person's ability to maintain independent functioning if her usual support mechanisms were absent. Without a holistic view, one might even conclude that Mrs. L.'s cerebrovascular insufficiency was worsening and that she should no longer be allowed to live alone. After all, wasn't she forgetting some things and overreacting to an everyday problem?

Healing includes any intervention that assists an individual to maintain or strengthen his or her coping abilities, self-esteem, self-care, and comfort and that promotes the individual's attainment of "desired wholeness." This is what we are challenged to teach our undergraduate students, along with the knowledge and understanding of pathology, pharmacology, and other scientific principles. Accomplishing this requires a special teaching and learning environment, in addition to a widely subscribed philosophy of healing by faculty.

RELATIONSHIPS BETWEEN STUDENTS AND FACULTY IN A HEALING ENVIRONMENT

Healing is never completely a "finished product," since perfect wholeness is rarely, if ever, achieved. (Perhaps it comes to some at the time of their death.) Healing is rather a desired destination or goal. It might be viewed as a "work in progress."

In a healing environment, faculty's relationship with students, then, can also appropriately be conceptualized as a developmental process, with the potential for mutual growth. Faculty who truly believe that healing is a worthwhile pursuit, and that the basic philosophy of healing can be taught, and learned, will strive to create an environment conducive to self-healing and healing of others.

The following are salient features of a healing environment in a school of nursing:

1. Mutual respect and trust between faculty and students.
2. Appreciation of the unique contributions of each individual, inclusive of faculty and students.
3. High standards for competence and integrity, for both students and faculty.
4. Clearly defined and communicated expectations and philosophical beliefs and values.
5. The willingness and ability to hear differing points of view and to criticize or disagree in a humanistic and constructive manner.

The teaching and learning environment described above will be most likely to flourish in an organizational climate that promotes healing.

Organizational Climate and Healing

The organizational climate must be supportive of a healing environment in order for a significant difference to occur in the outcome measures of student education and practice. One of the salient features of a healing environment resides in the quality of the relationships between and among faculty and administrators. The relationships must include mutual trust, respect, colleagueship, and professionalism. Just as the core of nurse/patient interactions is dependent on a mutual relationship, so too the quality of the organizational climate is highly dependent on the relationships between and among faculty and administrators.

Brown (1991) describes "healing through empowering" in an article that relates to nursing service administration. The key features that Brown describes are "authentic caring," which I see as being very closely related to our definition of healing and empowerment. Brown contrasts authentic caring to caretaking, wherein there are clear superior-subordinate relationships, and in which the ultimate power and authority rests with the superior. Caretaking may be very benevolent, even "motherly" and protective, but it is, by nature, also controlling. Because significant decisions are made at the top of the hierarchy, it does not encourage empowerment of the "rank and file."

In a school of nursing, authentic caring is operationalized, in part, through empowering individuals at all levels within the organization. Characteristics of empowerment within an organization include mutual ownership of problems as well as solutions and achievements. Mutual trust and respect are highly valued commodities. In order for healing to be taught, learned, valued, and practiced, such an environment is required.

REFERENCES

Brown, C. L. (1991). *Caring in nursing administration: healing through empowering.* NLN Press.

Benner, P., & Wrubel, J. (1989). *The primacy of caring: Stress and coping in health and disease.* Menlo Park, CA: Addison-Wesley.

Kritek, P. (1994). *Healing: A central nursing construct.* A UTMB School of Nursing Doctoral Program White Paper.

Leftwich, R. E. (1993). Care and cure as healing processes in nursing. *Nursing Forum, 28*(3), 14–15.

Mosby's Medical, Nursing and Allied Health Dictionary, (1994), 4th ed., St. Louis: Mosby-Yearbook.

Quinn, J. F. (1989). On healing, wholeness, and the haelan effect. *Nursing and Health Care, 10*(10).

Smerke, J. M. (1990). Ethical components of caring. *Critical Care Nursing Clinics of North America, 2*(3).

Watson, J. (1993a). Rediscovering caring and healing arts. *Nursing Standard, 7*(38).

Watson, J. (1993b). Interview by Eve Henderson. *AARN Newsletter, 49*(6).

PART FOUR

HEALING IN THE CARE OF SPECIFIC PATIENT POPULATIONS

PHYLLIS BECK KRITEK, RN, PHD, FAAN

I have for some time been fascinated by the idea that most academic disciplines in the United States have names that end with the familiar "ology," as in sociology, biology, or theology. This "ology" is a derivative from the Greek "logos," meaning discourse. In general, these disciplines translate this reference to "logos" as "the study of" some specified domain. Such study involves discourse, helping us trace our scholarship roots to our Greek role models.

In contrast to this pattern, some disciplines are not so named. Fine arts and architecture are useful examples, as are language studies and history. Here the referent is simply the domain itself. A few have a designation that is unique: they are neither "ologies" nor simple nouns. They are gerunds, nouns modified to function as verbs. Engineering, a very pragmatic problem-solving discipline, has this designation. So does nursing. I have always thought it said something important about us. We are first and foremost people who act, who do something, who study for the purposes of knowingly influencing our own behavior.

Predictably, then, for engineers, nurses, and like-minded professionals, the purpose of study is pragmatic, focused on the activity that will emerge guided by the outcomes of the study. We learn so we can do. Hence, Part Four of this book focuses on the pragmatic "doing" of nursing, on the care of specific patient populations.

Very early in my career, I did an evaluative study of job satisfiers for a local hospital. We were fascinated by the outcome. All the satisfiers were tied to direct patient care and most identified a specific patient population as the source of this satisfaction. While most nurses will simply report that they like to do nursing, its attraction to any individual nurse is often linked to the patient population of importance to that nurse. Hence, when we conceptualize our work, we tend to do so in light of the specific patient population of interest. It is here where we find that most of our passion and satisfaction reside. This part of the book provides some windows on the study of healing focused specifically on given populations. It is where the construct of healing begins to take on a concrete, practical utility.

Geraldine Dorsey-Turner opens Part Four with a reflective poem about the nature of healing, one that asks the questions that we all have about it, one that helps us get in touch with the mysterious dimensions it brings into our lives, the dilemmas, the hopes and the uncertainties. In asking these questions, her poem highlights the many remaining unanswered questions that this section of the book brings forth. If indeed we as healthcare providers wish to serve as persons who facilitate healing, we will need a good deal more wisdom on the art and the science of this activity and the roles we play in such service.

In the first chapter in this part of the book, Alice Hill provides an analysis of the possibilities inherent in creating a healing environment for the preterm infant. She analyzes existing data that demonstrate both the threats the environment presents to the preterm infant and the possibilities available for modifying that environment. She notes that these data are readily available, yet often unintegrated into the care of the preterm infant. In doing so, she reveals for us the impact of a constricted image of the "work" of nurses, where environmental management is not recognized as germane. Indeed, she further reveals that if we were to begin to see our work as inclusive of environment, we would alter our behaviors.

If our aim is to assure the preterm infant of wholeness, or healing, then any threat to that wholeness is within our purview. From this perspective, we would quite readily see that we need to take accountability for the environments we create, and assure that they are conducive to healing. Certainly, in the case of the preterm infant, it is unlikely that any other group of health professionals will assume this responsibility, and the environment, "left to the nurses," will be as healing as we elect to make it. With the construct of healing as our guide, we would be unable to ignore the impact of these environmental factors. Alice goes on to provide the reader with a proposal for a useful utilization model for studying the promotion of a healing environment . Thus, having identified an issue of import, she also provides a useful process for beginning to address an unmet need for preterm infants that could have a substantive impact on the outcome of their care, both in the immediate and in the long-term wholeness of the infant.

Jean Ivey explores the information we currently have available on families of a chronically ill adolescent, and the implications this information has for the nurse who seeks to assist these families in their healing. She notes that, while the available literature lacks organization, we do have enough information to demonstrate that family healing may have greater explanatory power than the impact of the chronic disease itself when we attempt to understand the adolescent response to the disease. In particular, family cohesion, expressiveness, communication patterns, and ability to normalize despite the disease appear to be useful predictors of the adolescent's outcomes. Her work provides a useful example of the impact of wholeness: family wholeness becomes a force determining the healing capacity of the individual.

Her exploration of the impact of the chronically ill adolescent on siblings further expands this understanding. An understanding of healthcare focused exclusively on the ill adolescent would ignore this factor, despite its obvious impact on the "identified patient." A parental couple unable to share this challenge is an equally important factor in understanding the effect on the adolescent. What becomes apparent in Jean's analysis is that the construct of healing would ask us to explore a wider range of issues, and would help us to better understand the holistic nature and complexity of the experience of chronic illness for the adolescent.

Kay Sandor also looks at an adolescent population; in fact, part of the patient population she serves at a nurse-managed clinic located in a housing project. In reviewing what is known about adolescence, Kay recognized that the disturbing array of problems and stressors confronting the adolescents in this housing project were considerable; she wondered if these young people had any place to simply talk out the challenges they faced, ones confounding to any human but rendered more troublesome by the impact of adolescence itself. To answer that question, she created a "psychosocial" group for adolescent young women, and provided them with a "container for healing." Her chapter describes this process.

Through her analysis of the characteristics and challenges facing the adolescent, Kay began to understand what kind of a container might be of value and what traits it might best possess. In addition, she created this container in context, in the real world where the adolescents lived and faced their life experiences. She acknowledges the impact of attempting this as one who was not an adolescent, not a member of this minority group, and not a resident of this community. These factors are important, and raise difficult questions about creating healing environments for any "outsider" in any role. Kay's commitment to keeping this container safe and standing by her word appear to have been powerful factors that helped modify the impact of her "outsider" status. Kay also describes the use of myth and storytelling, which transcends the kind of barriers that differences often create, and demonstrates the use of these tools in creating a healing experience for a group of young women in search of such healing.

Barbara Carnes also chronicles the lessons of a faculty practice experience, which she has been involved in for ten years. Her practice focuses on the psychosocial impact of HIV/AIDS. Barbara quickly grasped that for this population the scope of practice always includes the person faced with the disease and the family, friends, and caretakers. She conceptualizes her practice not from the perspective of the disease but from the reality of the human experience of HIV/AIDS and the many persons who play a role in that experience. This insight alone is a powerful one as we begin to understand the nature of healing. For Barbara, healing was a process that involved all these diverse persons, and all, each in their unique way, were involved in personal healing. She observes that they were both involved in their own healing and in contributing to the healing of others. Her paper is a personal description of the challenges and opportunities for healing "triggered by and associated with the HIV experience."

Barbara chronicles the many lessons learned during her work with a variety of patients, families, friends, and healthcare providers. She identifies the challenges faced by each, and notes the lessons learned, including experiences that have given her the "courage to examine and resolve some of my own issues." Hence, her discussion unveils for the reader the mysterious interactive quality of healing: to assist others to heal is in some real sense to learn how to heal oneself. This powerful dimension of healing work has only minimally been explored to date in nursing; this chapter begins to reveal the rich potential this insight holds.

Kay Branum provides a catalyzing reflection on healing in the context of terminal disease. She recounts her own developmental journey through nursing, curing, technology, and finally, healing. Combining candor with disciplined thinking, she is able to guide the reader toward an understanding of the impact of terminal disease, and the challenge that such disease presents to the healthcare provider who wishes to further healing in patients. She helps the reader define the differences between healing and curing, noting that one who is not cured from a terminal disease can nonetheless heal, the tasks being, as she identifies them, the restoration of hope and the relief of unnecessary suffering. Her analysis of suffering, which she describes as an underdeveloped concept in nursing, is particularly poignant in helping nurses to begin to reframe their understanding of healing in the face of imminent death.

In understanding the process of dying, and in being present to the dying patient and those who love this patient, the nurse is afforded a powerful opportunity to assist in healing, to further healing. Kay draws us into the stories of the nurse who participates in these profound moments. She explores the potential strategies the nurse can elect to operate from in participating in these moments, and concludes with a reasoned observation about the power of mystery in healthcare, and the respect it deserves from each of us.

Ruth Tucker's patient population is the childbearing family, and her interest in healing focuses on the complex array of experiences and the opportunities for healing that this family faces. Her interest is in identifying the ways in which this is also a set of experiences and opportunities available to the nurse providing care for such families. She starts with a description of the unique time of pregnancy, where there is greater intimacy with healthcare professionals, greater openness to assistance, greater awareness of one's body, greater introspection: a time of opportunity for healing. Using the mind-body connection as a starting point for her analysis, she chronicles the behavioral responses that may emerge if specific obstetric phenomena occur. She places this analysis within the context of stress.

Looking carefully at the attendant sociological, psychological, and physiological factors of import, Ruth notes that this is indeed a time where the stage is set for healing. She puts an emphasis on the connectedness between persons that is inherent to the healing process, and shows how the nurse can play a powerful role in preventing the complications of pregnancy by enabling healing of their stressful precursors. Interventions such as story telling and imagery are tools described to assist the nurse in this process, demonstrating that childbearing is "indeed a healing opportunity."

Mary Anne Hanley offers a prose poem as another way of discovering the importance of healing for a given patient population, in this case, the elderly person facing death, experiencing the desire to "go home." Mary Anne provides us once more with a glimpse of the power of healing, helps us see that in healing ourselves we are more available to others seeking healing, and in participating in their healing we further that process of healing ourselves. She also helps us recall the lessons of family, our personal lives, and their impact on our understanding of our role as healers.

Jeanette Hartshorn has a faculty practice with individuals with seizure disorders. Her contribution assists us in confronting the sharp difference between curing and healing. Her patients will not be cured, but through her advanced practice nursing interventions she is able to be a significant force in their journey toward healing. Jeanette describes the challenge of helping patients with seizure disorders manage their lives, their personal responses to seizures, and the meaning of this disease for their spirits, their sense of life's meaning. She faces with them a medical diagnosis with a distressing impact, and works with them toward their own healing solutions.

Jeanette gives focus to some dimensions of healing that are often neglected: that each of us has within us that which we need to heal, that the health care provider facilitates the process but the families and the patients do the healing, that the historic dependency model in Western medicine delimits patient opportunities to heal, and that nurses are called on to change that model of care if they wish to facilitate healing. She contrasts the reductionism of allopathic medicine to the holistic nature of nursing practice, placing the nurse in a key role—to assure that the healing process is furthered. Using Newman's model of life patterns, she demonstrates how the nurse can become the facilitator of healing during the process of changing life patterns, the creator of a healing environment.

Jeanette provides a series of case studies to demonstrate some of this potential. She notes that nurses can help patients reclaim portions of life patterns, identify options as life patterns shift, clarify the nature of patterns for patients, assist patients in identifying alternate patterns, and support the life pattern choices patients make. Her stories provide a rich picture of the many opportunities available to the nurse who approaches the patient from the perspective of healing.

Barbara Camune provides a glimpse at one very specific case study as a way of understanding the role a nurse might play in assisting others in their healing. She describes her experience with a couple who had lost their dream for their future. Their preterm infant twins were born over four months early, and thus unable to sustain life. They elected to not try futile extraordinary means to prolong their infants' lives, and instead, with Barbara's assistance, held their babies until they died. Barbara tells the story of their admission, their decisions, the labor and delivery, and the dying of the infants. Throughout this experience, Barbara is present as the nurse assisting in the process of healing. She shares with us the struggles, the stories told, the history and the loss for this couple.

Barbara shares the experiences, both hers and the parents, and the things she did to make this experience a healing one. In sharing this poignant experience, we glimpse the power of a nurse who understands the importance of healing. Barbara also shares her information on other healing resources, such as the organization called SHARE which helps such couples, and provides reflective advice on the needs of couples, such as the one she worked with, during this difficult time.

Patient populations readily capture the interest and attention of nurses. We relate to specific groups with a degree of consciousness not always noted by other healthcare providers. These papers begin to unfold the possibilities inherent in focusing on healing processes as we approach the populations of greatest interest to each of us.

Healing: A Poem

by Geraldine Dorsey-Turner

Healing, that is the word!

Can it be found in a book?
as a source of comfort within?
or is it a look in the skies
as one sees heavenly bodies
slowly passing by?

Is it a response, gently spoken,
at the end of the day,
that caresses your thoughts,
to soothe hurt's pain away?

Or is it the touch on the forearm
that eases muscles
so taut and drawn?

Is it the smell of fragrance
expelled by petals from flowers
blowing in the wind, or
the sound of roaring waves
rolling in?

Can one describe what healing is
or where it comes from,
or where it's been?

How it affects each and every one;
or is its response solely different to
everyone?

CHAPTER 27

The Promotion of a Healing Environment for the Preterm Infant: A Utilization Model

ALICE HILL, RN, PHD

Preterm infants enter into a world of turbulence and chaos. They are forced into an environment different from their natural surroundings. Their new exposures to inappropriate amounts of sound, light, touch, and movement are unlike their previous experiences, and impede growth and development (Deiriggi, 1990). The challenge that healthcare professionals face is the ability to identify and capture the positive aspects of these unfamiliar sensory exposures, and bring order into the infant's new world. The introduction of infants to appropriate amounts and types of sensory stimuli opens the gateway to a healing environment. The need for a healing environment is central to the care of preterm infants.

To understand the significance of a healing environment, we must first understand the events that alter the sensory world of the preterm infant, and the impact of these alterations on the health of the infant. Once there is a basic understanding of the sensory environment, either through research findings or clinical observations, we can begin to use that knowledge to improve the infant's health outcomes. Unfortunately, improvement of the sensory environment has not been a top priority for Neonatal Intensive Care Units (NICUs). To begin to understand why the available information is not used more widely, an exploration into the role of education, practice, and family units in the development of a healing environment for preterm infants must be undertaken. In this chapter we explore the nature of the sensory environment of the preterm infant, examine the nature of the organizations responsible for the promotion of a healing environment, and propose a utilization model as a mechanism for developing a healing environment.

THE ENVIRONMENT OF THE PRETERM INFANT

The sensory world of the preterm infant is best described in terms of sights, sounds, touch, and movement. Having lived in a light-deprived environment before birth, the preterm infant is forced into a world of high-intensity lights. For the infant born at 28 weeks, the retina is 50 to 60 percent developed. The intensity of the lights in the Neonatal Intensive Care Unit (NICU) makes it difficult for these infants to open their eyes to survey the surrounding, or to establish eye contact with the caregiver.

The literature suggests that term infants are fascinated with black and white contrast, rather than colorful pictures. Term infants fixate on colors of medium intensity rather than colors that are bright or dim (Ludington-Hoe, 1983). Much of the research on fixation and discrimination related to vision has been done with term infants. But given the intensity of the light in the environment, the ability for the preterm infant to discern these figures and/or their color would be difficult.

The sounds heard in the NICU vary in frequency and intensity. Some of these noises prove costly for the preterm infant. Infants respond to these stimuli with physiological changes, physical displays of fright, and perhaps developmental delays (Thomas, 1989). Because the central nervous system is immature, the infant cannot inhibit responses, and subsequently the energy needed for growth and to supply the brain with glucose and oxygen is used in response to the arousal.

The sound pressure levels in some Neonatal Intensive Care Units (NICU) have been found to be similar to those set for traffic on a street corner, or are equivalent to the noise level inside a motor car (Lawson, 1977). Hearing loss is known to occur in this range (Thomas, 1989). Nonspeech sounds of low frequency and high intensity account for the majority of the sounds detected in the NICU (Lawson, 1977; Thomas, 1989). Since speech is a low-frequency sound, damage to hearing in this range could occur.

Sound levels over 80 decibels (dB) are known to produce hearing loss in adults. And although preterm infants have a higher hearing threshold (40 dB for 28 to 34 weeks gestation) (Lary, 1985) than adults (10 dB), the noise level encountered in the NICU greatly surpasses that threshold. Dropping the head of a mattress inside an isolette or placing a plastic feeding bottle on top of the isolette produces an average of 88 and 84 decibels, respectively (Thomas, 1989). Other sounds such as the closing of solid plastic port holes on the isolette, closing an incubator cabinet, and tapping the hood of the isolette with fingers produce decibel levels greater than those known to produce hearing losses in adults. The seriousness of the preterm infant's condition usually dictates the use of complex equipment. This equipment, (that is, ventilators (Weibly, 1989), isolettes, and incubator alarms), is also a source of noise, and some of these sounds may be above acceptable levels.

In utero fetuses change position and constantly float in the amniotic fluid. The movement and position changes of the mother provide further postural changes, while contact with the uterine wall provides tactile stimulation (Blackburn & Loper, 1992). The preterm infant is often left to lie on a firm mattress or receive touch or handling that is invasive or intrusive in nature (Deiriggi, 1990; Solkoff, 1975). These infants may abruptly be moved from the bed to the scales for weighing or rolled briskly from one side to another. Although excessive or intrusive handling can cause changes in the infant's heart rate and oxygen saturation levels, systematic rubbing or massaging (Scafidi, Field, & Schanberg, 1993) are shown to have positive physical and developmental effects on the preterm infants. As is evident, preterm infants experience many stimuli, and many of these stimuli can be harmful or cause unsatisfactory health outcomes. Healthcare professionals may wish to examine a systematic plan for the promotion of a healing environment.

THE PROMOTION OF A HEALING ENVIRONMENT

Unfavorable outcomes are documented in the literature regarding the effects of noise (Philibin, 1994), light (Blackburn & Patterson, 1991; Shogan & Schumann, 1993), and excessive handling (Bhat, Abu-Harb, Chari, & Gulati, 1992; Jacobsen, Gronvall, Petersen, & Andersen, 1993) on the development of the preterm infant. However, many NICUs still do not vary the intensity of their light sources within a 24-hour period, the noise remains above acceptable levels, and excessive handling of these infants occurs. It is essential for healthcare professionals to examine comprehensive methods for using the research findings to promote a healing environment for the sensory needs of the preterm infant.

Failure by healthcare professionals to utilize the current research findings in practice may be symptomatic of the fragmented discussions of the sensory environmental needs of the infant in the literature. Although it is necessary to study each sensory stimulus separately, it is of equal importance that institutions responsible for the direct or indirect delivery of care utilize a holistic framework in the dissemination and utilization of these findings. One way to assure a holistic approach to the dissemination and utilization of the findings is to frame the need for a healing environment within the context of the arenas responsible for the preterm infant's care. These arenas include nursing education, nursing practice, and the family. This framework would guide the various arenas in identifying their individual and collective, direct or indirect, responsibilities for the welfare of the preterm infant. This framework would further provide a mechanism for studying "how" research findings are currently transmitted to potential and actual caregivers of preterm infants, and "how" current and future research findings can be utilized holistically to promote a healing environment. This framework would provide a method for studying "why" current research findings are not utilized on a broader scale.

Nursing Education

 As a part of the utilization model for the promotion of a healing environment, nursing education would focus on its students. The goal of this arena is to disseminate findings regarding the sensory needs of the preterm infant. Healthcare professionals could design their curricula so that sensory developmental needs of the preterm infant are integral to the neonatal educational programs. In the basic curriculum for nursing students involved in the care of preterm infants, healthcare professionals in educational institutions would include content in their programs on visual, auditory, and tactile stimulation as they relate to the sensory developmental needs of preterm infants. In these programs, special emphasis could be placed on the effects of touch, handling and movement, and students could be taught how to interact with the infants and their families.

Nursing Practice

In the utilization model, the practice arena would focus on the administrators and practitioners. The goal of this arena is to provide an environment sensitive to the sensory needs of preterm infants. First, the significance of a healing environment must be endorsed by those at the administrative level. Health professionals (i.e., nurses, neonatologists, occupational therapists, physical therapists) administratively responsible for neonatal units, would provide the support and set the tone for the establishment of a healing environment. For example, practice institutions have a responsibility to continue educating health professionals about the sensory needs of preterm infants. These institutions could provide workshops or conferences on sensory stimuli for all personnel responsible for the care of infants.

Second, healthcare professionals can critique the available research on sensory development and stimulation for preterm infants. Then a plan to incorporate these findings into practice can be developed. Although a majority of the research studies usually focus on one sensory need rather than a combination of the needs, healthcare professionals can identify ways to holistically apply these findings in practice. To ensure that future research efforts continue to target the needed areas of study, the practice arena has the responsibility to remain cognizant of the individual as well as the combination of sensory needs for preterm infants and identify topic areas for research that will address these needs.

Family

In the utilization model, the family arena would consist of parents, grand-parents, and/or legal guardians. The goal of this arena is to make the family member a key element of the healthcare team and thus contribute to the sensory needs of the preterm infant. NICUs would have a systematic format that will include family members in the care of the infants. A program to educate parents about the physical, emotional, and social capabilities of their infants can be developed by healthcare professionals (in consultation with family member advisors) and provided to all family members. Although it is possible to overload sensory levels of infants already exposed to high degrees of stimulation, a planned sensory developmental program for parents could include the significance of touch, and the infant's capabilities for sight and sound. The framework for including family members in the infant's care can contain the same elements for all families with infants in the NICU; however, the developmental plan could be individualized for each infant.

The sensory environment of the preterm infant has been studied in regard to the impact of individual forms of sensory stimulation on the developmental needs of these infants. While this method is certainly a valid process for determining how sensory stimuli affect the health of infants, perhaps the environment should be addressed in terms of those arenas responsible for utilizing the current research to promote a healing environment. A utilization model that promotes a healing environment by including the institutions responsible for the direct and indirect care of the infants could be developed and tested.

A Utilization Model for Studying the Promotion of a Healing Environment

A model can be used to depict a behavioral process that exists in reality, but is only observable through the indirect behaviors of those engaged in the process (Bush, 1992). The behavioral structures are nursing education, nursing practice, and the family, with observations made on the behaviors of the students, administrators, practitioners, parents, grandparents, and legal guardians. In order for research to be valuable in the care of the sensory needs for preterm infants, it must be utilized and disseminated to those individuals who are indirectly or directly responsible for promoting a healing sensory environment for these infants. The findings could be presented in such a fashion that a comprehensive holistic view is considered for the sensory needs.

Figure 27.1 depicts the model that could be used to promote a healing environment for the preterm infant. The purposes of the utilization model for the promotion of a healing environment are to: (1) provide researchers with a mechanism to study "how" sensory developmental research is disseminated to the different arenas responsible for the direct and indirect sensory environmental needs of the infant, "how" the three arena influence one another, and "why" the whole of sensory stimulation research is not incorporated into practice; and (2) provide healthcare professionals with a framework to incorporate and utilize research in practice and with family members.

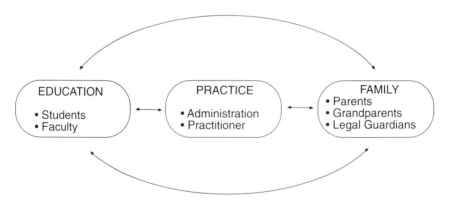

FIGURE 27.1.   Utilization Model for the Promotion of a Healing Environment for Preterm Infants

The major concepts of the utilization model for the promotion of healing in the preterm infant environment consist of nursing education, nursing practice, and the family. The education arena, which focuses on students, directly influences the practice and indirectly influences the family arenas. The direct influence of education on the practice arena is through the emphasis placed in the curriculum on sensory developmental needs of the infants. Graduates of these programs who function as practitioners or administrators will utilize their knowledge in the practice arenas to directly influence the sensory environment. The indirect influence of education on the family is through the practice arenas of graduates from programs with emphasis on sensory needs of preterm infants. The practice arena, which focuses on administrators and practitioners, directly influences the family arena. The direct influence of the practice arena on the family arena is through the teaching of family members about the sensory needs of their infants, and the involvement of family members as advisor members in the development of plans for the sensory developmental needs of the infants.

Researchers should continue to study the sensory environment of the preterm infant, and examine ways that all healthcare professionals can contribute toward a healing environment. While researchers have carefully addressed some of the individual aspects of noise, light, excessive handling and touch on the physiological and developmental outcomes of the infant, there is a need for researchers to also address the promotion of a healing environment.

Summary

It is important for all healthcare professionals to view the preterm infant's world from his or her view. One way to do this is to focus on the responsibilities of the arenas (i.e., nursing education, nursing practice, and the family) in the creation of a healing environment for the preterm infant.

References

Bhat, R., Abu-Harb, M., Chari, G., & Gulati, A. (1992). Morphine metabolism in acutely ill preterm infants. *Journal of Pediatrics, 120*(5), 795–799.

Blackburn, S., & Loper, D. L. (1992). *Maternal, fetal and neonatal physiology, a clinical perspective.* Philadelphia: Saunders.

Blackburn, S., & Patterson, D. (1991). Effects of cycled light on activity state and cardiorespiratory functioning of preterm infants. *Journal of Perinatal and Neonatal Nursing, 4*(4), 47-54.

Bush, H. A. (1992). Models for Nursing. In L. H. Nicoll (Ed.), *Perspectives on nursing theory.* 2nd ed. Philadelphia: J. B. Lippincott.

Deiriggi, P. M. (1990). The effect of waterbeds on preterm infants' sleep. In S. G. Funk, E. M. Tornquist, M. T. Champagne, L. A. Copp, & R. A. Wiese (Eds.), *Key aspects of recovery.* New York: Springer.

Ensher, G. L., & Clark, D. A. (1986). Sensory, motor, and psychological development of the high risk infant. In G. L. Ensher & D. A. Clark (Eds.), *Newborns At Risk.* Maryland: Aspen Publication.

Jacobsen, T., Gronvall, J., Petersen, S., & Andersen, G. E. (1993). "Minitouch" treatment of very low-birth-weight infants. *Acta Paediatrica, 82*(11), 934-938.

Lary, S. (1985). Hearing threshold in preterm and term infants by auditory brainstem response. *Journal of Pediatrics, 107,* 593-599.

Lawson, K. (1977). Environmental characteristics of a neonatal intensive care unit. *Child Development, 48,* 1633-1639.

Ludington-Hoe, S. M. (1983). What can newborns really see? *American Journal of Nursing,* 1286-1289.

Philibin, M. K. (1994). The effect of an intensive care unit sound environment on the development of habituation in healthy avian neonates. *Developmental Psychobiology 27*(1), 11-21.

Reynolds, P. D. (1971). *A primer in theory construction.* Indianapolis: Bobbs-Merrill, pp. 3-21.

Scafidi, F. A., Field, T., & Schanberg, S. M. (1993). Factors that predict which preterm infants benefit most from massage therapy. *Journal of Developmental & Behavioral Pediatrics, 14*(3), 176-180.

Shogan, M., & Shumann, L. (1993). The effect of environmental light on the oxygen saturation of preterm infants. *Neonatal Network, 12*(5), 7-13.

Solkoff, N. (1975). Effects of handling on the subsequent developments of premature infants. *Developmental Psychology, 1*(6), 765-768.

Thomas, K. A. (1989). How the NICU environment sounds to a preterm infant. *MCN, 14,* 249-251.

Weibly, T. (1989). Inside the incubator. *MCN, 14,* 96-100.

CHAPTER 28

Healing in Families with a Chronically Ill Adolescent

JEAN BELL IVEY, RN, MSN, CPNP, DSN

Chronically ill adolescents may have very few or no memories of a time when their "hurt" was not a part of their lives. They may even hurt more from others who did not understand their predicament than from the "hurt" itself. For others to whom the "hurt" came later after a period of being like others, the scar may still be new, tender, and easily disrupted. The family's history, experience, approach to their child's illness, and their expectations for this child and the family as a whole are important variables in evaluating what healing has occurred.

An understanding of how healing occurs in the family of a chronically ill adolescent requires an understanding of the changes in the family unit that allow the members not only to tolerate the illness of a child, but also to grow with the experience. Research suggests that dealing with a chronically ill child may stimulate family growth and solidarity. Surprisingly, this concept originated in studies investigating the unsupported hypothesis that such stress was often responsible for marital discord and divorce (Foster, O'Malley, & Koocher, 1981; Kemler, 1981; Lansky, Cairns, Hassanein, Wehr, & Lowman, 1978). Studies, however, have provided conflicting findings, and some investigators conclude that the ability of the family to survive the stress of a chronically ill child depends upon its previous overall coping ability (Dahlquist, Czyzewski, Copeland, Jones, Taub, & Vaughan, 1993).

There have always been some adolescents who were chronically ill, but previously many such children died during infancy or childhood. Advances in treatment and pharmacotherapeutics, understanding of disease pathology, and parent and community knowledge and awareness have resulted in increased numbers of chronically ill adolescents surviving into adulthood. Blum and Geber (1992) point out that in the past 25 years, the percentage surviving cystic fibrosis is up 700 percent; spina bifida: 200

percent, and congenital heart disease: 300 percent. As a result caretakers and healthcare professionals must deal with problems common in the adolescent age group such as: delayed or accelerated sexual maturation (Blum, 1992), impaired fertility, sexuality, appliances, or adaptive clothing different from that of peers, refusal or reluctance to comply with dietary restrictions, and restrictions on eligibility for a driver's license. Blum and Geber also observe that chronically ill adolescents must deal with the phenomenon of overprotection, as they attempt to separate from their families.

In stark contrast to some researchers discussed in this chapter (Magen, 1990; Tarvormina, Kastner, Slater, & Watt, 1976), Blum and Geber (1992) consider the "psychopathology" said to occur in chronically ill children to be a social phenomenon, not individual maladaptation. They state that the societal devaluation and limitations, and the environmental constraints chronically ill children must face on a daily basis result in the behavior society then labels as maladaptive (p. 364).

The family must cope with unexpected and often unfair conditions and somehow help the adolescent address the usual developmental issues, such as individuation, finding a vocation, sexuality and marriage, continuing medical coverage, but always with an eye to their adolescent's essential separateness from their peers. Any adolescent can be taught about sexuality and birth control, but the adolescent with a genetically transmitted disorder, such as cystic fibrosis or sickle cell anemia, must also be given genetic counseling and reproductive potential may be very limited. The adolescent female with insulin-dependent diabetes mellitus (IDDM) is just as conscious (or more so) of her appearance as her peers who diet frequently and exercise sporadically and strenuously, but her disease makes these behaviors dangerous. The adolescent female with heart disease must decide whether pregnancy and childbirth are worth the risks entailed and share her decision with potential mates. The adolescent male who wishes to participate in team sports but has sickle cell anemia or hemophilia must find a sport that is unlikely to result in physical contact.

During adolescence, the family unit that has successfully negotiated the crises of diagnosis, acceptance, and incorporation of medical restraints and regimens into their daily lives, explaining and offering reassurance to bewildered or guilt-bearing family members and friends, finding out what "mainstreaming" and "normalizing" mean for their child, comes up against an entirely new set of problems. Learning how to let go, how to encourage independence despite concern about the effects of acting out behaviors, how to discuss the realities of life with this disease, such as where a learning disabled child can get a college education, and how to set limits that are not limitations, are only a few of the challenges they must face.

A marker of the healing that occurs in families of chronically ill adolescents is positive adaptation, or the dynamic state of interpersonal and individual growth and development that occurs in the family that is able not only to survive the aforementioned stressors, but to be strengthened by the process. Such families can offer insights not only to other families, but to healthcare professionals, their communities and society at large. This chapter reviews several studies pertinent to this concept. This review is limited to those articles concerning adolescents with chronic illness and their families. This literature offers some insights and many questions.

REVIEW OF THE LITERATURE

Chronically Ill Adolescents

There is a vast body of work describing characteristics of chronically ill children (Graves & Pless, 1974; Kumar, Powars, Allen, & Haywood, 1976; McAnarney, Pless, Satterwhite, & Friedman, 1974; McCollum & Gibson, 1970; Mattson & Gross, 1966; Pless & Roghman, 1971; Pless & Satterwhite, 1975). During the mid-1970s, family theorists (Minuchin, 1974; Minuchin, Maker, Rosman, Liebman, Milman, & Todd, 1975) suggested that these children were "symptom bearers" of dysfunctional families, displaying that pathology through disorders such as migraine headaches, asthma attacks, and sickle cell crises. Other authors (Grey, Cameron, & Thurber, 1991; Hurtig, Koepke, & Park, 1989; Ivey, 1981; Kim, 1991) focused on correlates of a particular illness or disease entity.

Some authors have attempted to investigate unique characteristics of chronically ill adolescents. Howe, Feinstein, Reiss, Molock, and Berger (1993) reported a study of 165 chronically ill adolescents, using a group with "brain involvement" and "healthy controls," the latter known because they had recently been hospitalized with an acute illness or seen for dental work. They screened for I.Q. to "ensure that all adolescents" were capable of understanding the self-report instruments used. "Primary caretakers" and adolescents were interviewed and given "measures of adjustment." While brain impairment was significantly related to adjustment problems, other chronically ill teens "were no more at risk" than controls (p. 1164). Neurologically impaired boys were found to be more at risk than girls, but interview data did not support the questionnaire data.

Capelli, McGrath, Huck, McDonald, Feldman, and Rowe (1989) studied three matched groups of 31 adolescents each, with either Cystic Fibrosis (CF), Diabetes Mellitus (DM), or in good health. The standardized assessment instruments revealed no significant differences in the groups, but semi-structured interviews with the adolescents revealed important differences. Teens with CF and DM were concerned about family reaction to their health, their future health, complications and dying, stress from other family members and their own health.

Diagnosis Specific Research

Much of the literature has consisted of correlational studies, attempting to investigate relationships between a particular disease and various dependent variables. These studies are usually ex post facto, using no controls, matched controls, or presumably healthy age mate controls.

Ivey (1981) studied 19 school-aged children with Juvenile Rheumatoid Arthritis. She interviewed their parents, and administered a parental acceptance scale, as well as having the child with arthritis and his or her sibling closest in age complete self-concept, anxiety, and family relations measures. She found differences in children's and parents' perceptions of family relations, significant correlations between parents' and children's scores, and lower self-concept and higher anxiety levels in the siblings than in the children with arthritis.

Hurtig, Koepke, and Park (1989) limited their investigation to 8- to 16-year-old individuals with sickle cell disease and reported that adolescents were at greater risk than younger children and adolescent males in particular for problems such as poor school performance, personality disorders, impaired peer relationships, and behavior problems. They did not find a significant relationship between such difficulties and the severity of their disease.

Blakeney, Portman, and Rutan (1990) investigated the adjustment of 44 severely burned adolescents by administering three standardized instruments. They found that positive adjustment was more likely to occur when family cohesion, independence, and open expression were reported by the adolescents.

Grey, Cameron, and Thurber (1991) studied 103 8- to 18-year-old children with Insulin Dependent Diabetes Mellitus (IDDM). They used adjustment, self-perception, anxiety, and depression scales, as well as glycosylated hemoglobin levels to compare the subjects. They found relationships between the age groups and their respective "psychological, social, and physiologic adaptation." Adolescents were more anxious, depressed and in poorer metabolic control than the school-aged group (p. 147). Parental coping styles, self-care behavior, and current stressors were not predictive of diabetic control.

Walsh and Ryan-Wenger (1992) administered the "Feel Bad Scale" to 84 8- to 13-year-old asthmatic children, reading the items aloud to the younger children. They identified feelings of being left out in peer groups, being unable to participate in sports, and having parents argue in front of them frequently as major stressors (p. 461). No attempt was made to differentiate age-group responses.

Bartholomew, Guy, Swank, and Czyzewski (1993) administered a measure of self-efficacy expectations to parents and 199 children with cystic fibrosis (CF), 38 of whom were adolescents. Their conceptual framework was Bandura's (1986) social cognitive theory, specifically the concept of self-efficacy expectations. In this framework, "self-efficacy beliefs are related to whether the person will attempt to perform a task and to how long he or she will persevere" (Bartholomew et al., p. 1524). Self-efficacy was measured in the selected population for both the adolescents and their caretakers. During factor analysis, the caretaker data produced a five-factor solution and the adolescent data yielded a four-factor solution. Caretaker factors were: (1) medical judgment and communication, (2) compliance, (3) coping, (4) family communication, and (5) acceptance. Adolescent factors were: (1) communication with the healthcare team, (2) acceptance and coping, (3) medical judgment and communication, and (4) medical treatment. Both the caretaker and the adolescent forms dealt with medical judgment and communication, coping, communication, compliance, and acceptance of cystic fibrosis. The authors interpreted these loadings and the moderate correlations between factors to indicate that the behaviors of their subjects in relationship to self-management are "complex interactions of self-regulatory, problem-solving, and communication behaviors" (p. 1529). The authors further concluded that these solutions indicate the importance of "cognitive and behavioral processes of self-management" (p. 1529), rather than focusing on content alone in educational efforts. No distinction was made between age groups or severity of disease.

Families of Chronically Ill Children and Adolescents

Hymovich (1976, 1981, 1986, 1990, 1993a, 1993b) and Hymovich and Roehmert (1989) investigated the effects of chronic illness in families, beginning with instrument development to measure coping skills, responses, and perceived needs and culminating in work on adaptation in families with a child with cancer. Hymovich's Contingency Model of Long-Term

Care (Hymovich & Hagopian, 1992) for families with a chronically ill child up to 18 years of age states that the diagnosis of the illness results in changes in parental child-rearing practices, communication patterns, family cohesion and conflict resolution, and children's roles and levels of functioning. These variables are said to be mediated by family and individual family member characteristics (Hymovich, 1993b, p. 1356). The framework includes the expectation that family adjustment is dynamic, changing as the family and family members develop. Hymovich began developing a pencil and paper descriptive survey (the Chronicity Illness and Coping Interview: Parent Questionnaire) about parental coping strategies in the 1980s using specific diagnostic categories (osteogenesis imperfecta, cystic fibrosis, etc.) as well as general surveys of parents of children with chronic illnesses. More recently, Dr. Hymovich has used qualitative methods to investigate the phenomenon.

In a published study of 13 parents of 9-week to 20-year-old children with cancer, Hymovich used a grounded theory qualitative method. In these interviews, she investigated specific parental stressors and coping strategies related to child rearing as well as parental perceptions of child stressors and child coping strategies (1993b). Three categories of parental stressors were derived from the data: *knowledge, composure,* and *future.* Examples given were: having to talk about the child's illness with the child when they had insufficient information (knowledge); having to maintain composure by not crying in front of the children; and worrying about the future because of the child's illness or ultimate outcomes of therapy. Families of older children were also very concerned about communicating and maintaining a trusting relationship without devastating or depressing the child. The areas of relationships and communications were seen as critical by these families, and particularly avoidance of communicating about the threat of death and resultant tensions within the family were identified as critical to adaptation to cancer.

Hauser, Di Placido, Jacobson, Willett, and Cole (1993) report a series of studies of families who have an adolescent with diabetes, beginning with intensive interviews of two families, followed by an analysis of 79 two-parent families—42 with a diabetic child and 37 with an acutely ill child. Data were derived from "family discussions" about the family's coping strategies following a recent major event that changed or interfered with the family's usual activities. Independent raters analyzed the audiotaped data. The findings of this study were that the families of a diabetic child more often saw the illness as a family problem that could be managed by a family approach. Families of an acutely ill child on the other hand, stress overcoming the temporary set-back and being able to go on with their lives. Another distinction between the two groups was that acutely ill children's families were more likely to seek and accept adequate information and handle demands made on them, than were diabetic children's families. The latter group expressed avoidance of dealing with issues, frustration and feelings of futility, and having to find new ways of doing things that the other members could live with.

In their third study, using the data from the 79 families and correlating the coded interview data to an ego development test, they discovered relationships between coping strategies and parental and adolescent ego development. This demonstrated that families of chronically ill children may seek more support and approach problems more coherently than do families of acutely ill children. Also, lower levels of ego development were significantly related to decreased coping skills in adolescents, and a closed, simplistic approach to problems in families.

Ray and Richie (1993) studied primary caregivers of children 3-months to 16-years of age whose children had been diagnosed for at least 3 months with various chronic illnesses. They conducted semi-structured interviews and used measures of cognitive and behavioral coping strategies and the parents' perception of the burden of caring for the children and overall stress levels. The findings were that parents consistently saw the family unit and marital unit as the primary and irreplaceable source of support, and felt that maintaining a positive outlook was an effective coping strategy. In addition, families who felt most burdened by the care of the child were less able to use effective coping strategies, felt the illness was most restrictive to family activities and exhausting for the family members. This latter group's reported abilities to manage the child's care were lowest and their overall stress levels were the highest.

Burkhart (1993) reports a qualitative descriptive study of 3 mothers who had a child with a chronic illness that had been diagnosed at least two years prior to the investigation. The children's ages were 4 years, 8 years, and 14 years. The themes identified in the open-ended interview data were *acceptance* of the diagnosis, *relationships, coping, uncertainty, time perspective, heightened awareness, hope,* and *normalization.* All the mothers discussed the process of *acceptance* after shock, grieving, and information seeking, their need for family support (*relationships*), and the phenomena of uncertainty and fear that *time* with the child might be decreased or compressed by the course of the illness. *Hope* and *coping* were said to be expressed in the belief that while the chronic condition was hard to deal with, it was not impossible. This was reported by all the mothers, as was the desire to have the child participate in normal activities (*normalization*). This desire was described by one parent who put her immobile child in places that a child his age might crawl to, and provided things he couldn't reach so he could have similar experiences, such as shredding paper or spilling things onto the floor (p. 127). The mother of the 13-year-old discussed his need to be independent and able to conduct his affairs without the interruption of seizures or limitations of activities. She also stated that he was embarrassed when seizures occurred in front of peers and by his poor memory (p. 128). Another mother reported that she thought of little aspects of her life (*heightened awareness*) and what assistance her child would need just to accomplish those day-to-day tasks and how much she took for granted (p. 127).

Dahlquist et al. (1993) report a study of 67 pairs of parents of children aged 1 month to 17 years who had been diagnosed with cancer six to ten weeks before data collection. A battery of self-report standardized instruments measuring anxiety, depression, repression-sensitization, and dyadic adjustment were completed by the partners over a two-week period and returned by mail to the researchers. They found a positive predictive relationship between depression and anxiety and marital distress in the pairs and noted that as the discrepancy between the parents. As partners' anxiety levels or conflicting styles of coping (repression-sensitization) increased, so did the likelihood of marital distress. For example, one partner might express no anxiety and avoid talking about a child's prognosis, while the other expressed great apprehension and anxiety and approached the problem by discussing it with all their friends. This predicted marital distress. However, since this study was cross-sectional, the authors also suggested that after the initial crisis, differences in coping styles may be constructive and effective in long-term adjustment of the dyads.

Canning, Hanser, Shade, and Boyce (1993) interviewed 92 children from 9- to 18-years-old with various chronic illnesses and their mothers to compare the parents' and children's perceptions of the child's psychopathology as manifested by the presence or absence of DSM-III-R diagnoses. Maternal depression and distress were also measured using standardized instruments. There was marked disagreement between the mother-child dyads, and mothers whose scores indicated they were depressed or distressed tended to overestimate the child's problems. Other mothers were unaware of problems their children reported, and the authors suggested they might be "downplaying" their child's symptoms (p. 509). The authors suggest that these inconsistencies indicate the need for independent assessment of mothers and their children and careful interpretation of findings, preferably in longitudinal research designs.

Ecob, MacIntyre, and West (1993) also studied mother and child reports by interviewing 1009 15-year-old adolescents and either one or both parents for each. Two hundred and fifty (250) parents and 198 adolescents reported "long-standing illnesses" and 84 parents and 81 adolescents "limiting long-standing illnesses" (p. 1020). The data collected in the subjects' homes revealed that when two parents were interviewed they frequently disagreed about the child's illness, in addition to the fact that parents reported a higher prevalence of long-standing illness than did children. The authors concluded that one source of data about this population was not adequate and researchers should include not only multiple sources of information but ascertain the role of the family member in the care of and involvement with the child.

Copeland (1993) and Copeland and Clements (1993) report the findings of a survey of 124 individual parents of children with a chronic illness and a subset of 19 pairs of parents. The time since diagnosis for the child ranged from 1 to 15 years and the disorders were equally distributed between not severe, moderately severe, and very severe according to the parents. The time of diagnosis, increases in the child's symptomatology, and changes in the child's developmental stage were stated to be the most difficult for the individual parents. They reported a change in sources (unspecified) the family used for support and saw health professionals as not particularly supportive. Sources of support reported were categorized into *releasing, reasoning,* and *relating.* These categories included strategies used to cope when crises occurred in the child's condition: physical activities and diversional activities, reasoning about the solutions to problems, need for normalization, and dealing with the child about the necessary demands and limitations. They also reported that support groups, relatives, journaling, love, and God provided strength for living.

The parent pairs generally "perceived the child's chronic condition in a similar manner" (Copeland & Clements, 1993, p. 116), but reported different support strategies and responses. The construct of "chronic sorrow" long held to be present in such families was supported by the data. Fathers tended to submit incomplete questionnaires more frequently than did mothers and to answer more briefly. Finally, spouses were unable to accurately state what strategies their partner used to cope with the stressors.

Sibling, Teacher, and Peer Studies

Perrin, Ayoub, and Willett (1993) compared self-report and questionnaire data from children, aged 7 to 18 years divided into five "health statuses" ranging from health to chronic conditions which were both invisible and visible to that from one parent and one teacher to estimate their "adjustment" (p. 96). The researchers report that to the child, adjustment "depends on family environment, his or her health, and verbal intelligence" (p. 98). Findings for the mothers agreed, but additional variance was explained by the mother's own "locus of control" in regard to health. When mothers credit chance with changes in their own health, their beliefs about their child's adjustment is unrelated to their child's intelligence. When they have an internal locus of control, they believe that their child is better adjusted because of their ability to reason and understand. Teacher ratings for the children were also influenced by their perception of the family environment, but gender and verbal intelligence were more strongly related to the children's scores. Thus, girls who were more capable verbally were perceived as better adjusted than boys or those who were less verbal. Teachers' perceptions of a difference in adjustment was positively correlated with the mothers' locus of control in regard to health, and teachers scored children with invisible conditions (such as arthritis or petit mal seizures) lower on adjustment than peers with visible conditions.

La Greca (1992) suggests that comparisons between healthy and chronically ill adolescents have been sufficient, and that peer contributions to adjustment need further study. Her investigation of 74 adolescents with IDDM utilized a structured interview about family and peer support. Adolescents reported that families provided "tangible" support, such as meals, injections, equipment, and so forth. Friends provided "companionship" support, such as praise, or exercising together.

Williams, Lorenzo, and Borja (1993) report findings about 100 Filipino families with a chronically ill child from data collected in 1981. The school-aged ill children had neurological and cardiac conditions and had been diagnosed for from 6 months to over 5 years. Siblings were from 6- to 18-years of age. Mothers were interviewed about themselves and the sibling they thought was most affected by the ill child's illness using a structured interview schedule. No data were collected from the sibling directly. The mothers reported that siblings' household responsibilities increased and their school and social activities decreased and that their own involvement in care of well children, housework, social, and maternal role activities decreased after the ill child's diagnosis. The changes in sibling activities were most marked in female siblings and adolescent siblings. These changes included increased housekeeping and well-child caretaking, and significant decreases in school and social activities. Mothers of a child with a cardiac condition experienced more of the above changes than did the mother with a child having a neurological condition. Socioeconomic status, place of residence and family support were also related to the extent of changes required in the family.

Gallo, Breitmayer, Knafl, and Zoeller (1993) interviewed 10 mothers of chronically ill children about the adjustment of siblings and family life in general. The ill children and the siblings each were from 7 to 16 years of age. The pairs were selected from respondents to an earlier study of 28 healthy siblings. Five "very well adjusted" and five "poorly adjusted" subjects were chosen on the basis of scores on the Child Behavior Checklist completed by their mothers. Differences were found between the two groups as to the effects of the illness on the sibling, the ill child and the marital relationship, and the "perceived controllability of the chronic illness" (p. 321). Poorly adjusted siblings had brothers or sisters with poorer prognoses and were not able to express resentment toward that child, and the family often felt they had no control over the child's illness. Well-adjusted siblings had families which allowed expression of resentment and expected success in dealing with the child's illness.

Related Reviews of the Literature

Several pertinent reviews of the literature have been published in the past decade. Magen (1990) reviewed psychiatric aspects of chronic illness and adolescents and Kim (1991) reviewed psychiatric aspects in epileptic children and adolescents. These reviews suggest that there is a 10 percent to 20 percent higher incidence of behavior disorders in chronically ill children and adolescents than in others. Parents' and siblings risk factors were said to be increased as well. Magen points out that family isolation and lack of support are common, and that adolescents feel left out in peer relationships. Kim suggested that in order to understand the influence of sibling problems in families with an epileptic child, the whole family must be included in "interactive and systems" approaches (p. 879).

Quirk and Young (1990) reviewed literature on Juvenile Rheumatoid Arthritis (JRA) and it's impact on children and families. They stated that the lack of longitudinal studies, the predominance of small samples and retrospective designs not controlling variables that seem significant, and the lack of investigations of relationships between physiological, social and psychological variables are problematic. These reviewers also saw a need for studies focusing on positive adaptation and change in a family, as well as risk factors for families.

Patterson (1991) surveyed literature on youths with disabilities and their families. She found support for the idea that the most positive outcomes were in families where the needs of all members were valued, cohesiveness and flexibility were present, support systems were well-developed, there was open and direct communication, fathers were involved in the care of disabled members, and the family had developed "common beliefs" about "disability and life" (p. 139).

Faux (1993) reviewed literature about siblings of children with disabilities and reported few studies of adolescent siblings and, in agreement with Williams et al., found several studies suggesting that adolescent females were most often knowledgeable about the sibling's illness and likely to serve as leader and/or caretaker for the ill child. Siblings in general had more responsibilities at an earlier age than would be expected in families without an ill child and frequently did not received sufficient information about their sibling's illness or treatment, were more withdrawn, did more poorly in school, and suffered social isolation. Faux points out, however, that this literature has developed from case studies, anecdotal reports, small samples without comparison groups, and primarily parental or teacher reports, rather than from interaction with or observation of the siblings, and thinks this has resulted in overemphasis on problems and difficulties in the siblings. She advocates studies of communication patterns and coping strategies in these families and investigations incorporating reciprocity between ill children and their siblings.

Lavigne and Faier-Routman (1993) conducted a metaanalysis of literature about correlations between various factors and psychological adjustment to physical disorders, and located 38 studies for comparison. They concluded that previous work had demonstrated significant correlation with adjustment when considered collectively, and parent and child characteristics are more explanatory than are disease or disability risk factors, with child characteristics being most significant. They advocate more attention to risk and resistance variables for adjustment to such problems and that studies be conducted across diagnostic groups, rather than in disease specific designs.

FUTURE DIRECTIONS FOR RESEARCH

Some issues must be addressed for families with chronically ill adolescents, particularly those related to prolonged life expectancy, developmental process, family development, and adaptation. Longitudinal investigation of how families with chronically ill members develop over time, such as those begun by Hauser et al. (1993) need replication with other diagnostic groups and for chronically ill adolescents in general. Since several studies attempting to blend interview data and standardized instruments produced conflicting data, this phenomenon must be addressed. An approach might begin with more theory generating approaches, such as open-ended interviews and observations, rather than to continue the fragmented ex post facto correlational studies that have predominated to date.

Because the phenomenon of adolescence in itself is a significant source of variance in understanding healing, adjustment, and adaptation in family units, this age group deserves separate investigations. The validity and applicability of research findings are impaired when ages from 1 month to 18 years are grouped together and time since diagnosis ranged from 6 weeks to 10 years, ignoring the variability that can be attributed to these designs.

Family research requires separate consideration of family members, from their individual perspectives, not filtered through the perceptions of others. This can be augmented by independent sources (such as teachers, healthcare providers, or social workers), investigator observations, multi-member reports about a set of behaviors, actions, or characteristics, or by family discussions of the group's perceptions. But one-shot cross-sectional designs, second-hand reports or those utilizing one or two family members on one occasion cannot provide the validity needed to establish a firm research base for this area of study. Data triangulation and longitudinal designs are needed. Once this approach uncovers commonalties in families that demonstrate healing or the lack thereof in those living with the chronically ill adolescent, interventions designed to assist in achieving successful outcomes and more reliable measurements of these outcomes can be designed.

SUMMARY

The literature concerning chronically ill adolescents demonstrates several themes:

1. Families and their adolescents heal through the process of adapting to common personal and developmental stressors that are amplified by their problems and resources and unique stressors experienced because of the illness.

2. The process of healing occurs both in individual members and in the family unit as the family learns to modify approaches, substitute new ways of stimulating child development, and do new things they never felt capable of before.

3. Self-concept, anxiety, school performance, personality disorders, peer relationships, and behavior problems are a few of the many variables in chronically ill adolescents that have been studied. Most often, the children's problems in these areas could not be related to their illness. Very often the variables did seem to be related to their family cohesion, expressiveness, communication patterns, and ability to normalize despite the illness.

4. Siblings almost always were found to have increased responsibility, decreased support within and outside the family, and were less likely to participate in activities with their peers. Parents also felt stretched and limited by the demands of their chronically ill child and unable to properly balance their individual needs and the families' needs. Support groups, use of new sources of support, and adopting a positive attitude were effective ways of coping that promoted healing.

5. Concerns such as future outcomes for the chronically ill child, assuring that the child has similar if not equal experiences and opportunities, recognizing barriers and limitations, and maintaining composure, gathering knowledge and communicating so that trust and honesty are maintained were identified by parents who were interviewed.

6. Congruence and harmony between parents and an attitude of being "in this together" in the family were strengths reported by families who had achieved the solidarity and wholeness that typifies healing.

Healing occurs when a family has met the challenge of a chronic illness, accepted that this will be a part of their lives and engaged in a struggle to maintain their wholeness while meeting their individual needs. The coping mechanisms reported by families who are healing are as varied as the structure and patterns of relationships seen in society today. In order for caregivers to support these families in their attempt to normalize, caregivers need additional information about how this occurs, what supports families needs, what strategies work, and what outcomes are reasonably expected. An additional need is for healing in the relationships families with a chronically ill adolescent have with those caregivers so that trust and mutual respect replace antagonism and hostility. Studies that focus on longitudinal relationship focused inquiry and build upon each other, rather than on fragmenting persons into "variables" are most likely to yield that knowledge and that trust.

REFERENCES

Bandura, A. (1986). *Social foundations of thought and action; a social cognitive theory.* Englewood Cliffs, NJ: Prentice Hall.

Bartholomew, L. K., Guy, S. P., Swank, P. R., & Czyzewski, D. I. (1993). Measuring self-efficacy expectations for the self-management of cystic fibrosis. *Chest, 103:* 1524-30.

Blakeney, P., Portman, S., & Rutan, R. (1990). Familial values as factors influencing long-term psychological adjustment of children after severe burn injury. *Journal of Burn Care and Rehabilitation, 11,* 472-5.

Blum, R. W. (1992). Chronic illness and disability in adolescence. *Journal of Adolescent Health, 13,* 364-8.

Blum, R. W., & Geber, G. (1992). Chronic illness in adolescence. In E. McAnarney, R. Kreipe, & D. Orr (Eds.), *Textbook of adolescent medicine.* Philadelphia: Saunders.

Burkhart, P. V. (1993). Health perceptions of mothers of children with chronic conditions. *Maternal-Child Nursing Journal, 21*(4), 122-129.

Canning, E.. H., Hanser, S. B., Shade, K. A., & Boyce, W. T. (1993). *Psychosomatics, 34*(6), 506-511.

Capelli, M., McGrath, P. J., Heick, C. E., MacDonald, N. E. , Feldman, W., & Rowe, P. (1989). Chronic disease and its impact. *Journal of Adolescent Health Care, 10,* 283-288.

Copeland, L. G. (1993). Caring for children with chronic conditions: Model of critical times. *Holistic Nursing Practice, 8*(1), 45-55.

Copeland, L. G., & Clements, D. B. (1993). Parental perceptions and support strategies in caring for a child with a chronic condition. *Issues in Comprehensive Pediatric Nursing, 16,* 109-121.

Dahlquist, L. M., Czyzewski, D. I., Copeland, L. G., Jones, C. L., Taub, E., & Vaughan, J. K. (1993). Parents of children newly diagnosed with cancer: Anxiety, coping, and marital distress. *Journal of Pediatric Psychology, 18*(3), 365-376.

Ecob, R., MacIntyre, S., & West, P. (1993). Reporting by parents of longstanding illness in their adolescent children. *Social Science Medicine, 36*(8), 1017-1022.

Faux, S. A. (1993). Siblings of children with chronic physical and cognitive disabilities. *Journal of Pediatric Nursing, 8*(5), 305-317.

Foster, D. J., O'Malley, J. B., & Koocher, G. P. (1981). The parent interview. In G. P. Koocher & J. E. O'Malley (Eds.), *The Damocles syndrome* (pp. 86-100). New York: McGraw-Hill.

Gallo, A. M. , Breitmayer, B. J., Knafl, K. A., & Zoeller, L. H. (1993). Mother's perceptions of sibling adjustment and family life in childhood chronic illness. *Journal of Pediatric Nursing, 8*(5), 318-324.

Graves, G., & Pless, I. B. (Eds.). (1974). *Chronic childhood illness: Assessment of outcome.* Bethesda, MD: J. E. Fogerty.

Grey, M., Cameron, M. E., & Thurber, F. W. (1991). Coping and adaptation in children with diabetes. *Nursing Research, 40*(3), 144-149.

Hauser, S. T., Di Placido, J., Jacobson, A. M., Willett, J., & Cole, C. (1993). Family coping with an adolescent's chronic illness: An approach and three studies. *Journal of Adolescence, 16,* 305-329.

Howe, G. W., Feinstein, C., Reiss, D., Molock, S., & Berger, K. (1992). Adolescent adjustment to chronic physical disorders-I. Comparing neurological and non-neurological conditions. *Journal of Child Psychology and Psychiatry, 34*(7), 1153-1171.

Hurtig, A. L., Kowpke, D., & Park, B. P. (1989). Relation between severity of chronic illness and adjustment in children and adolescents with sickle cell disease. *Journal of Pediatric Psychology, 14*(1), 117-132.

Hymovich, D. P. (1976). Parents of sick children: Their needs and tasks. *Pediatric Nurse, 2,* 9-13.

Hymovich, D. P. (1981). Assessing the impact of chronic childhood illness on family and parent coping. *Image, 13,* 71-74.

Hymovich, D. P. (1986). Child and family teaching: Special needs and approaches. *Hospice Journal, 2,* 103-120.

Hymovich, D. P. (1990). A theory for pediatric oncology nursing practice and research. *Journal of Pediatric Oncology Nursing, 7*(4), 131-138.

Hymovich, D. P. (1993a). Designing a conceptual or theoretical framework for research. *Journal of Pediatric Oncology Nursing, 10,* 2, 75-78.

Hymovich, D. P. (1993b). Child-rearing concerns of parents with cancer. Child-rearing concerns of parents with cancer. *Oncology Nurse Forum, 20*(9), 1355-1360.

Hymovich, D. P., & Hagopian, G. A. (1992). *Chronic illness in children and adults: A psychosocial approach.* Philadelphia: Saunders.

Hymovich, D. P., & Roehnert, J. E. (1989). Psychosocial consequences of childhood cancer. *Seminars in Oncology Nursing, 5*(1), 56-62.

Ivey, J. B. (1981). *Psychosocial correlates of juvenile rheumatoid arthritis in children and their families.* Unpublished master's thesis: University of Texas, Galveston, TX.

Kemler, B. (1981). Anticipatory grief and survival. In G. P. Koocher & J. E. O'Malley (Eds.), *The Damocles syndrome* (pp. 130-143). New York: McGraw-Hill.

Kim, W. J. (1991). Psychiatric aspects of epileptic children and adolescents. *Journal of the American Academy of Child and Adolescent Psychiatry, 30*(6), 874-886.

Kumar, S., Powars, D., Allen, J., & Haywood, L. J. (1976). Anxiety, self-concept and personal and psychosocial adjustment in children with sickle-cell anemia. *Journal of Pediatrics, 88*(5), 859-863.

La Greca, A. M. (1992). Peer influences in pediatric chronic illness: An update. *Journal of Pediatric Psychology, 17*(6), 775-784.

Lansky, S. B., Cairns, N. U., Hassanein, R., Wehr, J., & Lowman, J. T. (1978). Childhood cancer, parent discord and divorce. *Pediatrics, 62,* 184-188.

Lavigne, J. V., & Faier-Routman, J. F. (1993). Correlates of psychological adjustment to pediatric physical disorders: A meta-analytic review and comparison with existing models. *Developmental and Behavioral Pediatrics, 14*(2), 117-123.

Magen, J. (1990). Psychiatric aspects of chronic disease in adolescence. *Journal of the American Osteopathic Association, 90*(6), 521-525.

Mattson, A. & Gross, S. (1966). Social behavorial studies in hemophiliac children and their families. *Journal of Pediatrics, 68*(6), 952-964.

McAnarney, E., Pless, I. B., Satterwhite, B., & Friedman, S. (1974). Psychological problems of children with chronic juvenile arthritis. *Pediatrics, 53,* 523-525.

McCollum, A. F., & Gibson, L. E. (1970). Family adaptation to the child with cystic fibrosis. *Journal of Pediatrics, 77,* 571-575.

Minuchen, S. (1974). *Families and family therapy.* Cambridge, MA: Harvard University Press.

Minuchen, S., Maker, L., Rosman, B. L., Liebman, R., Milman, L., & Todd, T. C. (1975). A conceptual model of psychosomatic illness in children. *Archives of General Psychiatry, 32,* 1031-1038.

Patterson, J. M., (1991). A family systems perspective for working with youth with disability. *Pediatrician, 18,* 129-141.

Perrin, E. C., Ayoub, C. C., & Willett, J. B. (1993). In the eyes of the beholder: Family and maternal influences on perceptions of adjustment of children with a chronic illness. *Developmental and Behavioral Pediatrics, 14*(2), 94-105.

Pless, B. I., & Roghman, K. J. (1971). Chronic illness and its consequences: Observations based on three epidemiologic surveys. *Journal of Pediatrics, 79*(3), 351-359.

Pless, B. I., & Satterwhite, B. B. (1975). Chronic illness. In B. I. Pless (Ed.), *Child Health and the Community* (78-93), New York: John Wiley & Sons.

Quirk, M. E., & Young, M. H. (1990). The impact of JRA on children, adolescents, and their families. *Arthritis Care and Research, 3*(1), 36-43.

Ray, L. D., & Ritchie, J. A. (1993). Caring for chronically ill children at home: factors that influence parents' coping. *Journal of Pediatric Nursing, 8*(4), 217-225.

Tavormina, J., Kastner, L., Slater, P., & Watt, S. L. (1976). Chronically ill children: A psychologically and emotionally deviant population? *Journal of Abnormal Child Psychology, 4,* 99-110.

Walsh, M., & Ryan-Wenger, N. M. (1992). Sources of stress in children with asthma. *Journal of School Health, 62*(10), 459-463.

Williams, P. D., Lorenzo, F. D., & Borja, M. (1993). Pediatric chronic illness: Effects on siblings and mothers. *Maternal-Child Nursing Journal, 21*(4), 111-121.

CHAPTER 29

Creating a Container for Adolescent Healing: The Group

M. KAY SANDOR, RN, PHD

Adolescence spans the second decade of life and encompasses a major developmental transition. During this developmental transition, the adolescent may experience disruptions as new and different patterns of behavior emerge. This period of disorganization may cause stress, leaving the adolescent more responsive and open to interventions aimed at coping with the stresses. Learning self-care during adolescence may provide teenagers with a key to life-long patterns of health and healing.

During adolescence, the young person experiences a period of rapid physical, social, cognitive, and behavioral change. Thus adolescents are continuously trying to cope with a variety of internal (emotional) and external (social) situations ranging from minor to extremely complex. As the young person copes with these situations using cognitive and behavioral responses to reduce, transform, or eliminate situational demands, they develop a repertoire of responses that may be the origin or continuation of life-long patterns. This process has been variously termed "real life problem solving," "personal problem-solving" (Heppner & Krauskopf, 1987), or "social problem solving" (Durlak, 1983; D'Zurilla, 1986).

Adolescence is often characterized as a time of great risk; only approximately one-half of all adolescents complete this developmental transition with healthy outcomes for adulthood (Jessor, 1993). Such findings have influenced the development of interventions for adolescents in recent years, directing the focus from deficit-reducing to competence-building interventions. Broad-based interventions designed to teach problem solving and enhance social competence focus on promoting healthy behavior rather than on solving a single problem. This appears to be the most promising approach since individual problems, such as drug and alcohol use, and increased risk-taking behaviors are often interrelated (Jessor, 1993; Kazdin, 1993).

COMPETENCE-BUILDING INTERVENTIONS

In a review of competence-building and competence-enhancement interventions, Gesten and Jason (1987) concluded that competence-building programs have been a productive area of intervention in recent years. Intervention programs usually have a multicomponent focus that includes an emphasis on communication skills, problem solving, assertive negotiation, and role-modeling exercises. Durlak (1983) conducted a review of current problem-solving intervention studies and indicated a lack of well-conducted studies showing long-term effects. However, a recent review (Pellegrini & Urbain, 1985) and a meta-analysis (Denham & Almeida, 1987) supported the relation between cognitive problem-solving skills and coping, concluding that problem-solving interventions clearly increase coping skills. Pellegrini and Urbain, however, caution that even though problem-solving programs are effective, the labor-intensive efforts involved in many such programs may put them in jeopardy for future research and intervention projects.

Psychosocial coping is often a key component of competence-building programs and a mental health strategy for primary prevention and health promotion with individuals. Mood state can be considered an indicator of mental health; however, the current status of mood state is rarely assessed in intervention programs (Petersen, Compas, Brooks-Gunn, Stemmler, Ey, & Grant, 1993). Broad-based intervention programs can be important in the prevention of depressive mood (Weissberg, Caplan, & Harwood, 1991), and Petersen et al. (1993) argue that it will be vital for future intervention programs to assess some measure of mood state. The diagnosis of depression appears to be underlying many of the issues that may bring an adolescent into therapy, such as substance abuse, conduct disorders, academic problems, and social withdrawal. Sadler (1991) suggests group therapy and cognitive interventions as methods to manage depression in adolescents. Dusenbury and Botvin (1992) suggest that competence enhancement programs for minority youths should also include information about positive life options, such as the identification of job opportunities. Just being able to consider future options may create an alternative to using substances to cope with uncertainty and despair.

INTERVENTION METHODS

There are numerous methods to present interventions for adolescents, ranging from individual therapy or group therapy to large classroom or community methods. Many of these interventions are labor intensive and/or expensive. They are often developed quickly in response to a perceived community need, but without proper development or testing, the effects of these interventions are not known. In some instances, the curriculum for a program will be of the highest quality, yet without proper teacher/facilitator preparation and training, sensitive material may not be presented in an appropriate manner.

Although group intervention with adolescents may be labor intensive, it may be the most appropriate method. Adolescents "hang" in groups. As they move away from the family group in the developmental stage of the "second individuation," they move into peer groups. A therapeutic group may offer the adolescent opportunities that do not regularly exist in their day-to-day lives. Privacy or confidentiality is one example. Home and school environments may not be able to give adolescents "private space" or the adults around them may not respect the concept of privacy or confidentiality. Another example is the ability to share their opinions or concerns that may not be given to them in a controlling, authoritarian school setting, or in a family setting where a parent(s) may be overwhelmed with responsibility and perhaps using drugs or alcohol to cope with or escape from that responsibility.

Adolescence is a time of paradox. Adolescents frequently experience loneliness and isolation as they strive for independence, yet at the same time want direction and structure. Therapeutic groups can be extremely useful in reducing isolation and loneliness for the young person while providing a safe, structured environment. In a group setting, adolescents will test the leader to find out if what he or she says about the group is really true. Will the group leader protect our privacy and our confidentiality? Will the group leader allow us to express our opinions and feelings in any language that happens to come along with the topic? Adolescents will quickly detect a leader's sincerity or facade. If one is honest and caring, nonjudgmental and nondefensive, an environment of trust and cohesion will likely develop within the group.

Yalom (1985) offers suggestions for the development of a specialized therapy group, such as a group for adolescents in the community. There are three essential steps: (1) Assess the situation to determine intrinsic factors and extrinsic factors. Examples of intrinsic factors include duration of meetings and attendance. Extrinsic factors are those that are to be developed, such as basic ground rules or "policy" for the group. (2) Formulate appropriate and realistic goals. Yalom emphasizes that this step is the most important one in group therapy. The therapist, as well as the participants, must participate in this process. (3) Modify techniques used in the context of the two previous steps. This step is one of discovery and creativity for the therapist as basic techniques are altered and modified to adapt to current situations and goals of the group.

Corey and Corey (1992) offer concrete suggestions for developing a group with adolescents, starting with a needs assessment, developing a proposal, giving a pre-test, conducting the actual group, giving the post-test, and finally ending with a follow-up and evaluation. Others suggest group configurations such as homogeneous or heterogeneous groups based on age and gender (Gaines, 1981; Kraft, 1968). Several authors recommended eating during group time, perhaps using this activity as a metaphor for nourishing the body as well as the spirit (Gaines, 1981; Lothstein, 1985; Moss, 1984). Considerations for selection of the therapist range from same sex therapists, to male and female co-therapists (representing the parents), to opposite sex therapists (Kraft, 1968). Although these various suggestions are worthwhile, issues of group composition and therapist combinations are not as clearly defined or managed in the real world. The issue of structured activity versus unstructured cognitive (insight) therapy for adolescents is not easily answered, but with openness and creativity the therapist can modify his or her approach to adapt to current situations and goals of the group as Yalom (1985) suggests with his third step.

PRACTICE-ORIENTED INTERVENTION

I currently have a faculty practice at a nurse-managed clinic in the Boys and Girls Club annex located in a local housing project. My interest in starting a therapeutic group came from history taking and assessments as part of conducting physicals for the adolescents. The physical exams of the teenagers revealed a few areas for intervention that could be "treated" very easily. However, I continued to hear about a variety of issues emerging from their daily experiences in the housing project, their schools, and the community, ranging from hunger to violence. I wondered if these adolescents had an opportunity to talk to anyone about these and other issues. I recognized the need for some type of practice-oriented intervention to assist the adolescents to sort out their day-to-day life experiences. I then had to ask myself if I was ready to descend into the "swamp" of the human condition and nonrigorous inquiry (Schon, 1990). The call was compelling and the answer was affirmative.

At a clinic meeting with the nurses, the housing authority officials, and housing project members, I mentioned my interest in starting groups for the adolescents to deal with a variety of topics that were important for the adolescents. One housing project official was quick to interject that there were already ongoing groups for adolescents, but the behavioral responses of some of the people living in the housing project told me the current groups were not meeting their children's needs. After the meeting, I was able to talk informally with a few mothers living in the housing project who encouraged me to begin the groups.

A formal proposal to the Boys and Girls Club to start "psychosocial" groups for adolescents during the summer was written and approved. The staff was able to get written parental consents for the adolescents to attend. Eight adolescent young women from 12- to 14-years-old attended the first group. Some had been in a group before at school. I wanted the first session to be quite unstructured to allow topics for discussion to emerge from the participants. My immediate goal was to offer the young women a safe place to talk about anything that was important to them, thus providing a "container" for healing. If the opportunity arose, I also wanted to use creative literature, such as fairy tales, myths, and poetry to weave together the themes emerging in the group. Bettelheim (1989) suggests that such tales show young people that struggle is an inevitable part of their daily lives, but that if one is strong and moves forward to tackle adversity, then one can reach one's goals. In the following section, I (a Caucasian) will describe several group sessions with eight female African-American adolescents and my experience as group leader. My intent is to describe the early phases of this community intervention and to focus specifically on group process. While outcomes are important, it is my conviction that process shapes results just as soundly as those activities directed specifically at outcomes. Thus, a focused review of group process and my interpretation of that process follows.

THE GROUP

During the group first session, I started out with introductions. Even though all the adolescents knew each other, I was still learning their names. The space for conducting the group was in the main clinic area

near where the receptionist sits, so I included the receptionist in our introductions. Then I asked the adolescents if the receptionist should sit in the
Club area with the portable phone during group time, or if she could stay
in the room. The adolescents answered spontaneously that the receptionist
could stay. I then spent some time talking about confidentiality and privacy. Shortly after our discussion about privacy, the male and female staff
members walked into the room unannounced and without knocking. The
young women reacted to their presence with mouth noises and body language (hands on hips, everyone turning toward the door, etc.). One vocal
participant told them, "Miss Kay said this group would be private." The
male staff responded with, "Watch how you talk to us." The female said,
"How do you think you got this group in the first place?" The staff members then seemed to became aware of their own behavior and responses
and reacted with nervous laughter, saying they just came in to see who was
attending and left. I chose not to say anything during this time.

After they left, I asked the young women what had just happened. They
were able to talk a little about their feelings and the importance of privacy. They watched me for my reactions and I reiterated that I would help
them keep their group time private. I asked them what we could do. They
talked about making a sign to put up on the door saying "Group in Session." In retrospect, I could feel something happen during this time—if I
had to name it I would call it the beginning of group cohesion.

After all that activity there was a period of silence. Someone asked what
they were going to talk about. I tossed the question back to them. The first
topic someone mentioned was sex (accompanied by giggles and careful observation of my reaction). The topic quickly changed to their shoes, to the
positions they played on baseball and basketball teams, to the teenage boy
who was killed (one young woman was his cousin), to how many had been
shot at (all but one young woman had experienced gunfire close enough to
run for safety or hit the ground), to exercise (a few did push-ups and cheers
on the floor), and then to a few other topics such as future goals (I want to
be a bus driver, I want to be a nurse).

Finally, they went back to the original topic of sex. When the topic returned to sex there was a sudden silence. One young woman responded,
"Everybody got quiet." They were all looking at me. I told them they
could talk about anything they wanted to talk about. There seemed to be
a collective nonverbal sigh. My hunch to begin with an unstructured format allowed topics to be generated spontaneously by the participants.

Someone then decided the group should have "rules." Everyone agreed.
The first thing they wanted was privacy (and confidentiality). Another rule
was "Don't talk when someone else is talking." Then someone said "No

food or drinks." Although I had been quiet as rules were being generated, I asked them if we could talk about this rule. I told them I thought it might be fun to eat occasionally during group time. After thinking about this for a while, they agreed. I told them I'd ask some local grocery stores to donate fruit or juices. This was my effort to nourish their bodies as well as their spirits. So the group concluded with only two rules: privacy and respect. This process took almost the full hour. I told the young women that it was almost time to close and then reviewed all the topics that had come up during the meeting. I asked them if there would be any conflicts with the time they wanted to meet. It seems they had chosen an acceptable time. I told them we'd meet again next week.

When I arrived at the Club the following week, I learned the Club staff had scheduled me to conduct a physical on a child during the group time. I was firm about the group start-up time and the physical was rescheduled for another day. This unintentional undermining of group time could be very crucial to the process of trust that was beginning for the group participants. During the second meeting, only three young women were available. Of the three young women attending, one was new to the group, although she knew the other teenagers from the Club and the neighborhood. I began the group with introductions again and asked one of the previous participants to explain the "rules" to the newcomer. I also reviewed the topics that were discussed in the previous week's session for the newcomer. Then I asked the young women if I could start with a story. They agreed and I began to tell the story. I explained that shoes was one of the topics that had come up early during the group time last week and I wanted to tell a story about shoes. I chose to tell a story about red shoes from Hans Christian Anderson (1992).

This story tells about a young motherless girl who makes her own red shoes from scraps she finds in the forest. Later an old woman finds the little girl and takes her home with her. The woman feeds, dresses, and cares for the little girl, but throws her old clothes and her special red shoes away. At first the little girl is happy, but she soon longs for her forest clothes and ways. Later, the little girl is able to get another pair of red shoes, but she does this through deception rather than her own creative effort. These red shoes, however, have a life of their own and make the little girl dance continuously whenever she wears them. The old woman sees that the little girl is "possessed" by the shoes, takes them away, and forbids the little girl to ever wear them again. One day, however, the old woman gets sick and the little girl sneaks into her closet to get the red shoes. This time the old woman cannot help the little girl. She dances over the countryside until she is almost dead from exhaustion. The little girl finally dances by the wood-cutter's cottage and she begs him to cut off her feet. He cuts off her feet to save her and the shoes dance off into the woods. The woodcutter then carves wooden feet for the little girl so she can walk again. The little girl never wishes for red shoes again!

As I told the story to the young women in the group, they sat forward in their chairs and listened intently. When I asked them what they thought about the story, they said they thought it was terrible. They were upset about the little girl getting her feet cut off! Then one young woman said, "She should have kept the first pair of red shoes." When I asked her what was special about those shoes, she said, "She made them." I told her I thought she was right—the first pair of red shoes were about the little girl's creative energy and the old woman didn't respect her creativity when she threw them away. One young woman responded that the story had made her feel sleepy. I asked her what she thought that was about, but she couldn't answer. I wondered if the young woman was doing some intro-spective work on the story and it felt as if she was getting sleepy. I asked them to think about the story during the week so we could talk about it again in group the following week.

Although I was not aware of it at the beginning of group, I soon learned the young women really wanted to talk about was the fatal shoot-ing of the son of one the Club's staff members. They were playing base-ball when they heard the shots and saw the young man fall to the ground with a wound to his leg. They then saw another young man walk up to him and fire two more shots—one to the chest and one to the head. Their coach told them to get down on the ground. They said that they thought the gunshots were firecrackers. They couldn't believe that someone was shooting in the park in the middle of the day. They talked about how the Club staff person rushed to the field to see her son before the ambulance took him to the hospital. They then talked about all the neighborhood sto-ries they had heard since the shooting and what others had seen about the details of the wounds.

One young woman then said that several days after the shooting she was just walking along the street and suddenly she "threw up." I asked her what she thought had happened. The young woman looked directly at me and said, "Maybe it was a virus." I told her that it could be a virus, but also explained that sometimes when we hold strong feelings inside it can make us physically sick. I asked if that could have happened to her. The young woman looked at me very carefully as she thought about this possibility. Again she dismissed her symptoms as a virus, but she was silent in the group for a little while. She was still thinking about what I had suggested. During this time, another group member had scratched a scab off her knee and was trying to mop up the blood with her T-shirt. I made no comment as I got her a tissue and bandage from one of the exam rooms, but wondered if the external pain and bleeding she was creating was a metaphor for the psychic wound and pain they all were expressing.

Next, one of the young women started to talk about instances where they had been called on to be strong. I thought this topic came in response to the stories they had just heard—one a grisly fairy tale, the other a frightening real-life tale. One young woman mentioned a time when she "broke up a fight on the street to save an old black man." She described his facial cuts and bleeding, but she explained that she couldn't stay on the street to help him any longer than she already had. I told her that it sounded as if she was telling me that being outside was sometimes dangerous, but that she could be strong when she chose to be.

They then talked a little about knowing when they could be strong and when they had to stay away. One young woman suddenly began to talk about something outside that had hurt her. I didn't understand her description of "green spikes that people have in their yards" so the young woman said she would take me outside after group to show me. Later, another young woman said she had once found some drugs that were supposed to have been hidden in a pipe on the street. When she found them, someone came out of a building and threatened her. She said she stood her ground and didn't run away. The person took the drugs and then she left and called the police. In another instance, one other young woman had been threatened with abusive language. She told the story emphatically nodding her head every time a foul word was spoken, but not actually saying the word. When she finished her story without once using a curse word, one of the young women looked at me and said, "Sometimes I swear." I responded, "So do I." They suddenly stopped speaking for a moment and stared at me, but then quickly moved on, seeming to understand that they had been given permission to express their emotions with words if they needed to.

At this point, the group was nearing the end of the session time. I asked the young women to help me summarize the whole group session. When they were finished, I added the theme of strength that I heard emerging at the end. I asked them to think about the "Red Shoes" story and asked if I could look for some more stories about women being strong. The young women agreed. I told them I would look for some stories about strong African-American women. They then took me outside to show me some plants that grow around the housing project that indeed did have spikes on them. One of the young women had been pushed into these bushes and another had backed into one when she was backing up to catch a fly ball in a baseball game. I was not sure why they insisted on showing me this. Perhaps they wanted to emphasize that there were many dangers outside—both animate and inanimate.

My goal was to create a container in the form of a group for adolescents to experience healing. Groups have historically been closely associated with healing, for example, when primitive communities called upon the collective power of the tribe or the family for energy and support (Greene, 1982). I also called on other ways of knowing (Belenky, Clinchy, Goldberger, & Tarule, 1986) and tried using myths and stories to help the adolescents find meaning and direction in this group endeavor. I shared this method with the young women in my group and found them eager to travel with me on this adventure. Although the group is in its infancy, and I cannot offer any empirical outcome data, I will continue to document the adolescents' paths and consult with other experienced group therapists for support.

REFERENCES

Anderson, H. C. (1992). *Fairy tales.* New York: Alfred A. Knopf.

Belenky, M. F., Clinchy, B. M., Goldberger, N. R., & Tarule, J. M. (1986). *Women's ways of knowing: The development of self, voice, and mind.* New York: Basic Books.

Bettelheim, B. (1989). *The uses of enchantment: The meaning and importance of fairy tales.* New York: Vintage Books.

Corey, M. S., & Corey, G. (1992). *Groups: Process and practice.* Pacific Grove, CA: Brooks/Cole Publishing Co.

D'Zurilla, T. J. (1986). *Problem-solving therapy: A social competence approach to clinical intervention.* New York: Springer.

Denham, S. A., & Almeida, M. C. (1987). Children's social problem-solving skills, behavioral adjustment, and interventions: A meta-analysis evaluating theory and practice. *Journal of Applied Developmental Psychology, 8,* 391–409.

Durlak, J. A. (1983). Social problem-solving as a primary prevention strategy. In R. D. Felner, L. A. Jason, J. N. Moritsugu, & S. S. Farber (Eds.), *Preventive psychology: Theory, research and practice* (pp. 31–48). New York: Pergamon Press.

Dusenbury, L., & Botvin, G. J. (1992). Substance abuse prevention: Competence enhancement and the development of positive life options. *Journal of Addictive Diseases, 11*(3), 29–45.

Gaines, T. (1981). Structured activity-discussion group psychotherapy for latency-aged children. *Psychotherapy: Theory, Research and Practice, 18*(4), 537–540.

Gesten, E. L., & Jason, L. A. (1987). Social and community interventions. *Annual Review of Psychology, 38,* 427–460.

Greene, T. A. (1982). Group therapy and analysis. In M. Stein (Ed.), *Jungian Analysis* (pp. 219–231). Boston: Shambhala.

Heppner, P. P., & Krauskopf, D. J. (1987). An information-processing approach to personal problem-solving. *The Counseling Psychologist, 15,* 371–447.

Jessor, R. (1993). Successful adolescent development among youth in high-risk settings. *American Psychologist, 48,* 117–126.

Kazdin, A. E. (1993). Adolescent mental health: Prevention and treatment programs. *American Psychologist, 48,* 127–141.

Kraft, I. A. (1968). An overview of group therapy with adolescents. *International Journal of Group Psychotherapy, 18*(4), 461–480.

Lothstein, L. (1985). Group therapy for latency age black males: Unplanned interventions, setting, and racial transference as catalysts for change. *International Journal of Group Psychotherapy, 35,* 603–621.

Moss, N. G. (1984). Child therapy groups in the real work. *Journal of Psychosocial Nursing, 22*(3), 43–48.

Pellegrini, D. S., & Urbain, E. S. (1985). An evaluation of interpersonal cognitive problem-solving training with children. *Journal of Child Psychology and Psychiatry, 26,* 17–42.

Petersen, A. C., Compas, B. E., Brooks-Gun, J., Stemmler, M., Ey, S., & Grant, K. E. (1993). Depression in adolescence. *American Psychologist, 48,* 155–168.

Sadler, L. S. (1991). Depression in adolescents: Context, manifestations, and clinical management. *Nursing Clinics of North America, 26*(3), 559–572.

Schon, D. A. (1990). *Educating the reflective practitioner: Toward a new design for teaching and learning in the professions.* San Francisco: Jossey-Bass.

Yalom, I. D. (1985). *The theory and practice of group psychotherapy.* New York: Basic Books.

Weissberg, R. P., Caplan, M. Z., & Harwood, R. L. (1991). Promoting competent young people in competence-enhancing environments: A systems-based perspective on primary prevention. *Journal of Consulting and Clinical Psychology, 59,* 830–841.

CHAPTER 30

The Potential for Healing: Living the HIV Experience

BARBARA A. CARNES, RN, CS, PHD

In 1986, I began an 8-hour-a-week faculty practice which focused on the psychosocial impact of HIV/AIDS. For the past eight years, I have been blessed with the opportunity to share the healing journeys of many very special people. Through these journeys, individuals, families, and professional caretakers infected or affected by HIV have been and are presented with many opportunities to heal themselves and/or to contribute to the healing of others. This chapter includes descriptions of the lived challenges—the opportunities for healing—triggered by and associated with the HIV experience.

WOUNDS

Healing is a process that occurs as a function of living. Society is a part of the healing environment and has impacted the HIV experience for many. The face of the HIV/AIDS epidemic is changing; the population initially affected was gay men. In this society, there is a stigma attached to being gay. Many of the patients I have worked with shared their childhood memories of feeling different from and being taunted by their peers. Others shared memories of being sexually abused by the same uncles, cousins, and neighbors who had mocked their being different. Being diagnosed as HIV positive refocused their attention on sexual orientation and re-opened the wounds of the past. Individuals who had hidden their homosexuality from family members feared joining the ranks of those gays who had been abandoned by families that would not accept their alternative lifestyles. Many shared their disdain for people who told them that "the gays were getting what they deserved." Some feared repercussions within their home communities. "They will burn my house down if they find out I've got AIDS. They've done it before to other people."

For gays and others, the issues related to intravenous substance use also arose. The second major cluster of cases resulted from the transfer of the virus via contaminated needles. Societal attitudes toward IV-drug users center around the misconception that those affected lack character and will-power. Many who were diagnosed as HIV positive were accused of being members of one or both of these disenfranchised groups and were faced with the stigma that went along with this association. The issue of "innocent" victims surfaced as individuals receiving blood products were found to be infected. However, even these families feared repercussions if members of their community discovered that their child or spouse was HIV positive. "I can't tell anyone. They'll fire my husband and torment the kids. Look at what they did to Ryan White." Realistic and unrealistic fears were pervasive in the environment surrounding the HIV experience.

Within the healthcare community, many individuals were dealing with their own fear of contracting a viral infection which they believed could end their careers and their lives. For others, working with HIV-infected individuals impacted not only their professional lives, but their private lives as well. Family members verbalized fear of their bringing the virus home; friends and neighbors questioned their having to work with "them." The potential for stigma, isolation, and feelings of abandonment was ubiquitous.

In addition to these issues, the HIV experience ultimately is associated with many losses. While there are those who survive, for the vast majority of individuals, HIV infection is a long-term, generally fatal condition. The initial diagnosis is viewed by some as a challenge that triggers their choice of healing approaches including complementary therapies, which can lead them to an even higher level of physical, mental, and spiritual well-being. Others choose to view the initial diagnosis as a death sentence. Some of these individuals who question their ability to deal with the reality of HIV infection and AIDS consider suicide. Many have watched friends and loved ones endure the losses associated with the disease process. As the virus replicates, there can be loss of energy, health, feelings of well being, physical appearance, mental capacity, and physical ability. Depending on the situation, there can be loss of independence, job, mobility, friends, and family.

Independence is lost when adult children have to return to live with parents; this is particularly troublesome when there is unfinished business from earlier in life. Employment has been lost when employers have reacted with fear after learning that an employee is HIV positive. Other jobs were lost as HIV-positive individuals chose to leave their work rather than face possible repercussions. Still other jobs were lost when disease progression robbed individuals of their ability to work. Deterioration of strength, muscle control, and vision has stripped individuals of their ability to negotiate their environment.

Members of the gay community are grieving the loss of multiple friends as they imagine the days of their own dying. Many members of the straight community are sharing these losses. Often the increased depression and anger associated with these losses can further strain already tense relationships. Questions of fidelity and trust are impacting more and more gay and heterosexual relationships. "I didn't know he was unfaithful much less that he had AIDS. Now he's dying. We've been married 15 years. What am I going to tell the kids?" Issues related to reproduction and orphans are relevant. Entire families are lost to this disease process. Women tend to take care of others before they take care of themselves, a practice that can lead to a more rapid deterioration of their own health and well being.

Healthcare workers working with HIV-infected individuals face the loss of multiple young, vibrant patients who have become like family. Those working in clinics express the sadness they feel watching their patients' health deteriorate as the virus replicates. At times there is a hopelessness as workers view the never-ending progression of "new cases." Staff members' feelings associated with their own unresolved issues related to infidelity, abuse, and death and dying are reawakened as they relive their experiences through their patients' stories. As members of society, more and more healthcare workers are living the HIV experience in their personal lives.

HEALING

Within this environment it is difficult to imagine healing. Nonetheless throughout the HIV experience there are many opportunities for healing and growth. Today, an ever-increasing number of individuals, families, and healthcare professionals have the opportunity to live and to grow through the HIV experience. As the epidemic progresses, the hope of finding a quick, easy, "magic bullet" cure diminishes. More and more heterosexual individuals and their families are having to deal with the disease that, in the past, only had affected "them." Borysenko (1989) suggests that, "Underneath our fears and worries, unaffected by the many layers of our conditioning and actions, is a peaceful core. The work of healing is in peeling away the barriers of fear that keep us unaware of our true nature of love, peace, and rich interconnection with the web of life. Healing is the rediscovery of who we are and who we have always been" (p. 189). The environment is changing slowly as more and more individuals and families are being forced by personal experience to get the real answers to what it is like to live with HIV. Accurate knowledge can diminish fear. As fear diminishes, the potential for healing increases.

Evidence of this healing has been present since the beginning of the epidemic when members of the gay community came together to care for one another. Many of the interventions were begun within this community. Based on their example, other communities, including churches, have established resources to assist those in need. I remember one client whose pastor gave him access to the musical instruments he needed but could not afford. A proud man, the client would not accept this gesture without "paying" for it. In return for his providing music lessons and playing his music for church services, this man achieved one of his life's desires: he could now hear the music he created. This individual chose to focus on and share his gift of music rather than on his disease process. He rejoiced in the fact that he accomplished this *his* way. Later, as his physical condition deteriorated, the support from church members changed and grew. It was not unusual to enter his hospital room and find church members with baskets of home-grown food and his "favorite" home-cooked meals. Through his journey, he was able to learn how to receive, unconditionally. His illness impacted not only his own well-being but also provided others the opportunity to appreciate their own blessings and to share these blessings with another.

While some complained that the services they needed were not available, others saw a need and worked to fill it. One client was angry about his HIV status and the injustice he associated with being HIV positive. He frequently complained about "all the support" available to gays and the lack of support for heterosexuals who were HIV positive. With encouragement, he used this energy to begin a support group for heterosexuals who were HIV positive. He frequently voiced his appreciation of the challenges and rewards associated with this endeavor.

Individuals and families have embraced the HIV experience and grown from it. One individual put it this way, "If I hadn't been HIV positive, I probably would have wasted another ten years going after material rewards. All that isn't important now. I wake up and rejoice in the sunrise. There is so much beauty all around me. I couldn't see that before." There are challenges associated with being a role model for living positively. One client in particular stands out. Everyone who knew and worked with him identified him as a role model for others. This man had met each new challenge associated with his HIV infection with courage and determination. One day he shared his belief that people expected him to be "up" all of the time. As his health deteriorated he said, "I'm tired; I've done all that I can. If I die, I'm going to disappoint everyone." A focus of our interactions became his challenge to accept the fact that it was all right for him to die, that he had made a major contribution to others, and that people would go on and live after his death. He did die peacefully, surrounded by those who loved him. His memorial service was a joyful celebration of his life.

During his experience with HIV, another patient verbalized his struggle with feelings of anxiety and panic about the possibility of his committing suicide and going to hell. He related this anxiety to his belief that he would not be strong enough to endure the trauma of living with Kaposi's sarcoma and of his own dying. Over the year and a half that we interacted, he verbalized his concerns and sought support when his fears escalated. There were also many occasions when he shared his joy that he had been strong enough to survive the previous impulses to end his life. When his treatment options had been exhausted, he decided that he wanted to die at home surrounded by his friends. He was discharged. After several days of struggling with his fears at home, he admitted himself to the hospital and died quietly in sleep six hours later. As I looked at his lifeless body, I remember feeling his presence as I celebrated his triumph over his fears and his ultimate victory over suicide. I remember the joy we shared.

HEALTHCARE COMMUNITY

People choose to enter the healthcare professions for a variety of reasons, both conscious and unconscious. Nurses often identify that they enter the profession because they want to take care of people. The choice of or assignment to caring for those affected by HIV presents an abundance of opportunity to care for others. Individuals also choose to work with the population as a visible way to support members of their own community and/or to honor the memory of others, including family members, who have died. Some identify the satisfaction they feel when they provide quality care for those who are living with the complex challenges of HIV, while others admit that working with this population satisfies their own need to feel needed.

Professional caregivers who work with those infected and affected by HIV face many challenges. In this era of downsizing and cost containment, only the "sickest of the sick" are admitted to the hospital. In addition to the challenges of providing physical care, these patients and their loved ones also present staff with challenging emotional and psychiatric problems. Those who are struggling to live with the effects of a life-altering disease process, to cope with losses, and to make difficult decisions express their thoughts and feelings in a variety of ways. Personal coping strategies can reflect both the effective and ineffective use of coping resources, extant personality disorders, and/or the physiological consequences of viral processes. Staff find it challenging to work with individuals who can be angry, demanding, and ungrateful. These clients often make choices different from the caregiver's. The belief that some of these choices are harmful to the client's well-being lead discouraged healthcare workers to ask, "What's the use?" The age and life experiences of both the clients and the staff put many of them in a position of having to deal with profound life and death issues while they are still struggling with their personal developmental issues related to identity and intimacy.

A major challenge facing the healthcare worker is to find a balance between caregiving and caretaking. Reflecting on her career as a nurse, an HIV-positive colleague shared her perception that nurses are humans *doing* rather than humans *being*. Working with individuals who are infected with and affected by HIV provides healthcare workers with a plethora of opportunities for doing to and for others. These activities can become a diversion from one's own issues, concerns, and pain, or they can provide healthcare workers with opportunities to recognize and to deal with their own unresolved issues related to grief, infidelity, childhood abuses, and the like. There is a constant challenge to find balance and to care for self.

Schwarz (1989) writes that the "common denominator of all healing methods is unconditional love—a love that respects the uniqueness of each individual client and empowers the client to take responsibility for his or her own well being" (p. 18). Many healthcare workers have chosen this path, demonstrating their ability to honor their clients in the choices that they have made. When healthcare workers view clients as individuals other than who they are, and when these workers meet their own personal need to be needed, then the potential for healing is compromised. Hay (1989) suggests that in order to heal, people need to learn to love themselves. My experiences working with those impacted by HIV have provided me with many opportunities to observe and to support courageous individuals meeting a variety of challenges. These experiences, particularly with those individuals facing death, have given me the courage to examine and to resolve some of my own issues. Making the journey with those living the HIV experience can be a life-altering healing experience.

REFERENCES

Borysenko, J. (1989). Removing barriers to the peaceful core. In R. Carlson & B. Shield (Eds.), *Healers on healing* (pp. 189-195). New York: G. P. Putnam's Sons.

Hay, L. (1989). Healer, heal thyself. In R. Carlson & B. Shield (Eds.), *Healers on healing* (pp. 22-25). New York: G. P. Putnam's Sons.

Schwarz, J. (1989). Healing, love and empowerment. In R. Carlson & B. Shield (Eds.), *Healers on healing* (pp. 18-21). New York: G. P. Putnam's Sons.

CHAPTER 31

Healing in the Context of Terminal Illness

KAY BRANUM, RN, CCRN, PHD

This chapter chronicles part of my journey toward understanding healing in relation to people who have been diagnosed with a terminal illness. Healing, within this context, is a matter of restoring hope and relieving unnecessary suffering. It is not the false hope of immortality, but the realistic hope of the soul for meaning and resolution in the time one has left for living. It is not avoidance of the necessary suffering that reveals possible meanings and resolutions, but the relief of meaningless suffering that endangers such revelation. Nurses must integrate the art and science of nursing in order to enter into a healing relationship with patients. I am convinced that the practice of nursing must have meaning and relevance for both the nurse and the patient and that anything less is a waste of time.

LIVING AND DYING

Living and dying are such huge concepts that I would never claim to comprehend all there is to them. However, in discussing terminal illness, it is essential to sketch in some experiences and beliefs about them in order to formulate a context for this discussion. For each person, culture, religious belief, and philosophy, there are attempts to understand the reason for our existence. We can only speak authoritatively from our own understanding, but there are enough commonalities between our understandings that if the basic beliefs and experiences are laid out clearly, we can share our knowledge and increase our comprehension.

The path we take to a particular perspective is as important as the worldview from that perspective because it serves the same purpose that method and design do in research. The path lends or detracts from the validity of the view and allows for reproducibility of the view for anyone willing to retrace the path for enlightenment's sake.

The Path

I don't remember thinking too much about living and dying before I became a nurse. In retrospect, living and dying were taken for granted, mostly because of the era, the rural area, and the culture in which I was raised. Deceased family members often laid in state in the home and children were taken to visitations and funerals. At age six, I accompanied my grandparents as they chose the casket for my great-uncle. Death was mourned, but was tacitly accepted as a part of life. Because I was raised by elderly grandparents, I knew a lot of old people and many of them died while I was growing up. There were specific rituals that provided order and structure to the grieving process and it was accomplished in an open, public way.

For whatever reason, life was accepted as a struggle over which individuals had little control. Just as there were death rituals, there were life rules. The life rules were handed down through the family, the church, the school, and the government. Living by the rules was very important in the community and punishment for breaking rules was swift. Questioning the rules or their source was actively discouraged.

My generation was better educated than our parents and grandparents, and through that education we were exposed to the world outside our community. That exposure planted within us the seeds of a desire to escape from what we saw as restrictive and binding rules. Work, college, or military service would enable us to escape from a community we then felt was all too small.

Our escape coincided with the social revolution of the 1960s that not only encouraged us to critically examine everything we had been taught, but required that we do so. Television, movies, music, and literature all influenced our ideas as they had no other generation. The pain, suffering, and grisly death, as imaged from Vietnam, seemed omnipresent. It was nothing like the death I experienced as a child. There was nothing peaceful about it. Instead of old people at the end of a full life, these were young people, my age. As a result, death itself became the scapegoat. If we didn't see death, or talk about it, perhaps it might not be so bad.

As in all wars, medical treatment was expanding exponentially and on television dramas patients were shown surviving against incredible odds. Surely death was a thing of the past, and if we ignored it and concentrated on life and medical intervention we would never have to deal personally with death. By 1979, such optimism received a public forum in Silverstein's *Conquest of Death*, where he asserted: "Today, for the first time, we are at the threshold of a new era in which death may no longer be inevitable" (p. 4). He outlined the latest advances in medical technology from nuclear medicine advances to genetic engineering and suggested that by the time our generation reached the age of terminal illness and disability, death from them would be defeated. The message was extremely attractive to a culture that worshiped youth.

I still remember the first person I watched die. I was in my senior year in nursing school and she was 14 years old. She had asthma and had been hospitalized for shortness of breath. Her physician made the decision to electively intubate her, and in the process she arrested and could not be resuscitated. I remember the anger the nurses expressed toward the physician and the blame they attached to him believing that he had not prepared adequately for this consequence. In fact, he had ordered the emergency cart in the room and sufficient personnel were in the room to handle the emergency. I think at that time I unquestioningly absorbed the belief that death was an aspect of failure and, therefore, someone's fault. The corollary here is also clear: if our work is done correctly, the patient lives. It was not until many years later that I became aware of my beliefs in this regard and began to question them.

After graduation, I entered the Army Nurse Corps as the war in Vietnam began to wind down. The physical, mental, and spiritual suffering I met had infinite variety and manifestation. Doctors, nurses, and soldiers expressed the belief that the dead were the lucky ones. Although this conflicted with my belief about good and bad care as the basis for life and death, there were many experiences that re-enforced those beliefs as well.

While in the military, I became addicted to my own adrenaline by working in critical care. The challenge of beating the odds, of constantly being ready to do battle, was both powerful and empowering. Once in civilian life I continued in adult critical care and even today feel that same powerful usefulness through "life and death" decisions. Critical care units were created specifically as the "Special Forces" in the war on death. Over the almost twenty-five years that I have been a critical care nurse, my ideas and beliefs have undergone tremendous evolution and revolution, but my need to be useful professionally has not changed in any way but in its intensity.

Much of the way I view the world and nursing has been and continues to be influenced by Dr. Martha Rogers. Her conceptualization of nursing and it's worldview have opened the door of my thinking to nontraditional ways of being a nurse and to reconceptualizations of old problems. Once this door opened and I stepped through, I could never return to my old way of thinking.

One of the advantages to a Rogerian view of nursing is that it opens dialogue on an amazing number of possibilities for which we currently have no scientific language or methodologies to explore. It is a science of the future as well as the present and a science as handicapped without the art of nursing as the art is without the science to inform it. It is an optimistic science because of the possibilities it proposes.

The Paradox of Life and Death

The appreciation of paradox is an especially liberating possibility in the worldview I have acquired. Webster's dictionary (1984) defines paradox as "an essentially self-contradictory statement based on valid deduction from acceptable premises." A paradox is a puzzle, a mystery to be apprehended, but never fully understood—life and death in constant tension, neither having any meaning without the other; life made more precious because it is finite, death more poignant because of the richness of the life that preceded it. When things no longer have to fit into one and only one category, I am free to consider many views or explanations for an event or phenomenon. I have choices or options and am empowered by what I choose to believe.

While the mystery associated with the paradox may not be completely understood, it can be explored. One method of exploration useful in the study of paradox is dialectic. Webster (1984) defines dialectic as "The Hegelian process of change whereby a thesis is transformed into an antithesis and preserved and fulfilled by it, the combination of the two being resolved in synthesis"—the merging of polarities into a cohesive whole that is greater than and different from the sum of the two parts.

Regarding terminal illness, a dialectic context is also clear: thesis, life; antithesis, death; and synthesis, living with a terminal illness. This exploration will form the foundation for examining healing when a cure is impossible.

Life and Living

Peck (1978) begins *The Road Less Traveled* with the assertion that life is difficult. This is not a negative assertion: It contradicts any notion that we are the passive victims of fate. Difficult has meaning only in relation to challenge, to puzzles, to problems that require solutions and decisions to be made. As nurses we see much of the difficulty in other peoples' lives while managing the difficulty in our own. Not only is life difficult, but there are various levels of difficulty as we progress much like a computer game where acquisition of a particular number of points passes one to the next level of complexity and challenge. Life is not for the faint of heart, however, like the computer game analogy, the reward is reflective of the level of complexity. If one chooses never to progress beyond the lowest level of challenge, then only the lowest level of reward is available.

Peck proposes four tools or techniques of discipline for experiencing and growing from the inevitable pain of living. Those tools are (1) delay of gratification, (2) acceptance of responsibility, (3) dedication to truth and (4) balancing. He acknowledges that some people don't seem to be damaged as much by the difficulties of their lives as others. This difference he attributes to grace which he describes as a powerful force that nurtures our spiritual growth. The motivation for using the techniques of discipline and accepting grace is love which he defines as "the will to extend one's self for the purpose of nurturing one's own or another's spiritual growth" (Peck, 1978, p. 82). Nozick (1989) in *The Examined Life* echoes this notion in defining love:

> *This extension of your own well-being (or ill-being) is what marks all the different kinds of love: the love of children, the love of parents, the love of one's people, of one's country. Love is not necessarily a matter of caring equally or more about someone else than about yourself. . . .The people you love are included inside your boundaries, their well-being is your own. (Nozick, 1989, p. 69)*

Love, discipline, and grace have been proposed as essential qualities of life, but one might ask, "Is there more?" Yes, I think there is. Hope, courage, joy, satisfaction with accomplishment, transcendence, and self-determination stand out in my mind as significant and essential qualities that make life worth living. And with the embrace of each of these qualities, we must embrace their shadows as well. For where is the fullness of love without the contrast of apathy, discipline without disorder, grace without abandonment, hope without fear, courage without cowardice, joy without suffering, satisfaction without anger and disappointment, transcendence without suffering, or self-determination without powerlessness? Just as the contrast of black ink against white paper dramatizes and emphasizes each letter, these opposites enrich and enlarge each other.

Jung said, "Emotion is the chief source of all becoming conscious. There can be no transforming of darkness into light and of apathy into movement without emotion." For me, a life worth living equates with be-coming conscious. It demands reflection and examination of everything.

Life and living are not the same thing. Life is the whole and can best be appreciated in retrospect either from the end or from the perspective of key landmarks along the way. Living on the other hand is day to day, minute to minute, experience to experience. Life is the domain of the spirit as it seeks after meaning. Living is the domain of the soul as it hammers out the shape of life in the present. Where life and spirit transcend, living and soul endure.

The hard and rewarding work of the soul is chronicled well in *Care of the Soul* by Moore (1992). He describes the soul as a quality rather than a thing and declares that care of the soul has to do with "modest care and not miraculous cure" (p. 5). He proposes that the work of the soul is to make us human and when we try to avoid human failure, "we move beyond the reach of the soul." Rinpoche (1992) says it well in *The Tibetan Book of Living and Dying:* "Whatever we have done with our lives makes us what we are when we die. And everything, absolutely everything counts" (p. 24). I submit that the harder one works at living, the more rich and complex the life that results. A rich and complex life is not dependent on the quantity of time one has to create it, but rather the intensity of the work and the receptivity to the experiences and the opportunity to do the work. One of the remarkable aspects of the living/dying paradox is that foreknowledge of one's death is a rare opportunity for soul work unavailable to most. It is the chance to make every second count.

Death and Dying

It is quite easy to get people to talk about their philosophy of life, even if they are not sure that that is what it is. Experiences of living are told hu-morously, and sadly and embarrassingly, but there is an underlying accep-tance of the stories. Stories of experiences of death and dying are reserved for only very special people or occasions, and storytellers who regularly overcome this inhibition are avoided or shunned. Few people will admit to a philosophy of death, but I believe it is as essential as a phi-losophy of life. Religion can be a part of it, but it is no substitute. Jung taught that growth and development of the human being, or individua-tion, required the embrace of the shadow or darker side in all aspects of one's being. I suggest that dying is the shadow of living. Dying is certainly characterized by the shadow qualities already described as the essentials of living. The refusal to examine death and dying and to formulate a set of beliefs about it is the chief source of the fear of death.

Death and dying are different. The death and dying of my grandfather led me to this constellation of thought and feeling. His dying was agonizing for him and for everyone who loved him, but his death was sweet release. In *The Fragile Species,* Thomas (1992) concludes that death is not a fearful occurrence and bases this conclusion on the fact that the only agonizing death he had seen was a patient with rabies. In *How We Die,* Nuland (1994) rightly points out that while this may be true of death, watching someone die often reveals tremendous agony and suffering.

Over the years, I have watched the approach to death and dying in the ICU evolve. Even in this intense battleground of lifesaving, I see the acknowledgment that sometimes all that can be done is not what should be done. In this one acknowledgment, the door is opened for aggressive intervention toward a different goal, a peaceful, comfortable dying. In retrospect, I can see that my grandfather's dying did not have to be agonizing for him or for us, but it was not the fashion then to use morphine drips for pain control and there were no benzodiazepines to control anxiety and produce amnesia.

We know little about death itself. Religion, philosophy, and science have all acknowledged death in their own way. Death might even be referred to as the ultimate mystery, about which we will never be able to do more than speculate. Religion divides neatly into those that guarantee an afterlife and those that do not. After that there isn't much agreement about what that afterlife, or lack of afterlife, is or how one experiences it. I don't think most people have any real confidence in any of the speculation, but are content to choose to believe what is most attractive to them. This is not a criticism, but an observation based on a need to choose a course that decreases not increases fear; in this case, the fear of death.

If we acknowledge that living involves some suffering, we may be quicker to acknowledge that dying requires some suffering as well. As in life, suffering has physical, psychological, and spiritual etiologies. Physical pain; fear of the unknown, of failure, of loneliness; loss of function, of dignity, of innocence are all more prominent in dying. The movement of dying from the public eye to the secret recesses of hospitals and intensive care units adds to the mystique but subtracts from its mystery. Our public denial of death makes it seem a failure, not only for the healthcare providers, but somehow for the person dying as well.

While the unknown and the uncertainty of death most often produce fear and avoidance, we are powerless to prevent death. Wisdom and maturation are found in the acknowledgment that everyone dies. We refocus from death to the process of living and dying. If we have no control over whether we die, might we have some control over how and when we die? With options comes empowerment and with empowerment, living. Living and dying, coinciding together.

Living with Terminal Illness

Because living doesn't stop when dying begins, the definition of terminal illness rests in two important characteristics or qualities with which it is associated. First, terminal illness hastens death and dying. Second, terminal illness reveals the imminence of death. These qualities are not mutually exclusive and their synergy heightens and intensifies every event, relationship, emotion, and process of being.

The focus on terminal illness changes death from a purely existential phenomenon to a personal reality. The case might be made that all illness hastens death, but perhaps it is more useful to think of a terminal illness as one that is associated with a particular diagnosis in which statistical survival is calculated in a limited number of days, months, or years. Nuland includes several disease categories such as ischemic heart disease, violence, trauma, AIDS, and cancer as the leading causes of death.

While all these diseases may hasten death, people live with some for many years and the presence of the diagnosis in a medical record is not sufficient to concede the imminence of death. By imminence of death I mean unavoidable, in-your-face confrontation with the reality that death is no longer some vague, ill-defined, future event for which there is plenty of time to plan.

In *Further Along the Road Less Traveled,* Peck (1993) writes about what he calls a "breaking moment," a point of realization that you need help. Twelve-step programs refer to this phenomenon as "hitting bottom." It can also be thought of as a fork in the road or a crossroads. The image is designed to convey the notion that whatever has been can no longer continue. Terminal illness is just such a breaking moment and provides the momentum for change. This is a tremendously positive concept, the idea of breaking a fall or pushing off from the bottom of the pool when you hit it. Not everyone sees the concept as positive, rather they see no way off the precipice that broke the path and only mud at the bottom of the pool that offers no footing to push against.

The issue here is more than the half full/half empty glass analogy. While optimism plays a role, the more important, determining factor in how one reacts to the diagnosis of a terminal illness is how one has reacted to other breaking moments throughout life. Basically, their dying is dependent on how they have lived.

HEALING

To heal is to make whole again. To make whole implies that something has become disconnected or broken. What better place to look for and expect healing than in a breaking moment? Making whole means reintegrating the parts into a recognizable entity much as individuation is integration of the shadow self into consciousness. Healing in the context of terminal illness is integrating the diagnosis and all its meanings and implications into the fabric of the self while reaffirming one's basic human value.

Healing and Curing

Although healing and curing are often used interchangeably, they are somewhat related constructs, but far from the same thing. Webster (1984) defines cure as a remedy, "something that relieves or corrects a harmful or disturbing situation." One may cure a headache, cure a wound, even cure a disease, but not a human being. Curing a disease does not reintegrate a person nor does integration of the diagnosis into the fabric of the person depend on, or guarantee the curing of the disease.

Healing is done *with* someone not *to* them. Healing is the work of the one who is broken and it cannot be accomplished by anyone else. The admonition "Physician heal thyself" is consummate. Although the task cannot be accomplished by anyone else, it can seldom be accomplished alone. For it is a mutual process where all are involved in healing—healer and healed.

What, then, are the tasks of healing in the context of terminal illness, by definition a diagnosis for which there is no cure? The tasks are the restoration of hope and the relief of unnecessary suffering.

Restoration of Hope. Most people react to the diagnosis of terminal illness with a certain amount of hopelessness. They vary only in the intensity of the hopelessness. No matter what one espouses about belief in an afterlife, death is certainly an end of what is. Fear of the suffering associated with the disease, the loss, and the unknown are powerful and leave the person and all who love and care for that person with a sense of powerlessness and loss of options. The focus of every thought and feeling zooms ahead to the time of death and there is no thought of events and experiences between the here and now and then. Viorst (1986) writes in *Necessary Losses* that for the person with a diagnosis of a terminal illness, the mourning begins immediately. The initial response of disbelief and numbness is often the place where the healthcare provider first becomes involved in terms of the patient's hope.

The healthcare provider involved in this experience can't help but feel and empathize with these feelings. We are so used to "doing" and so poorly prepared for just "being" in relation to patients and their families that we feel hopeless as well. Grief is the normal response to loss and should not be blunted or restricted. People need help to grieve. Ritual helps some, but especially for those without ritual, counsel and support from a therapeutic relationship are essential.

When I think of hope in relation to terminal illness, I remember the admonition of my instructors in nursing school many years ago not to create false hope in patients. While they weren't very clear about what constituted false hope, they weren't any clearer about what hope was either. I believe now that false hope is the unrealistic expectation that death is avoidable. Once the inevitability of death is accepted, where might one find hope?

In "The Politics of Hope," Havel (1990) gives this description of hope that I think is most applicable to this discussion:

> *Either we have hope within us or we don't; it is a dimension of the soul, and it's not essentially dependent on some particular observation of the world or estimate of the situation. Hope is not a prognostication. It is an orientation of the spirit, an orientation of the heart; it transcends the world that is immediately experienced, and it is anchored somewhere beyond its horizons . . . . Hope, in this deep and powerful sense, is not the same as joy that things are going well, or willingness to invest in enterprises that are obviously headed for early success, but, rather, an ability to work for something because it is good, not just because it stands a chance to succeed. The more unpropitious the situation in which we demonstrate hope, the deeper that hope is. (p. 181)*

I believe that we all have the capacity for hope and that this capacity can be developed. I also believe that the capacity for hope can be blunted by life events. The restoration of hope requires a diligent search for the roots of the capacity for hope and gentle nurturing and pruning as hope grows.

As a garden flourishes in the love of the gardener, so hope can flourish in the love and discipline of the therapeutic relationship.

What is realistic hope when cure is not realistic? There is the hope of deepened relationships with one's family, there is the hope of productivity in whatever time remains, there is the hope of symptom relief, there is the hope of legacy, the hope of understanding, the hope that one will not die alone. Spinoza said, "Fear cannot be without hope nor hope without fear." Anyone seeking to nurture hope must first search carefully for fear, embrace it, understand it. Only then can hope be sustained.

Relief of Unnecessary Suffering. Suffering is an underdeveloped concept in nursing. Kleinman and Kleinman (1990) posit that suffering, or the experience of the illness, has been medicalized out of significance as a professional issue. Within nursing, taxonomies of nursing diagnoses and standard care plans and protocols have sanitized suffering by reducing it to common denominators that are quantifiable and generalizable. While these are valuable tools for organizing the domain of nursing, they are often substituted for genuine entry into the patient's suffering. Relief of suffering integrates the art and science of nursing and absolutely requires that the nurse make a commitment, extend herself on behalf of the patient. By Peck's (1978) definition, this is love manifested in the courage to overcome our own fears and to enter into the hard work of healing in the hope of helping the patient, the family, and ourselves. In depicting the hard work of healing he says:

> *But more often than not, the most healing thing that we can do with someone who is in pain, rather than trying to get rid of that pain, is to sit there and be willing to share it. We have to learn to bear and to bear other people's pain. (p. 28)*

Suffering, the pain that accomplishes nothing, that wears us down beyond meaning and interferes with growth and work toward wholeness, is unnecessary. Physical suffering such as intractable pain, nausea and vomiting, draining wounds, and smells that isolate one from the community and society where love and support reside can and must be relieved. The specifics of the relief of such suffering are beyond the scope of this discussion, however, Lang and Patt (1994) in their book, *You Don't Have to Suffer,* describe in great detail and in lay language the repertoire of interventions available to relieve unnecessary physical suffering.

While pharmacology and technology offer some of the best options for physical suffering, other strategies must be found for other types of suffering, especially interpersonal suffering. I don't know anyone who is without loose ends in their lives; goals unachieved, loved ones unreconciled, feelings and emotions unexpressed, forgiveness unoffered. The imminence of death throws these loose ends into sharp relief against the background of self-examination. Reflection, examination, and Peck's concepts of love and discipline form a framework for relief of some of this interpersonal suffering.

Nursing, Healing, and the Dying Patient

Within the feminist literature, caring has taken on a new legitimacy and value in human interaction. Nursing, too, has begun to explore the construct of caring as a multidimensional aspect of the feminine nature of nursing. I am using feminine here as an essential quality rather than as gender. In this sense, feminine is not dependent on being female and is a characteristic of both men and women just as masculine qualities characterize both.

I believe that if nursing is to play a role in healing, then nursing must first heal its broken nature. Nursing must reintegrate science and art. This is much more difficult than it sounds. Addressing both art and science in the curriculum of nursing programs and celebrating nurses who are artists are important and sorely needed; however, this does not integrate them. The integration of the art and science in nursing can take place only within the nurse. The integration of the art and science of nursing can be demonstrated only in the care the nurse delivers to another person or group of people. It is an interpersonal endeavor, not an intellectual one.

The motivation for integrating the art and science of nursing is caring. Caring is an active commitment, an extension of one's self, and it is not entered into lightly. It is neither altruistic nor self-sacrificing. Altruism and sacrifice imply that the caring person receives nothing in return. Giving without receiving uses up the resources of the giver and extinguishes the giving. Reverby (1987) cautions that caring is not merely an identity; it is work. Caring in this sense equates well with Peck's definition of love.

Any artist must have knowledge of technique, equipment, skill, and perspective to do their art, but they are not enough to make the artist. Experience of life in the practice of the art enhances and refines the art and the artist. Nursing must have the science, technology, skill, and methods of critical analysis first to practice the art of nursing fully. Practice and life experiences catalyzed by the professional love we call caring allow the integrated nurse to emerge. This emergence is often evident in nurses' stories, poems, and art, but is most powerful in observation of the practice of a nurse who has made the successful integration.

No situation is more demanding of a caring, integrated nurse than the therapeutic relationship between a dying patient/family and the nurse. The science informs the nurse's ministrations that will hopefully restore hope and relieve unnecessary suffering, but beyond that the art of judgment, presence, wisdom, truthfulness, and discipline (Peck's definition) make the nurse a unique partner in this rich therapeutic relationship.

THE THERAPEUTIC RELATIONSHIP

A therapeutic relationship is made up of the therapist, the person or group seeking therapy, and some process that defines and structures the therapy. It is therapeutic because it is entered into to bring about some positive outcome. The nurse/patient relationship is a therapeutic relationship and for me the most important professional relationship. Traditionally, the outcome of this relationship has been limited to the patient with the assumption that the nurse is objective and unchanged, a facilitator but not a participant with the patient in the desirable outcome.

The origins of this tradition are described in detail by Reverby (1987) in *Ordered to Care*. The duty to care was equated with following orders. Total commitment to this duty made ethical dilemmas and questions of role implausible. Although the education and demands of nursing have changed, the myth of detachment has endured. I remember being a young ICU nurse, hiding in a supply closet shedding tears over the death of a patient we had worked diligently to save. The nursing supervisor found me there and asked if I thought I could get through the next one without crying.

As nursing pursued a scientific base in the interest of legitimization as a profession, the detachment of the logical, positivist philosophy of science was incorporated into practice to reenforce this tradition. The art of nursing was essentially abandoned in favor of a more scientific approach. Nursing "arts" became the skills lab where students learned to bathe and feed patients.

This traditional approach to the therapeutic relationship leaves the nurse in the position of constantly expending energy and never replenishing, a process that is incompatible with life. It is no wonder that so many who deal on a daily basis with patients, especially dying patients, become numb or burn out completely. To be effective, the relationship must nourish the patient and the nurse, it must be a reciprocal, mutual process. Marck (1990) has written in detail about reciprocity in the nurse/patient relationship. The question for the profession, then, is how to reframe the nurse/patient relationship so that it is a mutual process that can foster healing in both.

In contrast to my previous experience with hiding my tears over the death of a patient, my more recent ICU experience with dying patients reflects the evolution in our attitudes about professional detachment from the experience of patient and family suffering. I cared for a woman with liver failure from hepatitis B for six weeks as her primary nurse. Although the family held out hope that she would survive this crisis as she had others, even they came to realize that this episode was different and that intubation and dialysis would not be appropriate interventions. We developed a strong bond and when it was clear to me that her death would come in less than an hour, I was able to assemble all her family in the room and stay with them during her dying. I was able to "nurse" them in the most intense and active sense of the word through the process of her dying and the expression of their grief. No "Code" that pulled a patient back from the precipice of death for a long and fulfilling life ever produced a more powerful sense of success and satisfaction than the experience with this dying patient and her family. After the process was over and her body had been removed, I enjoyed the support and presence of my colleagues as I processed my own grief. Participation in healing with any patient, but especially dying patients, is a highly individual process. There are no useful nursing diagnoses, no standard care plans and no protocols, policies, or procedures to serve as a map or guide for this work. The nature and direction, the content and style of each process is a product of the people and circumstances involved. Techniques and strategies are available to the nurse, but when and how to use them requires the intuition, experience, and judgment of the nurse. Each patient the nurse enters into healing with is unique and leaves the nurse and the patient different than before.

Discipline as a Mutual Therapeutic Process

The application of Peck's tools of discipline as guidelines for the mutual process of healing will be discussed within a therapeutic relationship. While love is the energy that fuels the relationship, discipline is the mechanism that makes the relationship work. These guiding principles offer a foundation for the identification of strategies that are unique to the relationship as opposed to standard interventions for a standard problem label.

Delay of Gratification

Delay of gratification and a hastening of death may seem an oxymoron when time seems to be a precious commodity in short supply. In this case, however, it refers to setting priorities and doing the hardest part first. In essence, do not procrastinate. I must confess that this is a hard point for me to internalize since, like most of my generation, I am used to doing what makes me happy now and letting the future take care of itself. Intellectually I recognize that in the context of a foreshortened future and in fact, in life, this is ultimately self-defeating. It is hard to call that loved one, especially at a time of such vulnerability, but putting it off will not make it easier. Seeking or offering forgiveness is hard, but the potential reward is great. For the nurse, it may mean confronting one's own feelings about death and overcoming them in order to be able to enter the relationship with the patient. This internal conflict only points out how difficult it is within a therapeutic relationship to influence the course of healing and how impossible it is in the absence of hope. It suggests that discipline for the nurse is as crucial as discipline for the patient. The very hardest part for both the nurse and the patient may be to expose their vulnerability since the very work to be done here makes everyone involved vulnerable.

Accepting Responsibility

Accepting responsibility is a matter of reclaiming control of one's life and ultimately one's death. It is embracing the undesirable disease and its manifestations instead of being controlled by them. To accept responsibility is to become empowered by participating in the change that is occurring in one's life instead of becoming victimized by it. Barrett (1986) developed the Theory of Power as Knowing Participation in Change which makes a very effective model for empowerment within a nurse/patient relationship.

Knowing participation in change has three components: (1) awareness of choice, (2) perceived freedom to act on that choice, and (3) acting intentionally. Awareness of choice is a conscious process of choosing between viable options as well as the belief that one has choices or options. Often in terminal illness, the sense of hopelessness and powerlessness comes from the belief that one has no options; the sense that the imminence of death has somehow removed living as an option. The role of the nurse is to help the patient see that there are indeed options and to help and support the patient in making choices. Perceived freedom to act on the choice means identifying problems and working to solve them. Acting intentionally is taking public steps to follow through on the choice.

Assisting the patient toward empowerment empowers the nurse. Experience with each therapeutic relationship re-enforces and encourages the decision to commit to another with hope. Empowerment energizes the nurses as well as the patient and restores the energies necessary to continue such hard work.

Dedication to Truth

Within the context of terminal illness, dedication to truth takes on two very important aspects. The first is don't lie to yourself. The imminence of death is a reality that must be faced with great courage. Courage is not the absence of fear but action in spite of fear and demonstrated in the Bene Gesserit rite from *Dune:*

> *I must not fear. Fear is the mind-killer. Fear is the little-death that brings total obliteration. I will face my fear. I will permit it to pass over me and through me. And when it has gone past I will turn the inner eye to see its path. Where the fear has gone there will be nothing. Only I will remain. (Hebert, 1965, p. 8)*

Human beings are capable of great courage, but they are not infinitely courageous. There can be no standard of courage to which one can be compared, no courage goal toward which one can strive. Courage is not an outcome but a day-to-day, minute-to-minute struggle to live in the open, to come out of hiding. Courage is dependent on the context, the fear and the resources of the individual presented with the challenge. Just as hope is always present in fear, courage is irrelevant without hope.

Refusing to lie to yourself means reflecting on and reassessing your life. It is holding your life up to the light and being open to the failures as well as the successes. It means revising your conclusions and beliefs in the hope of transcending the mere experience in insight and meaning. Ultimately it means accepting the warts as enthusiastically as the beauty marks.

The second aspect is not lying to others. Nuland (1994) writes,

> *For it is the promise of spiritual companionship near the end that gives us hope, much more than does the mere offsetting of the fear of being physically without anyone. The dying themselves bear a responsibility not to be entrapped by a misguided attempt to spare those whose lives are intertwined with theirs. I have seen this form of aloneness and even unwisely conspired in it, before I learned better. (Nuland, 1994, p. 243)*

Dedication to the truth does not mean one cannot have secrets or that one cannot select from details to share with others. It does mean that one is open to those with whom loving relationships are vital and important. To do less deprives one of great comfort and peace.

The mutual nature of the nurse/patient relationship requires that the nurse be dedicated to truth as well. Withholding input in fear that the person can't handle it or will not make the "right" decision defies dedication to the truth. Let compassion be in the way truth is shared not in the way it is withheld.

Balancing

The essence of balance is surrender. Before one can be mended or healed, the inertia of remaining broken must be surrendered and with it the belief that the damage cannot be repaired. Hope is the surrender of fear that binds and gags the spirit. In the context of terminal illness it is the surrender of innocence in the experience of dying. It is surrendering the illusion of limitation of the future for the intensity of the present. The balance of surrender is the fullness of revelation.

FINAL THOUGHTS

One of the issues that I have not discussed and one that is seldom pursued in scientific discussions in nursing or medicine is that of miracles. I am convinced that they occur, but I am unable to even speculate as to why. In preparing to write this manuscript, I spent a good deal of time reflecting on past experiences with families and with patients that have been part of my search for understanding of both dying and healing. One experience stands out in my mind in that it is full of meaning, but remains a mystery to me almost forty years after it happened.

When I was seven or eight years old, my grandfather, who was probably the single most important person in my life, became quite ill. He was admitted to the small hospital in our community with what was diagnosed as pneumonia. Although he was in his fifties, he never seemed really old to me and since sickness, like death, was not hidden from children, my younger sister and I were allowed to visit him in the hospital just as we had visited other relatives.

Something caught the eye of the young physician who was substituting for our town doctor and as a result Grandaddy was sent to M.D. Anderson

Hospital in Houston. The concept of cancer and the modalities of diagnosis and treatment for that disease in the 1950s was beyond my comprehension, but he was gone several weeks. We made the 160-mile trip several times and, on occasion, my sister and I were allowed to go up and see him. He looked very fragile in the oxygen tent, but he reassured me that he was getting better all the time and would soon be home.

I was elated when I was told that Grandaddy was finally coming home from Houston. That is, until I overheard the adults talking about the fact that he was coming home because the results of all the tests and examinations was that he had lung cancer and there was no surgery or medicine that could make him better. I don't remember exactly how I progressed from this knowledge to the understanding that it meant he was coming home to die. The time frame eludes me a little, too, but I remember very soon after the real meaning of his homecoming came to me that I stopped in a private place and put my hands together like I was taught and prayed, "Please God, don't let my grandaddy die." That's all, no repeated pleas or churches called on, no penance or bargaining, just the request. I don't think I ever told my grandfather, or anyone else in my family about that prayer.

Several years later, my grandfather was again admitted to the hospital with pneumonia. Imagine everyone's surprise when there was absolutely no evidence of cancer, anywhere. He lived 14 years after his diagnosis before he died of cancer of the bladder. It is only in retrospect and from a considerable distance of years that the association between this innocent and faithful prayer and the result was identified.

What happened? I don't begin to know. It is unlikely that the doctors at M.D. Anderson made a mistake in their diagnosis, given that cancer was their specialty. Spontaneous remission/cure is the clinical answer, but it begs the question of what happened. Something wonderful, unreproducable and undeserved happened. No list of personal characteristics, qualities, or behaviors can be offered as justification for such a generous and unpredictable gift. Peck would suggest that it was a manifestation of grace. For me the mystery is intact and I am content as far as my grandfather is concerned.

The way this mystery is played out for patients and families with whom I enter therapeutic relationships is a source of some discomfort. How does one acknowledge the possibility of a miracle while acknowledging the tiny probability of one occurring? At this point, I go back to Peck's four tools of discipline, especially dedication to truth and balancing. I hope that at some point I will understand miracle cures with the same confidence that I have about the process of mutuality in nurse/patient relationships. Until then, the mutuality will have to be enough.

REFERENCES

Barrett, E. A. M. (1986). Investigations of the principle of helicy: The relationship of human field motion and power. In V. M. Malinski (Ed.), *Explorations on Martha Rogers' science of unitary human beings,* pp. 173-188. Norwalk, CT: Appleton-Century-Crofts.

Havel, V. (1990). The politics of hope. *Disturbing the peace.* New York: Knopf.

Herbert, F. (1965). *Dune.* New York: Berkeley Books.

Kleinman, A., & Kleinman, J. (1990). Suffering and its professional transformation: Toward an ethnography of interpersonal experience. *Cult Med Psychiatry, 14*(2), 275-301.

Lang, S. S., & Patt, R. B. (1994). *You don't have to suffer: A complete guide to relieving cancer pain for patients and their families.* New York: Oxford University Press.

Marck, P. (1990). Therapeutic reciprocity: A caring phenomenon. *Advances in Nursing Science, 12*(1), 49-59.

Moore, T. (1992). *Care of the soul: A guide for cultivating depth and sacredness in everyday life.* New York: Harper Collins.

Moore, T. (1994). *Soul mates: Honoring the mysteries of love and relationship.* New York: Harper Collins.

Nozick, R. (1989). *The examined life.* New York: Simon & Schuster.

Nuland, S. B. (1994). *How we die: Reflections on life's final chapter.* New York: Alfred A. Knopf.

Peck, M. S. (1978). *The road less traveled.* New York: Simon & Schuster.

Peck, M. S. (1993). *Further along the road less traveled.* New York: Simon & Schuster.

Reverby, S. M. (1987). *Ordered to care: The dilemma of American nursing, 1850-1945.* Cambridge: Cambridge University Press.

Rinpoche, S. (1992). *The Tibetan book of living and dying.* San Francisco: Harper.

Siegel, B. S. (1988). *Love, medicine and miracles.* New York: Harper.

Silverstein, A. (1979). *Conquest of death: A controversial look at the revolution in medicine and why we may be the last generation to die.* New York: Macmillan.

Thomas, L. (1992). *The fragile species.* New York: Scribner's.

Viorst, J. (1986). *Necessary losses: The loves, illusions, dependencies, impossible expectations that all of us have to give up in order to grow.* New York: Simon & Schuster.

Webster's II (1984). *New Riverside University Dictionary.* Boston: Houghton Mifflin.

CHAPTER 32

Childbearing: A Healing Opportunity

RUTH TUCKER, RN, RNC, PHD

How can this be—childbearing as a healing opportunity? At no other time do women have such intimate and continuous contact with healthcare professionals. At no other time are women more open to assistance. At no other time are women so in tune with their bodies. At no other time are women so introspective, allowing unresolved issues to surface. The stage is set for integration of body, mind, and spirit—a healing opportunity.

Though pregnancy is considered to be a normal, healthy state, it is a time of tremendous physiological, social, and psychological changes. A pregnant woman balances on a fine line between wellness and illness.

Physiologically, virtually all body systems are affected. Many of these changes are initiated by hormonal fluctuations and further affected by the growing fetus. These physiological changes are predictable with each trimester of pregnancy.

Socially, the woman begins to experience changes in her interactions with the father of the child, her family of origin, her peer group, and society at large. Her self-image changes to expectant mother and begins the transformation to that of mother.

Psychologically, she must cope with a multitude of issues. These are related to her ever-changing physical state, her altered social interactions, and her feelings about the pregnancy, childbirth, and motherhood. Issues from past life or obstetric experiences may surface.

Developmentally, pregnancy is viewed by many as a normal transitional crisis. Crisis, when written in Chinese characters, is translated as both *danger* and *opportunity*. The possibility that a person may become overwhelmed by changes and events places them in *danger*. Crisis may increase receptivity to learn new coping patterns, thus creating an *opportunity*. Therefore, childbearing as a crisis may be a healing opportunity.

We will review the mind-body connection during pregnancy, to identify psychosocial risk characteristics including their relationship to pregnancy outcome, and to propose healing interventions to facilitate more favorable obstetric, physical, and psychological outcomes.

HEALING POTENTIAL: THE MIND-BODY CONNECTION

Thought processes manifest in our bodies. "Inherent within this belief in the mind-body connection is the notion that our physical body takes on, holds, and manifests the emotions and thought patterns experienced within our mental and spiritual domains" (Keegan, 1994, p. 31). Contrasting results give a fuzzy picture of the repercussions of emotional state and pregnancy outcome (i.e., course of childbirth and impact on the health of the neonate). However, potential obstetric, physiological, and psychological consequences of psychosocial distress during pregnancy have been documented.

Obayuwana, Carter, and Barnett (1984) proposed a possible pathway for the effects of stress on pregnancy. Psychosocial stress coupled with the inability to cope effectively leads to psychosocial distress. This initiates the stress response in the body which triggers predictable immuno-endocrine and behavioral outcomes. The endocrine system responds by increasing the production of stress hormones (i.e., cortisol, aldosterone, epinephrine). Their study revealed that expectant patients in psychosocial distress had an 80 percent maternal and 44 percent neonatal incidence of less-than-optimum pregnancy outcome. The importance of assessing psychosocial stress as well as physical risk during pregnancy was supported. Resultant changes in the sympathetic and parasympathetic systems may be exhibited in behavioral responses and/or obstetric complications (see Table 32.1).

Omer and Everly (1988) report that cumulative or chronic environmental stress and high scores on psychopathology scales have been consistently linked to preterm labor. They propose a model that links preterm labor to a disorder of arousal manifested physiologically as a hyperreactivity of the limbic circuitry and its efferent components.

Understanding the relationship of stress and the subsequent development of illness has been a continuing quest. Obstetric complications, resulting from stressful life events and other factors including personality qualities (Rofe, Blittner, & Lewin, 1993; Tucker, 1988) have also been studied over several decades.

Research about stress and pregnancy preceded work done by Holmes and Rahe (1967) relating stressful life events to psychological and physical responses. McDonald (1968), in a review of obstetric literature spanning

TABLE 32.1.   Selected consequences of psychosocial distress.

Behavioral Responses	Potential Obstetric Manifestations
Non-compliance	Pseudocyesis (false pregnancy)
Drug/alcohol abuse	Habitual abortion
Poor hygiene	Hyperemesis gravidarum
Indifference	Intrauterine growth retardation
Depression	Preterm labor
Anxiety	Prolonged labor
Negative attitude toward pregnancy	Pregnancy induced hypertension
Mood lability	Labor complications
Poor body image	Low birth weight infant
Ineffective coping	Postpartum hemorrhage
Ineffective cognitive functioning	Poor maternal-infant bonding
	Postpartum depression/psychosis

15 years, explored the relationship between emotional factors and obstetric complications. No findings in McDonald's survey showed definitive causal relationships. However, consistent findings indicated psychological differences between subjects with obstetric complications and those with normal pregnancies.

Stress for a pregnant woman may be a reflection of the additive effects of the stress of pregnancy itself and stressors impinging on her from her own personality, her past, her anticipated future, and her environment. Pregnancy and labor are assumed to be events that require adjustment as do other events creating stress. A high-risk pregnancy with all its uncertainties creates additional anxiety (McCain & Deatrick, 1994; Penticuff, 1982; Rizzardo, Magni, Cremonese, Talamo-Rossi, & Cosentino, 1988).

The relationship of stressful life events and pregnancy has been studied singularly and jointly with other variables. Chronic stressors (e.g., financial and housing problems), negative life events, and inadequate social support were all linked to depression during pregnancy (Sequin, Potvin, St. Denis, & Loiselle, 1995). Clusters of life changes within one to two years increase the risk of a crisis situation. Recent life experiences may place a pregnant woman in a double crisis. She may be accommodating to events in her life that interrupt the normal emotional adjustments throughout pregnancy.

An early study (Gorsuch & Key, 1974) found the greater the stress caused by life events during pregnancy, the more likely it was that an obstetric abnormality would occur. This relationship was found to be true during the last two trimesters of pregnancy and did not necessarily pertain to those stresses occurring prior to the pregnancy. This suggests that an already taxed maternal system is less capable of coping with life stresses.

McDonald's review (1968) noted that anxiety throughout pregnancy increased in the presence of unresolved conflicts about that pregnancy. Higher levels of anxiety were also reported in women who had obstetric complications. Women with high anxiety levels during the third trimester of pregnancy have an increased incidence of hemorrhage and pregnancy-induced hypertension by three to four times (Crandon, 1979). Other studies also address altered psychological functioning in pregnancy and relationship to outcome (Condon & Ball, 1989; Cox & Reading, 1989; Lederman, 1990). Emotional arousal created by stress and anxiety may result in dysfunctional labor. Lederman, Lederman, Work, and McCann (1979) were able to show the relationship between anxiety and the body's negative physiological response during labor.

Women may have body image concerns related to the changes of pregnancy. These may accentuate behaviors reflective of body image concerns (i.e., anorexia nervosa, compulsive eating patterns). Women may be caught in a feminine identity crisis. Examples are those who have failed to separate emotionally from their mothers, who are revolting against mothers who are too powerful, or who are questioning their own sexual orientation. Women whose sexuality has been threatened by incest, rape, or sexual abuse are also at high risk during pregnancy.

Current researchers continue to study the stress phenomenon and its importance during the childbearing experience (Hickey, Cliver, Goldenberg, McNeal, & Hoffman, 1995; Lobel, Dunkel-Schetter, & Scrimshaw, 1992; Peacock, Bland, & Anderson, 1995; Perkin, Bland, Peacock, & Anderson, 1993; Steer, Scholl, Hediger, & Fischer, 1992).

WHERE HEALING IS NEEDED: ASSESSING PSYCHOSOCIAL RISKS

The complexities of life must be appreciated throughout the assessment process. Nurses are "guests" in a family's life during the childbearing process, sharing one of life's most intimate experiences. The intricacies of a person's life remain hidden even to the individual. They know only through their perceptions and at the conscious level. The subconscious has a way of revealing itself—sometimes gently, sometimes harshly. The childbearing period may be a time of revelation.

Pregnancy increases vulnerability to emotional disequilibrium and psychological disturbances. A broad relationship between psychological factors and obstetric complications has been confirmed. Women who report an increased number of ailments during prenatal visits may be providing clues regarding emotional stress and a need for additional psychosocial support (Forde, 1992).

Forde (1993) recommends clinical assessment of a woman's psychosocial condition using all accessible information. Social and psychological assessments as well as an obstetric history will provide insights into the pregnant woman's present psychological state. Suggested assessment areas are summarized in Table 32.2.

A person who optimistically appraises events and has decisive interactions with these events directed at decreasing their stressfulness seems to

TABLE 32.2. Summary of assessment topics.

Sociological Assessment	Psychological Assessment	Biological/Obstetric History
Support system	Intensity of recent life events	History of infertility
Ability to use resources	Clusters of life events	Unplanned pregnancy
Non-traditional mother	Personality characteristics	In vitro pregnancy
History of abuse/violence	Depression	Abnormal prenatal screening
Substance abuse status	Anxiety	Known fetal anomaly
Relationship with own mother	Locus of control	Prior birth defects
Sexual orientation	Prior psychological problems	Prior fetal/neonatal loss
		Prior preterm labor/delivery
		History of pregnancy or labor complications
		Previous cesarean delivery

have fewer stress-related illnesses (Kobasa, Maddi, & Courington, 1981). Peterson (1981) applies this belief to labor in her statement that "a woman who has developed a style during her lifetime of being able to meet and handle stress without creating distress for herself, will be less likely to create blocks for herself in labor" (p. 4).

Mediating variables are those that lessen the shock of stress when it occurs. Psychosocial assets that may serve as mediating variables include positive self-esteem, hardiness (Tucker, 1988), social support (particularly a supportive partner) and extended family and resources (Mills, Finchilescu, & Lea, 1995), coping style, positive perceptions of events, and internal locus of control.

LET THE HEALING BEGIN: SELECTED HEALING INTERVENTIONS

Setting the Stage for Healing

Progress in working through life's issues is a reciprocal process. When there is synchrony in the nurse's ability and willingness to be empathetic and the woman's ability and willingness to look within and to share herself and her life experiences with the nurse, there is also reciprocity. For the woman and her family, this is a journey of self-discovery and personal growth as they work through issues coming into awareness. The health professional serves as an advocate, facilitator, and cheerleader as this growth process evolves.

Healing takes more than high-tech and advanced diagnostic procedures. Healing begins with the giving of oneself to another, opening the opportunity for connection with another person. The most precious gift is that of self. Keegan (1994) encourages nurses to care for others as an extension of self and to consider the interconnectedness of human beings within the universe.

A second gift is the time spent with another. In our hurry, hurry world, time may well be the most important gift. Healthcare systems demand outcomes usually measured in numbers of patients seen, not necessarily the quality of care they receive. How can we meet the demands of healthcare management and the needs of our patients? These strategies have been chosen because they can be implemented within a managed care environment with minimal resources yet have proven effectiveness. Interventions can evolve with each visit. Activities for the woman to do between visits may be developed.

Person-Centered Approach

For obstetric care, a family-centered approach to childbirth, involving the expectant parents, their children, and other significant persons in the experience, is accepted as the norm. The family is viewed holistically as having biological, psychological, and social needs.

Consider a woman-centered approach to childbirth. Though the family is important and participates in the process, having the baby is the woman's experience. Her soul and spirit as well as her body are involved in the process. The experience is not bracketed in time by pregnancy and delivery. The experience begins early in her life and extends beyond the actual birth.

In a person-centered approach to childbearing, the woman is seen as a whole with mind and body intertwined and inseparable. Great personal resources reside within the individual who strives toward self-actualization. This striving is directed primarily from within the organism but is influenced by all that the individual has experienced. Social and cultural factors from the environment hold the potential for great influence in the woman's response to pregnancy and childbearing. An individual develops a self-concept as a sense of self made up of the experiences of how one functions within the existing environment.

During pregnancy, a woman's self-concept changes. She begins to see herself in new roles and as interacting with others in different ways. It is important to maintain or increase a woman's self-esteem and her feelings of self-worth.

Interactions with others influence the development of feelings of self-worth. If a woman receives positive regard from those around her whom she values, then she will develop a positive self-concept and self-esteem. Loss of conditions of self-worth can have a negative impact. Feelings of self-worth may be jeopardized by past unfavorable obstetric experiences such as feelings of failure resulting from premature delivery, fetal loss, or having a child with anomalies. Being a nontraditional mother in a culture where married motherhood is valued may also decrease feelings of self-worth. Nontraditional mothers include single heterosexual or lesbian women, lesbian couples electing motherhood via donor insemination, surrogate mothers, women with multifetal pregnancy reduction, and incarcerated women.

Assisting individuals to grow and to learn to cope with future as well as current problems are goals of a person-centered approach. Pregnancy may be a time of personal growth. Peterson (1981) provides insight into this phenomenon through multiple case reports. In a climate of acceptance and empathic understanding, this growth can be facilitated. A woman can learn to cope with current challenges presented by her pregnancy as well as the future. The nurse who displays congruence by matching of inner feelings and behaviors creates an aura of genuineness in which this growth can occur. No opinions or judgments are communicated. In this nurturing atmosphere, the pregnant woman senses unconditional positive regard and subsequently may experience increasing self-acceptance. It is important that she identify her inner strengths, physically, psychologically, and spiritually.

During the interactions with the expectant mother, the nurse identifies the personal meanings and feelings being expressed openly by her and senses those just below the level of her awareness. This process of identification and interpretation is based on perceptions and past experiences brought by the nurse to each encounter. These interpretations are communicated with the intent to support the woman in achieving greater understanding of and, therefore, greater control over her own world and behavior. Ideally, the sense of control becomes internalized. The stage is set for increased self-awareness, self-acceptance, less defensive behavior, and freedom to grow.

An individual is motivated by an inner drive toward health, growth, and adjustment. A discrepancy between self and an experience may cause tension and result in anxiety and increased vulnerability. When an occurrence is distorted, denied, or repressed, an incongruency exists. The role of the nurse is to make it possible for the individual to openly express feelings spontaneously without fear of judgment. By removing obstacles (incongruences), the woman can begin the healing process. The individual possesses the ability for self-understanding and for altering her self-concept and attitudes. Incongruences would be revealed and hopefully, could be resolved as the woman expresses her feelings about the pregnancy, labor and delivery, and past experiences. Her behavior changes as she strives for congruence between self and her lived experiences.

A woman may be seen alone, with a partner, or in groups. The purpose of these encounters might be loosely defined as an opportunity to talk to others with similar experiences. Participants would direct the group meetings with the nurse acting only as the facilitator. Cesarean birth support groups for families are an example. Edwards et al. (1994)

report a reduction in low birthweight babies in urban African-American, low-income groups by mediating maternal stress through providing an additional support system in a caring, sensitive environment.

Telling Stories

Nurses can assist in the healing process by simply listening. Healing for a woman may mean nothing more than retelling her stories to someone who cares. A nurse, identifying issues on a prenatal record, spends time with the woman encouraging her to explore her feelings and how that experience relates to where she is now, and then helping her to work through issues. Acknowledging the complexities and serious nature of some situations, the nurse may seek consultation or referral.

It is important for those who have experienced losses to tell their story over and over again. This is part of the healing process. Losses that may impact a current pregnancy include loss of a prior pregnancy, cesarean delivery rather than a normal delivery, or a baby with an anomaly rather than the expected perfect infant. Grieving may come up in new ways or at times that are unexpected—after the individual believes the grief is past. Family and friends may have worked through the experience and believe that the woman has or *should* have, too. They are no longer listening. New ears to hear the story retold can help as the woman works through remaining issues. She may never have told anyone about issues related to her family or her relationship with her mother or her husband. These individuals may knowingly or unknowingly make the pregnancy very stressful. Assistance can be given by creating a safe healthcare environment for telling their stories (Edwards et al., 1994), by helping them build a support network (Gjerdingen, Froberg, & Fontaine, 1991; Norbeck & Anderson, 1989), and by supporting them through what may be a crisis in their lives. Providing support to the partner and other family members is also important. Clement (1995) suggests that women with low emotional well-being be identified antenatally. Her research concluded that "listening visits" in pregnancy may be a useful strategy for preventing postnatal depression.

Imagery

The mind can be a powerful tool. Keegan (1994) suggests that "imagery allows you to create mental pictures that your holistic being can manifest on the physical plane." Visualization has been used for healing and has been

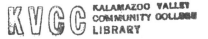
KVCC KALAMAZOO VALLEY COMMUNITY COLLEGE LIBRARY

suggested for use during the childbearing process (Keegan, 1994; Olkin, 1987; Peterson, 1981). The way we perceive things becomes our reality. The healing process can begin by changing the expectant mother's perceptions. Viewing things from a different perspective may alter the way pregnancy and the birthing experience are approached. Again, the complexity of any situation requires great sensitivity from the nurse.

The current pregnancy and future labor and delivery may be imaged with a positive ending. Past experiences impacting the current pregnancy may be revisited but with a different outcome visualized. For the woman who feels that her body has failed her in the past, either during pregnancy or otherwise, the visualization may include a conversation with her own body. This discussion can affirm and discover the inner strengths her body possesses, its ability to have a normal pregnancy, carry the baby to term, and have a positive outcome. For the woman who is experiencing a preterm labor, the conversation may be with the fetus, granting permission to remain in the uterus until maturity. For the woman who is experiencing a post-date pregnancy or whose labor process is blocked, the script may give the fetus permission to emerge.

Individualized audiotapes with background music selected by the expectant mother can integrate affirmations related to the pregnancy, to the labor, and to the outcome. Her ability to parent, to be in control of her responses to events, to make her wishes known, to stand up for her rights, and to describe the experience the way she wants it can be incorporated with her assistance. Building a personalized script requires asking her the right questions and listening to her responses. It is our self-talk (what each of us says to ourselves) and our interpretation or circumstances that creates anxiety, fear, anger, and depression. Dealing with automatic, distorted, or irrational thinking can be addressed directly and quickly. Self-talk can be redirected in more meaningful ways.

SUMMARY

Psychosocial risk assessment alone and in conjunction with biomedical risk assessment may significantly improve our ability to identify women who are at risk for perinatal complications (Herrera, Hurtado, & Caceres, 1992). Research has focused primarily on identification of causal relationships between psychosocial concerns and untoward pregnancy outcomes with little emphasis on prevention. Working with families to integrate the body, mind, and spirit during a developmental crisis such as childbearing is a challenging endeavor. The nurse through her encounters will also experience personal growth. Planned intervention during pregnancy may prevent or minimize the ever-increasing vicious cycle of psychological problems creating obstetric complications which may in turn trigger additional emotional difficulties. Childbearing is indeed a healing opportunity.

REFERENCES

Clement, S. (1995). "Listening visits" in pregnancy: A strategy for preventing postnatal depression? *Midwifery, 11*(2), 75-80.

Condon, J. T., & Ball, S. B. (1989). Altered psychological functioning in pregnant women: An empirical investigation. *Journal of Psychosomatic Obstetrics and Gynaecology, 10,* 211-220.

Cox, D. N., & Reading, A. E. (1989). Fluctuations in state anxiety over the course of pregnancy and the relationship to outcome. *Journal of Psychosomatic Obstetrics and Gynaecology, 10,* 71-78.

Crandon, A. J. (1979). Maternal anxiety and obstetric complications. *Journal of Psychosomatic Research, 23,* 109-111.

Edwards, C. H., Cole, O. J., Oyemade, U. J., Knight, E. M., Johnson, A. A., Westney, O. E., Laryea, H., West, W., Jones, S., & Westney, L. S. (1994). Maternal stress and pregnancy outcomes in a prenatal clinic population. *Journal of Nutrition, 124*(6 Suppl), 1006S-1021S.

Forde, R. (1992). Pregnant women's ailments and psychosocial conditions. *Family Practice, 9*(3), 270-273.

Forde, R. (1993). Clinical assessment of pregnant women's psychosocial conditions, prematurity and birth weight. *Scandinavian Journal of Primary Health Care, 11*(2), 130-134.

Gjerdingen, D. K., Froberg, D. G., & Fontaine, P. (1991). The effects of social support on women's health during pregnancy, labor and delivery, and the postpartum period. *Family Medicine, 23*(5), 370-375.

Gorsuch, R. L., & Key, M. K. (1974). Abnormalities of pregnancy as a function of anxiety and life stress. *Psychosomatic Medicine, 36,* 352-362.

Herrera, J. A., Hurtado, H., & Caceres, D. (1992). Antepartum biopsychosocial risk and perinatal outcome. *Family Practice Research Journal, 12*(4), 391-399.

Hickey, C. A., Cliver, S. P., Goldenberg, R. L., McNeal, S. F., & Hoffman, H. J. (1995). Relationship of psychosocial status to low prenatal weight gain among nonobese black and white women delivering at term. *Obstetrics & Gynecology, 86*(2), 177-183.

Holmes, T. H., & Rahe, R. H. (1967). The social readjustment rating scale. *Journal of Psychosomatic Research, 11,* 213-218.

Keegan, L. (1994). *The nurse as healer.* Albany, NY: Delmar Publishers.

Kobasa, S. C., Maddi, S. R., & Courington, S. (1981). Personality and constitution as mediators in the stress-illness relationship. *Journal of Health and Social Behavior, 22,* 368-378.

Lederman, R. P. (1990). Anxiety and stress in pregnancy: Significance and nursing assessment. *NAACOG'S Clinical Issues, 1*(3), 279-288.

Lederman, R. P., Lederman, E., Work, B. A., Jr., & McCann, D. S. (1979). The relationship of psychological factors in pregnancy to progress in labor. *Nursing Research, 28,* 94-97.

Lobel, M., Dunkel-Schetter, C., & Scrimshaw, S. C. (1992). Prenatal maternal stress and prematurity: A prospective study of socioeconomically disadvantaged women. *Health Psychology, 11*(1), 32-40.

McCain, G. C., & Deatrick, J. A. (1994). The experience of high-risk pregnancy. *Journal of Obstetric, Gynecologic, and & Neonatal Nursing, 23*(5), 421-427.

McDonald, R. L. (1968). The role of emotional factors in obstetric complications: A review. *Psychosomatic Medicine, 30,* 222-243.

Mills, E. P., Finchilescu, G., & Lea, S. J. (1995). Postnatal depression: An examination of psychosocial factors. *South African Medical Journal, 85*(2), 99-105.

Norbeck, J. S., & Anderson, N. J. (1989). Psychosocial predictors of pregnancy outcomes in low-income black, Hispanic, and white women. *Nursing Research, 38*(4), 204-209.

Obayuwana, A. O., Carter, A. L., & Barnett, R. M. (1984). Psychosocial distress and pregnancy outcome: A three-year prospective study. *Journal of Psychosomatic Obstetrics & Gynaecology, 3*(3-4), 173-183.

Olkin, S. K. (1987). *Positive pregnancy fitness.* Garden City Park, NY: Avery Publishing Group.

Omer, H., & Everly, G. S., Jr. (1988). Psychological factors in preterm labor: Critical review and theoretical synthesis. *American Journal of Psychiatry, 145*(12), 1507-1513.

Peacock, J. L., Bland, J. M., & Anderson, H. R. (1995). Preterm delivery: Effects of socioeconomic factors, psychological stress, smoking, alcohol, and caffeine. *British Medical Journal, 311*(7004), 531-536.

Penticuff, J. H. (1982). Psychologic implications in high-risk pregnancy. *Nursing Clinics of North America, 17*(1), 69-78.

Perkin, M. R., Bland, J. M., Peacock, J. L., & Anderson, H. R. (1993). The effect of anxiety and depression during pregnancy on obstetric complications. *British Journal of Obstetrics and Gynaecology, 100*(7), 629-634.

Peterson, G. H. (1981). *Birthing normally: A personal growth approach to childbirth.* Berkeley, CA: Mindbody Press.

Rizzardo, R., Magni, G., Cremonese, C., Talamo-Rossi, R., & Cosentino, M. (1988). Variations in anxiety levels during pregnancy and psychosocial factors in relation to obstetric complications. *Psychotherapy and Psychosomatics, 49*(1), 10-16.

Rofe, Y., Blittner, M., & Lewin, I. (1993). Emotional experiences during the three trimesters of pregnancy. *Journal of Clinical Psychology, 49*(1), 3-12.

Sequin L., Potvin, L., St. Denis, M., & Loiselle, J. (1995). Chronic stressors, social support, and depression during pregnancy. *Obstetrics & Gynecology, 85*(4), 583-589.

Steer, R. A., Scholl, T. O., Hediger, M. L., & Fischer, R. L. (1992). Self-reported depression and negative pregnancy outcomes. *Journal of Clinical Epidemiology, 45*(10), 1093-1099.

Tucker, E. R. (1988). *The relationships of hardiness and stressful life events to obstetric risks.* Eugene, OR: Microform Publications, University of Oregon.

CHAPTER 33

Going Home

MARY ANNE HANLEY, MA, RN

Every day she told her story; all day, morning and evening. She told everyone she met; some we knew and some we didn't; some we saw and some we didn't. Sometimes we listened and sometimes we didn't. She told her story when she was dressing, bathing, or eating, even when she was sleeping; alone or in company.

Her story was a simple one; its theme clear. We knew the story by heart. We were familiar with its rhythm. It was a story about going home, to a place in her heart. Going home to her family, where she loved and was loved. Thinking of going home gave her world meaning. In a dimension we could not see, her mother, sisters, and husband waited for her to rest in their love.

When we listened, her story told us how to get to that home filled with love. She imagined the way home, a road rising through waves of heather, blooming fragrant and heavy. The sky, slightly overcast, met the road. The heart of her journey was in the rhythm of her story. Her joy was her belief that she was on her way home; her desire was for peace at the end of the road and the rest she would find in her family's love.

Far from her lonely room, her only son rested in an unfamiliar place. On the wall was a painting of a familiar scene. A road, rising through blossoming heather, met an overcast sky and turned at the top of a hill. Following some ancient rhythm, her son traveled that road. He journeyed to the home she so long described; to the heart of the universe, to rest in the love of his children and his wife. We walked with him up that lovely road. Sharing his journey, we learned our way home and felt the rhythm of the universe.

Later, when she told her story of going home, we heard her. And we understood the truth of her story. The truth was in our letting each other go, releasing and being released. Barely born into this century, desiring to make her own homeward journey, our grandmother helped us travel with her son down the road of her dreams, to release him into the heart of her love.

We live the truth of her story each time a loved one travels home to rest in the rhythm of the universe. We lived the story as our mother released us to find the peace within our love.

Having gifted us with her story, showing us its truth, our grandmother's dream is complete. We walked with her once more. She has gome home to rest in the love of her family.

Traveling down that familiar road, on our way home, the heather and sky anchor us as we journey into the heart of healing, telling our story.

CHAPTER 34

Healing Processes in Individuals with Seizure Disorders

JEANETTE HARTSHORN, RN, PHD, FAAN

If healing is curing someone with an illness, then I am a failure. The patients for whom I care are chronically ill. Most likely, they will never be cured of these illnesses. Their lives will always revolve around visits to the clinic, management of medications and related effects and fears about their own safety. The patients I care for have epilepsy.

Epilepsy is a chronic illness that affects more than 2.5 million people in the United States. Although potentially severely disabling, it is not a condition one ordinarily thinks about in those terms. The management of epilepsy is a lifelong process and includes many levels. In some ways, the medical management is the easiest—manipulate drugs, do surgery, provide follow-up. Sometimes the challenges of medical management increase. For example, as new anticonvulsants are developed and released adding them to the existing regimen can be difficult. Some patients are intractable and despite the medical care given, the seizures are not controlled.

While this is a particularly troublesome and frustrating experience, the challenges of medically managing the seizures pale in comparison to the challenge of managing the patient's life and his or her response to the seizures. One of the toughest parts of caring for patients with seizures is to help them grapple with the meaning of the illness in terms of their spirit and looking for ways to help them heal. In this context, healing refers to helping them deal with the seizure disorder within the greater whole of their life, no matter how that life may have been redefined by the medical diagnosis.

Seizures offer a unique look at the mind-body connection. Something happens in the brain—multiple neurons fire and the body responds. Imagine the sensation! Your body does something you did not intend for it to do. You cannot exert enough control to stop it. That's the feeling, total loss of control over functions many of us take for granted. Pollock (1993) observes that seizures are unpredictable and as such are perceived to be more of a burden than chronic illness with a progressive, predictable course. In her work, Pollock studied people with hypertension as an example of those who have a disorder that does not include physical disabilities. In many cases, seizures do not coexist with physical disabilities. Adaptation to physical illness was easier for conditions that were constant as opposed to those that are progressive or unpredictable. One of the major components of seizure disorders is the unpredictable nature of the condition. How can healing be approached when one cannot even control the physical response of the body or the times it will fail to respond?

The purpose of this chapter is to review the concept of healing within the framework of a chronic illness, epilepsy. If curing is not possible, healing can still take place within the context of a seizure disorder. Further, the role of the advanced practice nurse as a provider of care within the healing environment is critical.

HEALING AS A CONSTRUCT

An underlying assumption about healing is that each of us (patient and nurse) has what we need to heal. What is needed differs among us and the goal of nursing care is to create an environment that helps to identify these unique features which can then, in turn, promote healing. We seek to move toward wholeness utilizing the patient and family as not only the focus of our attention, but also as the resources to make healing possible. For healthcare provider traditionalists, this is the most difficult part; recognizing that the patient and families do the healing and our job is one of facilitation of that process.

One of the challenges in operating from this paradigm is that people with a chronic illness often have been schooled in dependence on a system. More often than not, their input into their own care or the responsibility for that care has been focused away from the individual and placed directly with the providers. In the traditional system, the provider's goal is to fix the patient's problem. The patient has a passive role, while the provider's role remains active. This system serves to increase the powerlessness perceived by the individual patient. Such patients continually experience an external source making decisions for them. How then can a nurse provider approach care of these individuals within a healing framework?

Advanced Practice within the Context of Healing

The goal of all nursing care is to create a healing environment. The advanced practice nurse structures the concept to include appropriate aspects of medical management within the healing context. Traditional medical management is reductionistic in nature; that is, isolate the problem, treat it, and refer anything else. Nursing management moves toward a sense of wholeness. The goal of the advanced practice nurse is to assist the patient and family in recognizing life patterns and how they are manifested in the patients daily life and health. We seek to help the patient's see and make choices relative to those patterns. According to Newman (1986), this pattern recognition is the heart of human interaction. It is basic to responding to the individuality of another person and therefore basic to the nurse's effective use of self and therapeutic interaction.

Within this context, even the most serious of medical diagnoses (i.e., terminal cancer) is an expression of a person's life patterns. Hence, resolution of the issues that precede and produce the patterns have been credited with "curing" these diagnoses.

The Uniqueness of Seizures

A seizure disorder represents for many people a life-changing as well as a life-encompassing experience. No matter when within the life span the diagnosis is made, the challenges are numerous.

Individuals with epilepsy experience an unusually high number of problems in psychosocial functioning (Gehlert, 1994). The issues include social isolation, impaired learning, employment problems, and dysfunctional family relationships. Among all of the potential psychosocial issues, the concepts of "locus of control" related to perceived powerlessness along with perceived hopelessness are central to our understanding of the experience. An external locus of control and perceived powerlessness has been implicated as etiologic factors in the development of psychosocial problems in epilepsy (Gehlert, 1994; Hermann, Whitman, & Wyler, 1990).

Studies have shown that individuals with epilepsy have an external locus of control. One hypothesizes that with the generally unpredictable nature of seizures, individual's rely on external sources (i.e., the medical establishment), to control their seizures. This lack of control spills over into various aspects of these person's lives, and they begin to deal with other aspects of their life in exactly the same way (i.e., expecting others to be in the central role of problem solvers). The external locus of control is seen to be a fairly constant personality trait. Its outgrowth concept, powerlessness, is seen as a reaction to an event which potentially can be managed. Powerlessness is actually a reflection of an inability to cope with a chronic illness (Miller, 1983).

A related concept, "learned helplessness" has been linked to many of the psychosocial problems associated with epilepsy. Studies of patients with pain have shown that perceived helplessness is positively associated with noncompliance, passive coping-style, physical impairment, and pain intensity (Jensen et al., 1995). In addition, a decreased level of perceived helplessness over time is associated with decreased passive coping and pain intensity (Stein, Wallstone, Niccasio, & Castner, 1988). Perceived helplessness in the individual with epilepsy will make their medical management difficult as they struggle with noncompliance and passivity. In clinical practice, passivity and noncompliance are common variables linked to medical instability.

With these variables in mind the following several case studies are presented to explore the application techniques for healing.

CASE STUDIES

Mr. L.

Mr. L. is a 58-year-old man who has had seizures since he was 30 years old. The probable cause for his seizures is a head injury which occurred following a motor vehicle accident. He has been well controlled with medication for more than 10 years. Recently, however, he has begun to experience new "blackout" spells which most likely represent a new form of seizure. Following the onset of the blackout spells, a repeat MRI and EEG were performed and no evidence of a new abnormality was found. To control the immediate events, a new medication was added until seizure control was achieved. In response to this turn of events, Mr. L., because the seizures had now become unpredictable, stayed within his home and was afraid to continue with his normal social activities. He became very isolated from friends and family and his normal routine had been drastically interrupted. His response to these changes was surprise and eventually anger since he grieved for the way things had been. On clinic visits, he was sad and withdrawn. Once the medications had been altered and he was again seizure free, Mr. L. was able to return to his normal activities. However, his basic assumptions of normalcy had been challenged and the old "spunk" which had characterized him was now greatly subdued. Because of the number of seizures, his life pattern had been interrupted and although medically he had returned to his previous state, he was in need of opportunities to heal. Once medically stable, the focus of care was on developing an understanding of how his life pattern had been altered and how this alteration had precipitated seizures. Another important variable to consider included his current reaction of withdrawal and the potential effects of the withdrawal on future development of seizures. To help him develop the needed insight, Mr. L. was asked to bring his family in for a few visits. The discussions which followed with his daughter helped him to see that while he had experienced a setback, he was returning to equilibrium and that he did not need to focus on a worsening health picture. With that recognition and the support of his daughter, he was able to regain some of his old "spunk."

Miss W.

Miss W. is a 35-year-old woman with a history of tuberous sclerosis as an infant and a resulting intractable seizure disorder. She is cared for, almost exclusively, by her 70-year-old mother. She has an older brother who is married, and lives in the area. Miss W. is moderately retarded. She has received some education, but functions at a level consistent with moderate mental retardation. She is able to feed herself, but requires assistance with dressing. She is able to walk for short distances only and utilizes a wheelchair for long distances. It is not possible to leave her alone. At the current time, her mother has been able to take advantage of home health services that assist with Miss W.'s daily care. On each visit, time is spent with Miss W.'s mother attempting to discuss realistic future plans for her daughter.

This family system has survived for many years and has kept Miss W. as a focal point of their activities. As her mother ages and the family grapples with the notion of "other arrangements," the system goes into disequilibrium and the opportunities for healing are rather extensive. The goal of the advanced practice nurse's interventions is to assist the family in the exploration of all of the options for Miss W.'s care. Preplanning will help the family members to come to terms with her needs and to be at peace with their decisions before the time for implementation arrives. In this way, healing will be possible.

RM

RM is a 34-year-old woman with a seizure disorder since childhood. Every time she has a seizure, she calls me. More often than not, my major role is to reassure her that all is well and that no change in therapy is indicated. During one clinic visit, we carefully took her recording of seizures and placed it on a calendar. We also listed all of the other events which occur during the month. Before long a pattern emerged: The seizures only occurred during her menstrual cycle. This is not an unusual finding and one that can be medically managed very easily.

What was significant about this visit was that RM "saw" the pattern. She then began to recognize the variables surrounding it and was able to fully participate in the decision to increase medication during this time. She saw the pattern. Recently, RM called in a panic to say that her seizures were worsening and that she needed to come in right away. When she didn't come for her appointment I called to check on her. She said that after she called she researched her calendar and noted that she had missed seeing her "patterns." She started her medications as we discussed and she felt safe. Her ability to see the pattern increased her sense of control to the extent that she took care of the situation and did not need to seek reassurance from the provider.

A far more complex pattern is a life time of events which lead to the production of "nonepileptic seizures." Individuals with this diagnosis are noted to be difficult to manage since the evidence of any physical basis for the seizures is not available.

BG

BG is a 24-year-old woman with a history of seizures for the past 12 years. Despite numerous EEGs, no evidence of seizures could be found. Her seizures, atypical in nature, continued and were difficult to control. Due to her increased anxiety, she was referred to a therapist. While working on the issues which were related to her anxiety, a past history of sexual abuse was discovered. BG's ability to recognize the abuse coincided with the onset of the atypical seizures. Based upon this evidence, the seizures were diagnosed as nonepileptic seizures. It was discovered that BG used the seizures as a way to withdraw during any emotionally painful event. During clinic visits when the subject included discussions of her father, BG would always have a seizure. Once this pattern was obvious, she began to deal with the issue of past abuse and to begin the healing process. The seizures were a representation of a disrupted life pattern. Resolution of the pattern lead to a seizure-free life. Although the link between past abuse and nonepileptic seizures has been identified, few patients are able to see the pattern of the escape which the seizure provides. BG's willingness to see this pattern is the only way the healing process could begin.

Conclusions

For true epileptic seizures, cure is not a reasonable goal. However, healing is. As an advanced practice nurse, the traditional medical care of these individuals can be strengthened by an approach which is directed toward creating a healing environment. By assisting patient and family to analyze the patterns that surround the seizure disorder, an honest attempt toward healing can be made. As a provider, the advanced practice nurse strengthens patient management by providing an environment that will improve the patient's situation through a variety of techniques. When reviewed from this vantage point, even patients with intractable seizures can progress toward some level of healing.

References

Gehlert, S. (1994). Perceptions of control in adults with epilepsy. *Epilepsia, 35*(1), 81–88.

Hermann, B. P., Whitman, S., Wyler, A. R., et al. (1990). Psychosocial predictors of psychopathology in epilepsy. *British Journal of Psychiatry, 156,* 98–105.

Jensen, I., Nygren, A., Gamberale, F., Goldie, I., Westerholm, P., & Jonsson, E. (1995). The role of the psychologist in multidisciplinary treatments for chronic neck and shoulder pain: A controlled cost-effectiveness study. *Scand. J. Rehab. Med., 27,* 19–26.

Miller, J. (1983). *Coping with clinical illness: Overcoming powerlessness.* Philadelphia: F.A. Davis.

Newman, M., & Marchine, J. (1986). *Health as expanding consciousness.* St. Louis: Mosby.

Pollock, S. E. (1993). Adaptation to chronic illness: A program of research for testing nursing theory. *Nursing Science Quarterly, 6*(2), 86–92.

Stein, M. J., Wallstone, K. A., Niccasio, P. M., & Castner, N. M. (1988). Correlation of clinical classification schema for the arthritis helplessness sub scale. *Arthritis Rheum, 31,* 876.

CHAPTER 35

Healing the Loss of a Dream for the Future: Preterm Twins

BARBARA CAMUNE, RN, RNC, MSN, COGNP, CNM, DRPH(C)

"Congratulations Ms. Smith, you are going to have a baby." Even for a planned pregnancy, this statement will probably evoke mixed emotions for the pregnant couple. Ambivalent feelings surrounding role changes, personal expectations and physical discomforts are common.

If the diagnosis of more than one fetus is confirmed, the ambivalent feelings are increased. Many couples and families are delighted, but the majority are initially in shock and wonder (Gilbert & Harmon 1993). At the onset of the diagnosis, there may be denial of the reality of the situation. Anxieties expressed by pregnant mothers of twins focus on worries of premature birth, survival of one or both twins, financial support for both sick and well babies, need for a larger home, coping with raising two babies at a time and concern over the difficulty of delivery (Spillman, 1987). Gradually these anxieties can be replaced with excitement about the pregnancy and the eventual birth.

Both mothers and fathers need to accomplish the developmental tasks of pregnancy. For the mother, accepting the pregnancy, establishing a relationship with the fetuses and preparing for the birth are paramount (Gay, Edgile, & Douglas, 1988). Developmental tasks for the father involve announcement of the pregnancy (usually with pride), adjustment to the loss of social freedom, privacy, and financial security, and the redefinition of his future role as a father (Diamond, 1986). Once progression in these steps occurs, attachment to the fetuses can begin.

Traditionally, fetal movement (quickening) has signaled the beginning of bonding to the baby. With the advent of numerous prebirth technologies, such as visualization of the fetus early in the first trimester, audible fetal heart tones by ten weeks' gestation and various genetic screening tests, the attachment process can be accelerated. Snapshots of fetal outlines by ultrasound personify the developing fetuses. Each fetus can be identified in utero by its own activity patterns, heart rate patterns, and position (Gilbert & Harmon, 1993). Each of these technological advances has helped parents not only adjust to the reality of two babies, but also to dream about the appearance and personality of each as an individual.

Education about the possible factors involved in high-risk pregnancy can be discussed by the nurse and the couple at the antepartum visits. Coping mechanisms successfully used by the couple in the past can be developed for further use. The couple's perceptions of events need to be grounded in reality, being positive about the pregnancy, yet not offering false hope of a successful outcome if this is warranted (Aguilera, 1990). Significant people in the pregnant woman's life should accompany her to the hospital for any preterm visits. Flexibility of the staff to accommodate the pregnant couple is paramount and minimizing separation ensures adequate emotional support.

THE STORY

Mr. and Mrs. J. came to Labor and Delivery during the 3 to 11 PM shift on a warm November evening in 1980. Mrs. J. was 26 years old and pregnant for the first time with twins. Mrs. J. stated that while she was watching television, she felt her legs get damp and when she went to the bathroom her panties were wet with clear fluid. She told us that she wasn't due for 4-and-a-half months (about 22–23 weeks' gestation). Both Mr. and Mrs. J. were very anxious when they arrived on our unit. They wanted to know what the chances of survival were for their twins. The neonatologist discussed options available for bigger babies, but basically told them little could be done for such small and immature babies. Mr. and Mrs. J. decided that they would like to hold and see the babies at birth and that they would not try extraordinary means to prolong their lives, since most of the treatments were painful and probably would be futile in their case.

After admission, Mrs. J. was placed on bedrest to prevent the cord coming out the vagina and cutting off circulation to the twins. This could possibly aid in resealing the bag of waters. Mrs. J. was not experiencing uterine contractions and the twins were too immature to use a fetal monitor to trace the heart rate. She was left to rest. It was evident that Mr. J. was very concerned about Mrs. J. and the imminent loss of his "family." The obstetrician had discussed use of potential medications to postpone labor temporarily, but after hearing about the probable death of the twins and the risk to Mrs. J. of infection and/or blood clotting problems, Mr. and Mrs. J. agreed to "trust God in whatever happens." Although Mr. J. didn't vocalize his thoughts, his facial expression and posture reflected grief.

We decided to send Mr. J. home to sleep, since Mrs. J was resting and there really was not a comfortable place to sleep in the birthing room. I decided to stay with Mrs. J. to answer any questions she might have had and to lend support. After performing routine lab procedures and admission assessments, I listened again to the fetuses' heart rate by Doppler (a very sensitive electronic stethoscope). Mrs. J. cradled her abdomen with her hands and began to describe her guilt about the pregnancy and this "bad" situation.

Mrs. J. explained that she had been very unhappy early on with the pregnancy because they had only been married six months. However, she felt she had just about adjusted to being pregnant when her obstetrician suggested an ultrasound. Both Mr. and Mrs. J. went together for the ultrasound where they had discovered a twin gestation. They experienced shock, happiness, and anxiety. She perceived that Mr. J. had been very proud and in awe of the whole situation. After the initial shock wore off, Mrs. J. worried that she would be unprepared for all the possible complications of this pregnancy. She felt that all the stress (worrying about money, coping, and parenting ability) led to the ruptured bag of water. I assured her that all those feelings were normal and common to pregnancy and that the cause of premature rupture of the bag of water was inconclusive. As she began crying, I just sat there silently and waited for her to continue.

After about twenty minutes, Mrs. J. began describing her feelings after seeing the ultrasound and hearing the babies' heart beats. Feeling the flutterings from kicks made the babies real to Mrs. J. Although the sex of the babies was not distinguishable, names were picked out for them and preparation for a unisex nursery was initiated. Encouragement from friends and family had pushed them to buy baby furniture already. Mrs. J. described the last several weeks as being happy and busy. As she spoke, Mrs. J. stated that she felt God was punishing her for her previous upset with the pregnancy and denying her now that she had reconciled her doubt. I sat with her, holding her hand, rubbing her shoulder, and continued to listen.

After about an hour, Mrs. J. decided to rest for the night. Mrs. J. said she did not want medication because she wanted to be totally lucid for the twins' delivery if that occurred during the night. She expressed a wish for a natural (no medications) labor and delivery. It was agreed that her husband would be called if labor started. Mrs. J. fell into a restless sleep.

About 2 AM, Mrs. J. awoke with severe pain. She had a gush of blood and an urge to push. I immediately phoned both the physician and her husband to come to the hospital. Mrs. J. squeezed my hand and watched me breathe through the contractions with her. Before either her husband or the physician could reach the hospital, the birth was imminent. Since no other physician was available in the hospital, Mrs. J. asked if I would deliver her twins. I had delivered babies in such a situation before, but this made me feel both honored and nervous. As the first twin started to appear, I placed my hands to receive the baby. She was born quickly without difficulty, but her eyes were fused shut and she didn't try to breathe. After I cut the cord, we wrapped her in a warm blanket and handed her to her Mrs. J. At that point, both Mr. J. and the physician entered the birthing room.

Doctor M. took over to deliver the second twin who came out bottom first about 5 minutes later. The second little girl was smaller than her sister. She also had her eyes fused shut and didn't breathe. The physician cut her cord and delivered the placenta almost immediately. We (the nurses) wrapped the second twin up in a blanket and handed her to the husband. Both babies had heart beats so they were considered alive even though they didn't have mature enough lungs to take a breath. There was no episiotomy, so Dr. M. finished quickly. Throughout the whole delivery process, Mrs. J. had been crying very softly. Through her tears she asked the physician if she could hold the babies until they died. Although surprised at the request, Dr. M. agreed to let her.

We were all going to leave the room to allow Mr. and Mrs. J. some privacy, when I heard Mrs. J. call my name. I was embarrassed because I had been crying too and now she would know. However, I went back to the bedside and Mrs. J. asked if I would stay to help them. She asked for help in placing both twins on her breasts so that "they could feel her skin just one time and be fed just once before they went to heaven." My heart was in my throat, but we prepared Mrs. J.'s breasts for feeding and placed the babies with their lips on her nipples. The first twin had her mouth open so we were able to get part of the nipple in. The look on Mrs. J.'s face was excruciatingly beautiful while exhibiting a very deep sadness. She continued to cry softly. I showed Mr. J. how to lightly stroke the babies' heads and cheeks to soothe them. After about 15 minutes, the girls died while both their parents lovingly held and nurtured them. Although all three of us were grieving in different ways, we were bound by this very private and special experience.

Mr. and Mrs. J. were Catholic and expressed a desire to have their girls baptized. While they were being held prior to dying, I did this for them.

After the girls had died, together we said a prayer for them. Perhaps it was more for us. Then Mr. and Mrs. J. started weeping loudly. I placed the babies on the warmer and told Mr. J. to sit on the bed so he could hold his wife. They sat there for about 30 minutes.

During that time, I made bracelets out with the mother's name, date, time of birth, sex, and Dr.'s name. I also made footprints and handprints of the girls for them to keep. Each baby was weighed and measured. I filled out small identification cards with the names, time of birth, date of birth, weight, and length. We kept a small Polaroid camera in the department to take pictures of sick babies for their parents. I found this and took pictures of the babies together in their blankets in the warmer. All the while I was trying to act professionally and handle the girls matter-of-factly, but inside I was raw with emotion. I decided to give these parents keepsakes that I would want if these were my babies.

When these duties were completed, I realized that Mr. and Mrs. J. were quiet, so I asked if they would like to see how beautiful their daughters were. At first they were hesitant, but Mr. J. decided that it was important to see the babies closer. I unwrapped the babies on the bed and encouraged Mr. and Mrs. J. to examine the fingers, toes, facial features and other aspects of their daughters' bodies. Although the girls' skin was transparent and bruised, it was soft, warm, and fuzzy with soft baby fur. The facial features were distinct and it was obvious that the twins were not identical. The parents were able to identify distinguishing features that made the girls individuals. Mr. and Mrs. J. commented on the beauty of the girls and I was able to agree with them.

The most difficult time after this tragic event was signing the release of body permits. Neither parent had thought about burial nor the expense entailed. I found the name of a funeral director that helped bereaved parents with inexpensive plots and services and provided Mr. J. with that. We also discussed feelings and resource people to provide support for them including the parish priest, social worker from the hospital, and the local visiting health nurse. I helped Mrs. J. bathe herself, then presented them with the bracelets, pictures, footprints, and cards that I had made for the babies. They told me that they "would treasure them always." They also asked for my picture!

The rest of the night went quickly and Mrs. J. was discharged by the time I returned the following evening. I never saw them again, but I will never forget them. I know I helped the healing process begin.

Several very well-known national perinatal support organizations such as the Pregnancy and Infant Loss Center in Wayzata, Minnesota, SHARE in

Bellville, Illinois, and Resolve Through Sharing in LaCrosse, Wisconsin, have developed protocols for in-house follow-up after perinatal loss. Ilse and Furrh (1988) have written an article on how to organize a community follow-up program after perinatal loss. All of these programs include many of the interventions that I tried and lend credibility and respectability to those interventions. Carr and Knupp (1985) have written about a community hospital approach to support grieving families. An excellent book called *"Empty Arms: Coping with Miscarriage, Stillbirth and Infant Death"* by Sherokke Ilse (1985) describes parents' reactions to the sudden loss of a child and is a very thorough reference to own.

Few formal research articles have been published on the subject of infant loss and parental follow-up for emotional adjustment. One study has indicated that bereaved parents have a marked reduction in symptoms of mental illness over the first eight months after the loss, with mothers suffering from anxiety and depression more often than fathers (Vance, Najman, Thearle, Embelton, Foster, & Boyle, 1995). Reval-Lutz and Kellner (1994) have described paternal involvement after perinatal death in minority, lower socioeconomic families. Presence at birth, holding the infant, and presence at follow-up visits were indicators of paternal grief. Fathers definitely needed to be included in the support services offered the mothers. Lilford, Stratton, Godsil, and Prasad (1994) conducted a randomized trial among bereaved couples to determine if routine psychological counseling improved emotional well-being for the parents after perinatal loss. Overall, women who underwent termination of pregnancy did slightly worse than women who experienced stillbirth or neonatal death. Routine counseling did not appear to be cost effective. In a study that examined social support received by women following a perinatal death, many women experienced social isolation and did not receive the support that they needed from partners, friends, and health professionals (Rajan, 1994).

Both parents need to be involved in the nursing interventions in the hospital as well as at home. I grew from the giving of myself to help this couple initially cope with the tragic loss of their premature twins and they benefited as well. Most importantly, those tiny babies died in the loving arms of parents who will remember them always as fleeting precious gifts.

REFERENCES

Aguilera, D. (1990). *Crisis intervention: Theory and methodology.* St. Louis: MO: Mosby.

Carr, D., & Knupp, S. (1985). Grief and perinatal loss: A community hospital approach to support. *Journal of Obstetric, Gynecological and Neonatal Nursing, 14*(2), 130-139.

Diamond, M. (1986). Becoming a father: A psychological perspective on the forgotten parent. *Psychoanalytic Review, 73*(4), 41-64.

Gay, J., Edgil, A., & Douglas, A. (1988). Reva Rubin revisited. *Journal of Obstetrics, Gynecology and Neonatal Nursing, 17*(6), 394-399.

Gilbert, E. S., & Harmon, J. S. (1993). *High risk pregnancy and delivery.* St. Louis, MO: Mosby.

Ilse, S. (1985). *Empty Arms: Coping with Miscarriage, Stillbirth and Infant Death.* Long Lake, MN: Wintergreen Press.

Ilse, S., & Furrh, C. B. (1988). Development of a comprehensive follow-up care plan after perinatal and neonatal loss. *Journal of Perinatal & Neonatal Nursing, 2*(2), 23-33.

Lilford, R. J., Stratton, P., Godsil, S., & Prasad, A. (1994). A randomized trial of routine versus selective counseling in perinatal bereavement from congenital disease. *British Journal of Obstetrics and Gynaecology, 101*(4), 291-296.

Rajan, L. (1994). Social isolation and support in pregnancy loss. *Health Visitor, 67*(3), 97-101.

Revak-Lutz, R. J., & Kellner, K. R. (1994). Paternal involvement after perinatal death. *Journal of Perinatology, 14*(6), 142-224.

Spillman, J. R. (1987). The emotional impact of multiple pregnancy. *Midwives Chronicle Nursing Notes, 100*(190), 58-62.

Vance, J. C., Najman, J. M., Thearle, M. J., Embelton, G., Foster, W. J., & Boyle, F. M. (1995). Psychological changes in parents eight months after the loss of an infant from stillbirth, neonatal death, or sudden infant death syndrome—a longitudinal study. *Pediatrics, 96*(5), 933-938.

HEALING INTERVENTIONS

PHYLLIS BECK KRITEK, RN, PHD, FAAN

One way of understanding our work as nurses is to conceptualize that work as the assistance we provide to specific patient populations. Part Five provides an alternate approach to this conceptualization. It focuses on the interventions that nurses might elect to implement to assist their patients and their families. While all interventions eventually will include a focus on the unique needs of a given population, conversely, all analyses of patient population needs will eventually turn toward appropriate interventions for the problems of that population. Thus these two perspectives serve as complementary dimensions of a common enterprise. And, like Part Four, these chapters give a variety of perspectives on potential interventions. They also reveal some of the inherent complexity and promise embedded in the nature of healing interventions.

In her four poems about healing after loss, Nonie Mendias provides another window on the interventions that heal. She first demonstrates that with her own action: writing the poem, expressing the hurt and the healing. She shares with us the importance of taking the time to heal, the struggle to commit to healing, the newness of life after healing, and the gratitude we feel for those who help us to heal. In all these perceptions, there are clues to the interventions of choice, the ones that assure us that we too can heal and that guide us in helping others in their quest for healing.

The first chapter, by Michele Clark, aptly exemplifies these observations. She describes the intervention of story with elderly women and its healing impact. Michele is interested in elderly caregivers and the challenges that they face. While she has studied and worked with both men and women, since the numbers of women are substantially larger, she has focused her work on this group. Her goal was to assist them in meeting the demands of their role as caregivers, yet balancing this with care of themselves. She describes the use of story to assist them, and the utility of this intervention. In the process, she reveals the healing aspects of this intervention.

Michele describes the depression and burden that accompanies the effort to assist elderly family members to remain at home. She also describes the power of story to help us make sense of our life experiences, to provide us with alternate perceptions of those experiences, to stimulate new behavior, and in becoming more whole to heal. In sharing stories, we share these possibilities with others. Using cost-effective available media technology, story sharing can become a formal intervention that can be used conveniently in homes. Hence, Michele develops such a story, videotapes it, and creates an intervention for others confronted with the challenges of caregiving for the elderly. She demonstrates the impact of this intervention and provides a comprehensive analysis of the uses of storytelling as a therapeutic device that enhances healing processes.

Audrey Chadwick is also interested in the elderly, but her approach is quite different. Audrey describes the healing power of gardens. She begins with an analysis of the central role of gardens in the history of humanity, showing that her approach to the healing power of gardens is rooted in our nature and our past. She then describes the move from agrarian to urban living and livelihood, and the loss of gardens as a dimension of that process. Finally, she describes recent attempts to create city gardens that can bring us back to their healing potential, as a resource not only for relaxation and community building, but also for mental and physical therapy.

Audrey provides this analysis as a backdrop to her healing interventions. She teaches gardening, and she develops gardens with the elderly. She involves her student nurses in this activity and has given them a new perception of this timeless intervention. She provides us with some of the comments of her elderly "students" to show us how this intervention, so compatible with our inherent nature, can help us to become and to feel whole. In her commitment to gardening as therapy, she serves as an example of creative nursing intervention and its capacity to further healing in others.

The next chapter explores conflict resolution as a healing intervention. I wrote this paper in part to explicate my experience of the convergence of two central activities in my own career: developing a doctoral program focused on healing and working as a trainer and mediator in healthcare conflict resolution. This convergence is not described in the nursing literature or the healthcare literature in general. Indeed, when the effort is made to bring the healthcare and the conflict resolution communities together, the congruence between the two is often startling. Hence, conflict resolution is described as an intervention that furthers healing processes.

The chapter describes current practices that are common in nursing concerning conflict, ones that focus on smoothing over, appeal to a higher authority, manipulation or avoidance. These are dysfunctional, but commonplace. In identifying and understanding these practices, however, we can begin to get a grasp on the shared realities of two enterprises: facilitating healing and resolving conflicts. Indeed, we may discover, as I have, that to be a skilled healer in healthcare today calls upon us to become skilled resolvers of conflict. The chapter attempts to explain why the interdependence between these two enterprises is both intrinsic and promising.

In this chapter on conflict, relationship is given a central focus. So too is relationship central in the next chapter by Nonie Mendias. Nonie places her emphasis on reciprocity, and explores in a comprehensive and thoughtful manner the importance of such reciprocity in achieving a healing relationship between the nurse and the patient. She first provides a thorough discussion of the concept of reciprocity which undergirds her understanding of professional-patient relationships, including in this a review of nursing literature on this topic. From this base of conceptual clarity, Nonie goes on to describe some personal experiences as a practicing nurse that helped her better understand the nature of reciprocity in her relationships as a nurse.

Having provided a rich analysis of reciprocity, Nonie then clarifies her personal views: that indeed reciprocal interactions between nurses and patients are not problematic, although they can be empowering, and thus are "normal, necessary, healing, desirable, and useful." Her position stands in sharp contrast to the historically recommended role of the objective and impartial observer, and changes the nature of how one does nursing. For Nonie, it is the key to creating a healing milieu, one that would heal both nurses and their patients.

Gerry Dorsey-Turner provides yet another intervention that speaks to one of the troubled arenas in nursing in need of healing efforts: the successful recruitment and retention of minority students into nursing programs. She describes Project Hope Alliance, a program initiated at UTMB to address this need. Gerry starts from an analysis of grade point average as a commonly used measure of academic achievement and competence, and explores its limitations. She notes that a primary emphasis on this measure may lead to overlooking other important measures such as "motivation, leadership, commitment, and past personal achievement" that may indicate promise of achievement in nursing school. Lacking the necessary grade point average, however, some students may never get admitted or only be admitted with a deficit that leaves them feeling at risk, in need of healing. Their prior experiences in other educational institutions may have exacerbated these feelings, or they may lack family support. Whatever the causes, the need for healing exists.

Gerry then reports on the efforts of a group of faculty to address these healing needs, to enable these students to achieve in nursing school and to graduate, and in the process to heal the wounds of prior deprivations. She describes the effort to create a healing environment for the students where caring is the guiding principle. She describes her role, as director of the program, as one of motivating, providing support and encouragement—a role of healer. It is her contention that while there are substantial challenges in the efforts asked of everyone in a project like Hope Alliance, it can be accomplished if barriers are removed and a healing environment is created.

"Soul Image: A Healing Metaphor" is a poem I wrote when I was attempting to express the soul as home, and its healing processes. It attempts to capture the sense of complexity and multiplicity of the human, and therefore the healing of the human. Wholeness, it has seemed to me, is one of those words used without adequate sensitivity to the scope of intention. If indeed we mean wholeness when we talk of assisting others in their healing, then inevitably we find that the task is complex, multifaceted; a large mansion of rooms, each with its own story, memories, hopes, and fears. The search for wholeness serves more as ideal in the human condition, and it seems wise to me to know this when we respectfully approach an other in the hope of serving them in their efforts at healing. This sensitivity to and respect for reality is often the first and most powerful step in intervening with an other in search of their own wholeness.

The final chapter in this part of the book describes an approach to psychotherapy that has served for the author, Patricia Romick, as a wonderful intervention to help others in their search for healing. Patricia describes her work as a nurse psychotherapist, and her discovery of psychosynthesis as an approach to her work that is not only highly congruent with nursing but provides a set of understandings, tools, and opportunities for her to facilitate the healing processes in others. She summarizes the key concepts and resources of psychosynthesis, and then describes how these might be used by the nurse psychotherapist to craft an approach to therapy that furthers healing in her patients.

Of particular note is the emphasis on the impulse and potential for healing as residing within the patient, not the provider of care. Patricia is careful to note that this approach carefully honors the patient's internal process and views the therapist as a guide, one who serves as a pathfinder and assists in the journey of the patient. This is an important consideration in evaluating any intervention that purports to further healing processes. Psychosynthesis is also holistic in its outlook, and acknowledges all dimensions of the person's humanity. It includes a strong attention to the spiritual dimension of therapy without prescribing the nature of that spiritual dimension for the patient. These philosophical premises are not only congruent with the history and traditions of nursing, but essential elements in approaching others as one who wishes to assist in healing. Patricia's description is also useful in that it discusses stages or phases of therapy, and thus highlights the fact that healing is not so much an event as an on-going process. She is careful to note that this process enriches both the patient and the therapist, pointing back to the issues of patient patterning, reciprocity, and mutuality already discussed in other chapters. As she concludes, "persons interested in holistic health care and healing practices would greatly benefit from the use of psychosynthesis in clinical practice." Her paper is an apt closure to this section on the interventions congruent with the basic nature of healing.

HEALING AFTER LOSS: NOTES FROM MY SPIRIT

Elnora (Nonie) P. Mendias, RN, CSFNP, PhD

Go on with Your Life

"Go on with your life"
Is good advice.
Easier to give,
Than to live.

When I can, I'll go on.
For now, give me time to heal.

A Butterfly Experience

I wish I could make
Something beautiful out
Of this awful experience.

I wish I'd emerge—
Greatly improved—
Like a butterfly from its cocoon.

Now *that* I could see
Would give this a purpose,
Making it—almost—worthwhile.

Healing

For every pain, there is a healing.
Bones can knit, and wounds can
    mend.
Spirits can find freedom again.

Even death wipes clean the past
And creates a new beginning.

To a Healer, with Love

When I was hurt, you reached for me
With healing hands and words.
You listened with your heart and
    head.
You shared your thoughts and
    honored mine.

You offered hope and kind concern,
Took tender care of all of me.
You saved my life—you gave me life!
I took your gifts and healed.

Because of you, I will reach out
A loving hand to those in need.
I will repay this debt I owe
By passing on the gifts you gave.

CHAPTER 36

The Healing Effect of Story with Elderly Women

MICHELE C. CLARK, RN, PHD

Story allows us to be still and listen, like
A good traveler (who) has no fixed plans
and is not intent upon arriving.
A good artist (who) lets his intuition
lead him wherever it wants.
A good scientist has (who) freed himself of concepts
and keeps his mind open to what is.

(*Tao Te Ching*)

Like the journeyman in the *Tao Te Ching* we are carried by the story, allowing ourselves to suspend judgment and wait for the events to unfold. As we become transformed into travelers "not intent upon arriving," we enter the story to receive the insight we need. It is the story that shifts us away from old concepts and opens the door through which we can slip, away from the mundane and familiar, into another world to receive the insight we need to transform and heal our lives. This chapter explores how story affects the unconscious and facilitates healing by changing attitudes. Particular attention will be given to how therapeutic story facilitates elderly caregivers in transforming their attitudes of depression and burden into a healthy acceptance of assisting dependent elderly family members to remain at home.

THE POWER OF STORYTELLING

How do stories allow us to let go of old patterns and deal more realistically and kindly with ourselves, allowing a deep healing of the spirit to occur? There are numerous explanations that elucidate how storytelling affects the attitudes of the listener.

Baker (1985) discusses numerous possibilities that are noted else-where in the literature (Hensel & Rasco, 1992; Larkin & Zahhourek, 1988; Sandelowski, 1991). He feels that the power of storytelling lies in its magi-cal ability to encode and transmit the human experience. The story allows the listener not only to see things differently but also to feel differently about them. Because stories often deal indirectly with difficult issues and have meanings that are veiled by metaphors, they are less threatening, al-lowing listeners to interpret stories in their own ways and apply them to their own situations. By presenting several different choices for con-fronting difficult situations, listeners are provided with options that they can selectively adapt to their individual situations. This process ultimately allows them to see things in a new and different way.

Also, human experiences that connect us to a story have some interest-ing and common elements that seem to make them powerful and meaning-ful to our individual experiences. MacDonald and Runge (1993) maintain that important growth of the human spirit happens as a sensate journey in which the three elements of "disorder," "irreversibility," and "neverthe-less" always occur. If one can move through these three stages successfully, a profound sense of "I matter" evolves. Stories help us discover ways in which we "matter" despite the disorder and irreversibility brought on by events such as aging or the death of a spouse. When such human circum-stances move physical and/or mental functioning out of their usual pat-terns of operating, we often experience confusion, discomfort, insecurity, uncertainty, and loss of control. These feelings can help us begin to pay at-tention and look for new ways of dealing with problems so that we can feel that we "matter" in spite of our losses.

The circumstances that often introduce disorder create an event that shatters all old ways of being. When this shattering occurs, issues of final-ity become a reality, destroying the invincibility of our youth. Characters in all great stories experience this chaos when a life event has forever ended old ways of being. However it is the character's struggle with "nev-ertheless"—that challenge to live life in the face of the limits set by the "ir-reversibility" of an event—that haunts and inspires us. Understanding the meaning of their struggle and how they continue "to matter," despite life's irreversible changes moves us to address our problems in new ways.

Stories allow sharing the experiences and knowledge without which we often feel limited in our choices. The magic of stories is that they can remove us from our personal situations and allow us to relate to the prob-lems the characters face from a different perspective. With this distance, the construction of reality can become more flexible, expanding beliefs and feelings to develop a new range of possibilities for action.

CAREGIVER BURDEN

Unfortunately, few stories exist within individual families or on a broader cultural level to guide the new caregiver through the common frustrations and problems often experienced in caregiving. Although it is commonly believed that our society typically abandons its elders to extended care facilities, studies show that it is the family that usually bears primary responsibility for the care of the chronically ill and dependent elder (Montgomery, Gonyea, & Hooyman, 1985). Unfortunately, when family caregivers are themselves elderly, care burdens can overwhelm them (Brody, 1981; Cantor, 1983).

Recent studies have focused on gaining a better understanding of the concept of caregiver burden by relating the subjective interpretation for caregiver burden to the life-specific problems of the elder's impairment (Hadjistavropoulos, Taylor, & Tuokko, 1994; Markides & Cooper, 1989). For instance, Montgomery (1989) distinguished the objective components of the concept of burden from the subjective components. She defined objective burden as the concrete events, happenings, and activities of the caregiving experience, whereas subjective burden encompasses the caregiver's feelings, attitudes, and emotional reactions to the caregiving experience.

Findings have shown that individual counseling and support groups are relatively successful methods of assisting caregivers to restructure their individual interpretation of the caregiving experience, thus diminishing the experience of burden. Although these studies indicate that those caregiver behaviors and attitudes toward caring problems are amenable to change, interventions such as counseling and support groups are costly and require that the caregiver leave home to use such services. Healthcare providers who work with elderly caregivers need to consider other creative and cost effective interventions, like stories, to assist caregivers in restructuring their lives and attitudes so that they "matter." These caregiving stories can be told through visual media at convenient times in the caregiver's home.

THE CAREGIVER STORY

There is a need for stories about meaning and the caregiving experience, stories that emphasize caregivers' shared struggles as well as the values and attitudes often brought to their encounters with the dependent elder in their lives. Since stories often stimulate listeners' imaginations, as well as their emotions, it is essential that stories designed to help caregivers use images that reflect their realities. Creating a context that is familiar, realistic, and authentic to the listener can help bring the story to life and make it meaningful.

In response to these needs, I undertook the project of creating a therapeutic story for use with elderly caregivers. Previous research demonstrated that women's caregiving experience differed from their male counterparts (Clark, 1989). Interestingly, though men, like women, complained of feelings of depression with the caregiving experience, it was primarily women who complained of feeling angry, pressured, and often overwhelmed by the caring experience. These findings emphasized the importance of considering different interventions for men and women. Women became the focus of this first intervention study.

The first step in developing this story included asking healthcare professionals involved with caregivers to share their professional experiences, to identify important themes in the caregiver's story. The context of the caregiver story evolved from the clinical practice of professional home healthcare nurses. Through the review of a number of home healthcare cases of elderly caregivers who were women, important patterns began to emerge. Caregivers often complained of feeling overwhelmed, confused, tired, and disorganized. Caregivers also spoke about the irreversible losses they experienced daily. These common themes became the structure on which the caregiver story was built. Through these interviews it became apparent that successful caregivers possess crucial information about caregiving that others without the experience lack. Consequently, those caregivers who had been identified as successful by professional nursing staff were interviewed.

Using ethnographic methodology, I found that caregivers using home healthcare services for their dependent elder were applying similar empowerment strategies to assist them through some of the difficult caregiving experiences. Further analysis of the caregiving experience highlighted other important gender differences that existed between men and women. Specifically, men had less difficulty dealing with role changes and formulated the caregiving experience so that it would have measurable goals similar to their employment experiences. Women, on the other hand, had greater difficulty with role changes, especially when the changes related to assuming a leadership role in the relationship. They also felt less supported by family and more isolated from their community of relatives and friends (Clark, 1989). Though both men and women felt the burden when caring for an elder, women's experience was significantly different. After considering some of these gender differences in the caregiving experience, I decided to create a caregiver story oriented toward women's caregiving experience. The empowerment strategies that women identified as important included social nurturing, love/affection, increasing leisure activities, normalizing negative emotions, diminishing stress, and improving their outlook (Clark, 1992).

The caregiving story was shown to 120 caregivers who were elderly women taking care of a family member in the community setting. The story was structured around two friends discussing some of the feelings and responsibilities related to the care of a dependent elder at home. One of the characters, Martha, has just begun caring for a dependent elder while her friend, Louise, had actively been involved in this experience for six years. The empowerment strategies are embedded in the storyline with the hope that the ongoing crises that often occur with the changing care needs of a dependent elder would make caregivers more open and receptive (Larkin & Zahhourek, 1988). While receptive, it was hoped that the empowerment themes embedded in the story would be more effective and relevant.

In this caregiver story, the initial fears, frustrations, losses, and disappointments associated with care of a dependent elder are dramatically presented by Martha to her friend Louise. This realistic presentation style allows the viewer to feel the intensity with which events can be experienced by the caregiver. For example,

> **Martha:** I feel like I'm spinning out of control. I had no idea it would be like this.
>
> **Louise:** Most people don't know. It's very difficult to take care of someone around the clock. Especially at our age. When I started caring for my husband after his stroke, I never imagined that I would be learning so much when I turned 70.
>
> **Martha:** I know that I didn't. You've been taking care of Larry for six years, and I never realized how difficult it's been for you. Now, I'm beginning to understand. How have you managed?

This story was also fashioned to highlight events common to the caregiving experience, thus allowing the listener to interpret it in terms of her own worldview. When this connection between caregiving circumstances and caregivers' own worldview is made, the listener can more easily identify with key characters.

Caregivers who viewed this videotape reported that they felt better immediately following the viewing and showed a greater acceptance of the empowerment strategies six to eight weeks after seeing the videotape

(Clark, 1992). Incorporating the strategies presented in the story into the caregiver's everyday life expanded the range of possibilities for action, thus allowing attitudes toward caring problems to change. Consequently, caregiving mastery and caregiver satisfaction improved (Lawton, Kleban, Moss, Rovine, & Glickman, 1989). Understanding how story can initiate change that facilitates the development of the human spirit is an important adjunct in using stories in clinical practice.

UNDERSTANDING THE HEALING POWER OF STORYTELLING FOR THE CAREGIVER

Before change can be initiated, it is important to understand what motivates behavior. These caregivers, like most people, employ a personally developed map of reality to guide their behavior. This structure, representing reality, is created through generalizations, experience, and modeling (Grinder & Bandler, 1976). For most people, all these processes are adaptive. However, when there is a distortion between one's representational structure of the world and reality, burden and dissatisfaction can emerge through abusive behavior. This often occurs, for example, when caregivers misjudge the dependent elder's abilities and motives. Such misjudgment can instigate what will then be judged by others as neglect and/or abuse.

One therapeutic component of this videotaped story is that what begins as the private agony of a caregiver becomes a collective story that reveals common problems. The irreversibility and chaos in this therapeutic story can be compared to the caregivers' limited representation of the world. However alternative ways of looking at problems that are provided by the caregiver story can be contrasted to the caregivers present situation. Caregivers are thus provided with options in care that may not have been obvious (Fazio, 1991).

More importantly, therapeutic relief can transpire for the caregiver when he or she no longer has to carry the problems of the caregiving experience alone; the load is shared with the characters in the story. Consequently, a community develops, as everyone who watches the story becomes connected to it, even though they are connected in different ways. Caregivers begin to understand that their individual problems are common to the community of caregivers and are part of the human condition. Therefore, by participating in the story, caregivers can establish their bearings in difficult caregiving situations. Thus, this therapeutic story guides caregivers beyond feelings of incompetence and loss and helps them begin to assess problems with a more balanced perspective.

When caregivers connect with the videotaped story, a period of engagement occurs and the activities of the story's characters give options to the caregiver for therapeutic change. Also, the story is told in the third person, so that suggestions embedded in the storyline are more likely to be accepted. Shulik (1979) found that men and women are more willing to change attitudes and behaviors if suggestions are made indirectly and in the third person rather than directly and in the second person (e.g., his arm is heavy versus your arm is heavy). Giving advice is frequently perceived as intrusive and minimizes the caregiver's specific situation (Baker, 1985). Therefore, the third-person nature of the story provides a safe emotional distance from the presenting problems and expands the influence of the indirect suggestions revolving around the empowerment strategies. With the storytelling approach, the caregiver becomes simultaneously an observer and evaluator of the presented options. This reduces the defensive posture of the listeners and establishes their connection with significant elements of the caregiving story. The caregivers are allowed to use the content of the story in their own way and take from the story those meanings that apply in their particular situation. Thus in this story about caregivers, the characters don't argue that options are real but demonstrate change is possible.

This approach provides caregivers with more choices on how they behave or respond emotionally in various situations. The caregiver story does not tell people what to do but rather helps them to see things differently and to feel differently about them. The story frees them of the restrictions created by their thought patterns and becomes an avenue to enlarge their world view.

However, it is the embedded messages that have the greatest impact on listeners. Embedded statements and metaphors are the language of the right cerebral hemisphere, and in order to resolve a person's emotional or behavioral problems, one needs to change how the right side of the brain processes its input (Baker, 1985). It is not an improved understanding of their difficulties that changes the way caregivers feel about their situation but rather an acceptance and reframing of their caregiving reality. Caregivers frequently mentioned that they did not need a better understanding of their situation or a logical explanation of why they were feeling or behaving a certain way. They identified a need to develop a different way of interpreting their caregiving experience. Storytelling through the videotaped story facilitated this process.

CONCLUSION

As dependent elders become more frail, caregivers struggle to maintain a healthy relationship with their life as the responsibilities to the elder become more complex. In attempting to maintain themselves and the elder, caregivers often feel as if their choices and possibilities become less optimal. Also their life becomes less supported and more isolated as well as their understanding of how they "matter" becomes more veiled. Understanding that mind and emotions play a central role in one's sense of well-being, storytelling becomes a bridge to the unconsciousness. The caregiving story, whose intent was to change the distressed patterns of the caregiver's thoughts, became the bridge for healing. The story allowed the caregiver to give up the familiar but less useful information concerning the caregiver experience, to connect with other positive possibilities that would substantiate their potential for wholeness and well-being.

Healthcare providers need to look for new and economical ways in which to facilitate the care of community elders. Using visual media in the caregiver's home is an effective way of reducing some of the burdens frequently seen in this experience. The visual medium of videotape is a convenient and economical medium for healthcare providers to present stories as an intervention strategy to help improve or change the attitude of their clients.

REFERENCES

Baker, P. (1985). *Using metaphors in psychotherapy.* New York: Brunner/Mazel.

Brody, E. M. (1981). Women in the middle and family help to older people. *The Gerontologist, 25*(5), 471–479.

Cantor, M. H. (1983). Strain among caregivers: A study of experience in the United States. *The Gerontologist, 23*(6), 597–604.

Clark, M. C. (1989). *Caregiving functional learning model: Preliminary testing,* Unpublished doctoral dissertation. Tucson: University of Arizona.

Clark, M. C. (1992). *Final report: Impact of a structured nursing intervention on caregiving burden.* Post Doctoral Fellow, National Research Service Award, Department of Health and Human Services, Public Health Service, No. 5 F32NR06387-02 NRRC.

Fazio, L. S. (1991). Tell me a story: The therapeutic metaphor in the practice of pediatric occupational therapy. *The American Journal of Occupational Therapy, 46*(2), 112–119.

Grinder, J., & Bandler, R. (1976). *The structure of magic 11.* Palo Alto, CA: Science and Behavior Books.

Hadjistavropoulos, T., Taylor, S., & Tuokko, H. (1994). Neuropsychological deficits, caregivers' perception of deficits and caregiver burden. *Journal of American Geriatrics Society, 42*(3), 308-314.

Hensel, W. A., & Rasco, T. L. (1992). Storytelling as a method for teaching values and attitudes. *Academic Medicine, 67*(8), 500-504.

Larkin, D. M., & Zahhourek, R. P. (1988). Therapeutic storytelling and metaphor. *Holistic Nursing Practice, 2*(3), 45-53.

Lawton, M. P., Kleban, M. H., Moss, M., Rovine, M. & Glickman, A. (1989). Measuring caregiver appraisal. *Journal of Gerontology.* 44(3), 69-71.

MacDonald, C. B., & Runge, A. (1993). *Spirituality and aging: A perspectival view.* From the Sojourner Counseling Services, 4615 Post Oak Place, Suite 140, Houston, Texas 77027.

Markides, K. S., & Cooper, C. L. (1989). *Aging stress and health.* New York: John Wiley.

Meade, M. (1994). Once upon a time, once under a time, before digital time. *Inquiring Mind A Semi-Annual Journal of the Vipassana Community, 10*(2), 17-19.

Montgomery, R. J. V. (1989). Investigating caregiver burden. In K. Markides & C. Cooper (Eds.), *Aging, stress and health* (pp. 201-218). New York: John Wiley.

Montgomery, R. J. V., Gonyea, J. G., & Hooyman, N. R. (1985). Caregiving and the experience of subjective and objective burden. *Family Relations, 34,* 19-26.

Sandelowski, M. (1991). Telling stories: Narrative approaches in qualitative research. *Image: Journal of Nursing Scholarship, 23*(3), 161-165.

Shulik, A. (1979). Right versus left hemispheric communication styles in hypnotic trance. Ph.D. Dissertation, California School of Professional Psychology, Fresno, California. *Dissertation Abstracts International, 40,* 2445-B.

CHAPTER 37

The Healing Power of Gardens

AUDREY L. CHADWICK, RN, MS

There is a corner of my garden where I can find a measure of peace and mental refreshment that has no equal in my life. My awareness of this healing power of gardens has grown steadily over the years and has been reinforced both by reflections on the history of Western culture and by my clinical experience especially among the growing class of senior citizens. Out of these latter experiences has grown a conviction that horticultural therapy is an extremely valuable resource for all concerned with community health.

In this chapter, I will show how closely our lives are intertwined with gardens and the world of nature. The radical changes of urbanization and industrialization that overtook the lives of Western people in the 19th and 20th centuries have brutally interrupted this relationship. While these changes are considered largely irreversible, there is also a growing recognition that gardens and gardening will have a significant role not only in mental and physical therapy but in health maintenance in the urban communities of the 21st century.

I first review how gardens, manmade enclaves in the dangerous world of nature, have played an important role in the aspirations of mankind from the earliest recorded times. Then, I will discuss the revolutionary changes that took Western people from the countryside to the city and from agriculture to the often meaningless activities of factory labor. Finally, I will discuss recent attempts to find in city gardens opportunities for relaxation, community building, and physical and mental therapy.

In the scientific world, only proven theories are accepted as useful truths. In the field of horticultural therapy, little quantified research has yet been done. Organizations like the American Horticultural Therapy Association and its European counterpart, the Society of Horticultural Therapy (England), however, are documenting the great variety of experimental programs being established in psychiatric hospitals, and in children's and senior's centers as potential spaces for healing.

GARDENING AND OUR PAST

The roots of our civilization lie in the great river valleys of the Middle East, India, and China. Those who gathered there more than 5000 years ago did so to practice a hard and monotonous agriculture. They dreamt, however, of gardens, a gentler and more creative culture, the property of gods and kings (King, 1941).

> *And the Lord God planted a garden eastward in Eden, and there he put the man whom he had formed. And out of the ground made the Lord God to grow every tree that is pleasant to the sight and good for food . . . and a river went out of Eden to water the garden. . . . (Gen. 2:8–10, King James Version)*

A true Eastern paradise—a garden of trees and living waters whose beauty and spiritual peace is echoed in the vision of the Prophet Mohammed and recorded in the Koran. It was the reward of the faithful and the aspiration of every person from that already harsh landscape of the Middle East who longed for shade, fragrance, and cool water. Few poems have exceeded the rich imagery of the Song of Solomon, that rare female voice in a patriarchal world.

> I am the rose of Sharon and the lily of the valleys,
> as the lily among the thorns, so is my love among the daughters. . . .
> For lo, the winter is past, the rain is over and gone;
> The flowers appear on the earth. . . .
> (Solomon 2:1–12, King James Version)

Solomon's garden was an elaborate one with many rare plants and spices

> *an orchard of pomegranates, with pleasant fruits, camphire, with spikenard . . . and saffron; calamus and cinnamon, with all trees of frankincense; myrrh and aloes . . . (Solomon 4:13–14, King James Version)*

This garden contained many flowering and aromatic shrubs, exotic spice plants from the Far East and other plants possibly brought by the Queen of Sheba. From Persia and Egypt, Solomon is said to have borrowed floriculture; lilies and crocuses are mentioned among the flowers of his garden. It is described as a place of fountains and living waters and when the wind blew the air was filled with spicy fragrance (Shewell-Cooper, 1977).

To modern Western minds, the word garden suggests a garden of flowers, but gardens of the older civilizations were gardens of trees and scented shrubs. Shade, scent, and water were the chief requisites in gardens of the ancient world, water being the soul of the Eastern paradise and shade the essential luxury. The mystic garden of Eden, like the palm groves of Anu, was a garden of trees and living waters (Sandars, 1972).

A garden was essential to man's life, and in death he was often buried there. If gardens were sometimes the scenes of forbidden sacrifices surviving from heathen worship, they were also pleasant gathering places for friends and places of rest for wayfarers. Jesus and his disciples often went into gardens to rest and pray. It was in the garden of Gethsemane that Jesus made his decision to allow himself to be taken before Pilate, and it was in the garden of Joseph of Arimathea that his body was laid in its sepulcher.

There is evidence that 5000 years ago the Egyptians already had a highly developed gardening tradition. In Mesopotamia, this river civilization surrounded by desert clearly valued both formal and informal gardening since both are to be found on its tomb paintings (Jellicoe, 1989).

An early tomb illustration at Thebes, that of a general of the pharaoh Amenhopis III, shows a garden enclosed by a wall. Its entrance is through a high door covered with hieroglyphic inscriptions (Rhode, 1967). The same kind of illustrations record a love of flowers. Garlands of flowers were worn on festive occasions, guests were given flowers and food at banquets and the table was decorated with flowers. Even the sleeping chamber of the great Pharaoh Akhnaton had walls covered with flower paintings (Rhode). We have an unusually fine record of the Pharaoh Tutankhamon (ca. 1347 BC) and flowers feature prominently among his remains. He was buried with wreaths of olive and willow leaves, lotus and cornflowers, wild cherry, nightshade and devil's apples. He and his wife are illustrated in a garden, their images carved on the front of a funerary casket. The queen hands her husband two bouquets of papyrus, lotus, and poppy. The scene is framed with poppies, cornflowers and mandrake. On another face of the casket, the king sits by a fishpond with the queen at his feet surrounded by a garden "densely planted with the by now familiar species" (Manniche, 1989).

The great hanging gardens of Nebuchadnezzar, ruler of Babylon in the sixth century BC, became one of the Seven Wonders of the ancient world. Built to ease the loneliness of his young wife, who grew up in the hills of the north, these gardens survived into the Christian era and were described by Diodorus Siculus, a contemporary of Julius Caesar:

Since the approach to the garden sloped like hillside and the several parts of the structure rose from one another tier on tier . . . it resembled a theater . . . the uppermost gallery, which was fifty cubits high, bore the highest part of the park. . . . The roofs of the galleries were covered with beams of stone. . . . Over this there were layers of bitumen, reeds, brick lead and then earth sufficient for the roots of the largest trees; and the ground when leveled off, was thickly planted with trees of every kind that could give pleasure to the beholder. . . . The galleries contained many royal lodgings and there was one gallery which contained openings from the topmost surface and machines for supplying the garden with water. (Thacker, 1979)

The Persians were the conquerors of the Babylonian Empire and the inheritors of the traditions of horticulture in Mesopotamia. Their horticulture became the models and origins of both the gardens of Islam and, through the Greeks, of the Roman Garden. From these two sources eventually developed the enclosed garden of the modern world.

The Greek conquerors of Persia brought back a more sophisticated concept of the garden than can be found in the legends of their forebears. The "Dark Age" warriors of the Iliad and Odyssey worshipped their Gods in forest and wooded groves as, later, the Germanic tribes were to do. The Greeks were quick learners and the Hellenistic successors of Alexander the Great recreated in the Mediterranean world the closed gardens of Persia. These refined gardens became a model for the villa gardens of Rome. Some outstanding examples of villa gardens can be found in the remains at Pompeii. The eruption of Vesuvius in AD 79 buried the town completely. Through relatively recent excavation, we are able to glimpse the gardens and the way of life of their owners in the first century. Houses were built about a central enclosed garden, open to the air. The gardens contained statues and sculpture in abundance. Even the walls of the garden were decorated with frescoes of trees and flowers. Descriptions of similar villas and their gardens are recorded by Pliny the Younger (AD 62-113) and his uncle Pliny the Elder (AD 23-79), whose famous book *Naturalis Historia* combined traditional teaching with his own experience of trees, flowers, plants, and fruit with information about their use. They both practiced the art of topiary, the regular clipping and shaping of trees.

After the fall of Rome in the 5th century, the development of gardening virtually stopped in Western Europe. It was preserved, with the Persian tradition of the closed garden, by the Arab conquerors of the Middle East. With the rapid spread of Islam from the 7th century onwards, the closed garden of Persia was transmitted to all corners of the Islamic world—from Egypt to Spain and later from Istanbul to the gates of Vienna. In the middle of every Persian garden a reservoir was to be found from which canals or streams flowed in four directions. This symbolic quartering of the gardens by running water was a direct reference to Paradise, the Garden of Eden from which supposedly, the four rivers of life flowed. Also characteristic of the Islamic garden are pavilions and covered seating placed around the reservoir, or most picturesquely, on a small island at their center. Much of our knowledge of Persian gardens comes from carpets just as the delicate porcelain of China bears the traditional outlines of the gardens of ancient China (Wengel, 1987).

In the Christian West, the Barbarian heirs to the Roman Empire settled to grinding, subsistence agriculture, and the defense of their hard-won land. In small rural communities, they struggled with nature and periodic invaders to survive. For most people this was to be their lot until the onset of industrialization broke the harsh mold of rural life. This feudal society had no great gardens and indeed rare opportunities for peace or leisure. For a few, however, who took monastic vows, horticulture survived both as a supplement to diet and as a source of medicaments. Despite the sometimes stern discipline of the monastic orders, these religious communities offered a measure of peace, security, and culture available no where else. The monasteries were the only centers for medical attention and their herb gardens played a very important role in providing medication for the sick. The monks were often physicians and care for the sick was seen as part of their Christian duty. The monasteries were a vital link in the spread of medical knowledge. The monks were skilled copyists and, until the invention of printing, were the most important source of books. Contacts between monasteries of the same order no doubt led to an interchange of information and of actual plants. It was monastic scholars like Gerald of Cremona (1114-1187) who translated the work of Arab scholars and thus brought Eastern knowledge into the West. Similarly monks like John of Gaddesden combined their knowledge of plants and their properties into books known as herbals (Stuart, 1987).

The shape of the medieval garden followed the square or rectangular shape of the cloister. The cloister itself was modeled after the Roman villa garden (hortus conclusus) and the Persian garden of ancient times. In religious houses, the walled garden acquired a special Christian symbolism as the virgin bride of Solomon's Song of Songs, and by implication the Virgin Mary:

A garden enclosed is my sister, my spouse: a spring shut up, a fountain sealed. (Solomon 4:4-12, King James Version)

Medieval paintings show Mary, the mother of Jesus, in a garden—almost always an enclosed garden with a wall, a fence, or a paling, and often the means of enclosure is the most carefully depicted part of the background. Once again it is the safety and peace of the enclosed garden that is portrayed (Thacker, 1979).

This pattern of life began to change when the insecurity of life in the West gave way to the relative peace of developing nation and city-states. In the 13th and 14th centuries, communications both within and without Europe improved, trade began to recover and cities began to grow again for the first time since the Roman era. Italian cities were especially prosperous since they stood at the heart of the trade routes between Northern Europe and the East. Wealth, security, and the recovered culture of the East, of Greeks, and of Arabs brought about the rebirth of learning that we call the Renaissance. At its heart were new humanistic attitudes that became the guiding light of a great explosion of cultural and artistic activities. Life acquired a new meaning for the individual, whose thoughts no longer concentrated on the transcendental, on the world to come, but on the realities of the world around us. This was accompanied by the awakening of a new attitude in people toward their environment. The desire of Renaissance people to shape and decorate the areas around their homes was, in due course, enhanced both by scientific research, itself a product of the new humanism, and by the products of overseas exploration. As Europeans began to explore both East and West they brought back an increasing volume of exciting new plants and shrubs.

The gardens of Renaissance Italy are typically large and elaborate expressions of the wealth and confidence of their creators. In 1580, the Villa d'Este was completed. Its famous gardens are an architectural extension of the villa itself. In the Roman fashion, it combined water features, sculpture, and huge areas of geometrically arranged plantings. It is a triumph of man over nature. In the Boboli gardens at Florence and in the Villa Medici in Rome equally spectacular effects were created. Their style was carried northward over the Alps by the princes, nobles, and merchants who were impressed by the new humanism. In France, the French kings created the still famous gardens of the Luxembourg palace, those at Fontainebleu, and at the end of the 17th century the most elaborate of all at Versailles. In England, kings and rich nobles copied them. At Hampton Court, at Richmond, and at Greenwich, Henry VIII built both formal gardens and parks which now serve the people of London as a whole. At Chatsworth and Syon and many other great noble Houses formal gardens, stonework, and statuary were imposed on the fertile English countryside. Less spectacular were the small city and suburban gardens that the merchants of London and Paris, of Flanders and Germany began to build. The walled garden was preserved with its intimacy and its peace.

The formal gardens of Europe in the 16th and 17th centuries remained a secure refuge from the wilderness of a harsh world and an even harsher nature. Within their walls nature was contained and controlled and along their gravel walks people could stroll safely in an artificial and orderly world. This fear of physical nature began to recede in the 18th century as a growing understanding of its laws began to spread. This knowledge came on the one hand from scientists like Newton and from the reports of naturalists and explorers like Captains Cook and Bougainville on the other. As fear ebbed western man began to find in nature not only physical solace and recreation but moral renewal. Romantics like Rousseau and Wordsworth saw that in unity with nature man could give his life a wholeness unattainable in the artificial world of urban civilization:

> One impulse from a vernal wood
> May teach you more of man,
> Of moral evil and of good,
> Than all the sages can.
>> *Wordsworth (as cited in Clark, 1969, p. 279)*

Romanticism was more, however, than a reawakening to nature. It was often a bitter attack on the threat of industrialization. We need nature and beauty, Wordsworth argued, to restore ourselves:

> But oft in lonely rooms and mid the din
> Of towns and cities, I have owed to them
> In hours of weariness sensations sweet
> Felt in the blood and felt along the heart
> With tranquil restoration . . . .
>> *(Wordsworth, Tintern Abbey, 1975, p. 171)*

The effect of 18th-century romanticism and its worship of nature on gardens was spectacular. The work of C. L. Hirschfeld in Germany and of William Kent (1685-1745), Lancelot "Capability" Brown (1715-1783), and Humphrey Repton (1752-1818) in England began a rapid retreat from formalism. The aim of gardeners became increasingly to recapture the natural landscape and to incorporate it in the domestic environment. The poet Goethe wrote of the famous German garden Worlitz, near Dessau:

> *It is beautiful here beyond description . . . it is like a fairy tale unfolding. In it, oh so gentle manysidedness, all melts into one. Goethe (as cited in Wengel, 1987, p. 219)*

GARDENING AS THERAPY

The English style of gardening, which Kenneth Clark claims to have been the "most pervasive influence that England has ever had on the look of things in Europe" (Clark, 1969, p. 271), remained dominant in Europe throughout the 19th century. As the level of affluence rose and gardens became more widely available to the bourgeoisie as well as the gentry, the natural style evolved to accommodate smaller scale and an increasing concern for intimacy and privacy. These are the concerns of city dwellers and in the 19th century there had occurred the greatest single change in mankind's way of life since the end of the Paleolithic era. Man, for more than thirty or forty thousand years an agriculturist, became an urban industrial worker. Men and women who had lived within the slow cycle of the agricultural year, from seed time to harvest, were suddenly made to conform to the strict disciplines of a factory's working day. "The chief difficulty," wrote Andrew Ure (*The Philosophy of Manufacturers,* 1835, Book One, Chapter One) lay "in training human beings to renounce their desultory habits of work, to identify themselves with the unvarying regularity of work of the complex automation" (as cited in Clark, 1969). In short to make farm workers into "mechanical" men and women, these workers were forced to live in close contact with millions of their fellows—separated from nature and all its salutary gifts. It was a renunciation only marginally less severe for human beings than those sacrifices of instinctual gratification which Sigmund Freud identified in *Civilization and Its Discontents.* The therapeutic properties that Wordsworth and his contemporaries identified in the simple life of the countryside have never been available to the mass of city dwellers. For the fortunate among them, small yards and vegetable gardens can offer an alternative and creative form of labor and moments of peace in the working week. (*Note:* They were not always successful as Henry Thoreau relates in his account of the bean field at Walden or in the adventures of George Ripley and Nathaniel Hawthorne at Brook Farm which collapsed in 1847.) For many more, city parks alone can provide a brief taste of the space and natural growth that so recently surrounded us. In the United States in 1900, 70 percent of the population lived in rural areas and were involved in agriculture. Today less than 10 percent do so.

City parks, whose construction began seriously in the last decades of the 19th century, were an important recognition of the therapeutic property of the natural world but they were essentially passive. Only recently have therapists begun to recognize that a recovery of the rhythms and rewards of garden work can be of real value both mentally and physically in the recovery and maintenance of wellness.

If the 19th century saw the establishment of nature and the countryside as a positive source of recreation and preventive medicine it also began to see its therapeutic possibilities. As early as 1798, Benjamin Rush of Philadelphia, the father of American psychiatry, reported that digging the soil had a curative effect on the mentally ill. At this time, indigent patients were required to pay for their care by working in the institution's gardens, dairies, and fields. It soon became apparent that such patients improved faster than those who did not need to work. This convenient observation no doubt saved money for the institutions involved, but it also began a very beneficial tradition.

By the turn of the century, horticulture was a well-established method of treatment in both physical and mental disablement. During this century, a major source of such problems were the two world wars and after both the Veterans Hospitals used garden therapy for the treatment and rehabilitation of disabled service men. Their efforts were reinforced in the 1950s by the National Federation of Garden Clubs who sponsored volunteer programs in hospitals throughout the country. This practical work led to professional and academic involvement and soon to two important university training programs at Michigan and Kansas State Universities. The former offers a master's degree program in Horticultural Therapy for occupational therapists. The Menninger Clinic in Kansas traces its Horticultural program to its founder, C. F. Menninger. He was a keen gardener who instilled the love of nature in his staff as well as his patients.

In his walks around the gardens, Menninger invited patients to accompany him. Very soon these walks developed into a regularly assigned part of the therapy program. The garden club met once a week on Wednesday afternoons for two hours and Dr. Menninger taught the patients how to identify plants and to use botanical as well as common names for them. This program continued to grow and the result, in 1971, was a formal program of training leading to a Bachelor of Arts degree in Horticultural

Therapy under the joint auspices of the Menninger Foundation and Kansas State University. Today there are colleges offering Horticulture Therapy courses in Texas (Texas A&M), New York, Rhode Island, Maine, Pennsylvania, Wisconsin, Oklahoma, and Virginia.

A professional organization for this new, multidisciplinary, activity was founded in 1973. The American Horticultural Therapy Association (AHTA) has developed into a dynamic and influential professional body with over 700 members and an annual budget of nearly $500,000. It is matched by similar organizations in Canada and Great Britain. These activities have begun to attract the attention and support of government and substantial federal grants have been awarded for the administration of the Horticulture Hiring the Disabled and HIRE programs.

Horticulture allows the disabled to work at their own pace and follow simple rhythms. It has satisfying outcomes in the development of plants and the gardens in which they grow. The skills necessary are often relatively easy to learn and gardening can thus become a basis for an independent way of life. However, there is happily a much larger group of clients for whom horticulture offers a different kind of promise. Senior citizens are a fast growing segment of our society. As recently as 1900 only 5 percent of the population, they now account for more than 15 percent. Maintaining physical and mental wellness among this group has become a major public health goal and horticulture is a highly appropriate means of addressing it. Not only does gardening help maintain bodily activity, but it also helps seniors socialize and, since it is "goal oriented," it gives them something to look forward to when such objectives are often hard to find. "The exercise and camaraderie are all delightful and I love to be busy," said one 78-year-old student at a gardening class. "I like to learn—even when I can't always remember the day and time," she added. "I would like to tell you how I feel about gardening," said another 74-year-old student. "It's a love affair with nature . . . it gladdens the eye and refreshes the spirit." "Why do I take horticulture classes?" asked another 78-year-old and, answered himself, "First it's spring and I just need contact with the earth, hands digging in the dirt—to see what I can make grow!"

These activities seem certain to expand. As urban centers continue to drain population from the countryside, the social and medical problems which such lifestyles promote will get worse. Access to affordable leisure in green and uncrowded areas will become increasingly rare. Such leisure areas as we presently have will become overcrowded and, like so many public parks and gardens, unsafe and unattractive to use. The problem is not one merely for therapists, it is for society as a whole to replan and renew the tradition of gardening which is so deeply implanted in our western culture. When Rachel and Stephen Kaplan (1989) summarized the results of their recent research into a range of recreational opportunities, they identified the key importance of nature in physical and mental well-being. They concluded:

> *The immediate outcomes of contacts with nearby nature include enjoyment, relaxation and lowered stress levels. In addition, the research results indicate that physical well-being is affected by such contacts . . . . The longer term impacts also include increased levels of satisfaction with one's home, one's job and with life in general. (p. 153)*

CONCLUSION

In these past pages, I have tried to explain how gardens have been an integral part of human civilization, of mankind's experience of living in cities. These roots are the source of the deep meaning which the garden has established in our memory. We do not exist alone but are part of the natural cycle around us. Our development from embryo through birth, childhood, and adult life to old age and death mirror the life cycle of the plant. Growing and nurturing a garden from bare earth, tilling the soil, planting the seeds and enjoying the reward of fruition is to achieve a very basic fulfillment. In a recent senior's garden program which I taught, it is exactly this sense which these senior students captured in their final reports on the course. "I call it my quiet time with God" wrote one 76-year-old lady. Another elderly town-dweller explained that for her gardening had been "a love affair with nature." "Neither rainfall nor feeding can nourish plant-life and flowering things as much as a gardener's work of love and praise," said another. Giving and taking from nature we can, indeed, find in a garden a true "healing source."

REFERENCES

Clark, K. (1969). *Civilization*. New York: Harper & Row.
Ebersole, P., & Hess, P. (1994). *Toward healthy aging*. St. Louis: Mosby.
Freud, S. (1961). *Civilization and its discontents*. New York: W. W. Norton.
Jellicoe, G. (1989). *The landscape of civilization*. E. Sussex, England: Garden Art Press.

Kaplan, R., & Kaplan, S. (1989). *The experience of nature.* Cambridge, England: Cambridge University Press.

King, E. A. (1941). *Bible plants for American gardens.* New York: Dover Publications, Inc.

Manniche, L. (1989). *An ancient Egyptian herbal.* Austin, Texas: University of Texas Press.

Rhode, E. (1967). *Garden craft in the Bible.* New York: Books for Libraries Press.

Sandars, N. K. (1972). *The epic of Gilgamesh.* Middlesex, England: Penguin Books.

Shewell-Cooper, W. E. (1977). *Plants, flowers and herbs of the Bible.* Connecticut: Keats.

Stuart, M. (1987). *The encyclopedia of herbs and herbalism.* New York: Crescent Books.

Thacker, C. (1979). *The history of gardens.* Los Angeles: University of California Press.

Wengel, T. (1987). *The art of gardening through the ages.* Leipzig, Germany: The Slotterg.

Wordsworth, W. (1975). *The selected poems of William Wordsworth.* London, England: Oxford University Press.

CHAPTER 38

Healing Possibilities in the Practice of Conflict Resolution

PHYLLIS BECK KRITEK, RN, PHD, FAAN

Healing as a theme that ties together diverse perspectives is increasingly recognized as an awareness whose time has come. Publishers often inform me of this, as we see a sudden potpourri of readings emerge on such a theme. The Putnam Publishing Group's *New Consciousness Reader,* involving, as they term it, "a new series of original and classic writing by renowned experts on leading-edge concepts in personal development, psychology, spiritual growth, and healing," is one example among others. In 1989 they published one of the series called Healers on Healing which was edited by Richard Carlson and Benjamin Shield. In this book twenty-seven authors, including two nurse authors, Dolores Krieger and Janet Quinn, provide a cornucopia of insights into the concept of healing. The perspectives are diverse and international in character, and are introduced by the publishers explanation provided above.

Nonetheless, among the many perspectives presented in such literature, none focus directly on the relationship between healing and conflict resolution, the subject of this chapter.

I became interested in the relationship between healing and conflict resolution for very personal reasons. Since 1986, I have worked to understand the scope and skill base that could bring the resources of conflict resolution to healthcare issues and environments. The outgrowth of a three-year Kellogg Leadership National Fellowship, I, with two colleague fellows, Leonard Marcus and Timothy Dutton, struggled to build a bridge spanning the two worlds of conflict resolution and healthcare. We discovered that few experts in conflict were working in healthcare, and few healthcare providers knew of or recognized the opportunities afforded to us by the tools of conflict resolution, despite escalating costs and harms that were emerging due to conflict in our environments.

In the ten ensuing years we have learned a great deal. Tim became the administrator of the Albert Schweitzer Hospital in LaChapelle, Haiti, moving his household and family members into this environment, practicing his skills in this conflict-ridden country. Lenny and I, knowing that Tim had found a pathway for his ideas and ideals, carried on our dialog and efforts in the United States, with Lenny emerging as a national expert in the field of conflict resolution in healthcare. I learned to give voice to the issues of difference, diversity, and powerlessness in healthcare conflicts. Lenny's efforts eventually gained him a post at the Harvard School of Public Health, where he leads a very successful program on healthcare negotiation and conflict resolution.

As an adjunct faculty member to the Harvard program, I continue to do mediation, training, and workshops both alone and with colleagues. From our sharing of experiences with our healthcare colleagues, we have all learned much. We have also recently discovered that one impressive outcome of applying conflict resolution to healthcare issues involves substantial savings for those who access this resource. This has given conflict resolution a new relevance in today's healthcare climate.

Four years ago, I was hired to provide leadership in the development of a doctoral program in nursing, at the University of Texas Medical Branch in Galveston. I had done this once before, and believed my skills and competencies would be of value. Philosophically I believed and experientally I had validated a key consideration in developing a doctoral program: inclusiveness. A doctoral program is as strong as its capacity to include the whole school, all faculty and students and all other school programs, in its worldview and purpose. A strong pervasiveness of a doctoral program's theme and commitments throughout the institution changes the experience for everyone: administrators, faculty, staff, and students. It makes what can become a "Lone Ranger" experience into a collective enterprise where everyone contributes and benefits, and the strength of many synergistically generates more than any one or few people might have generated.

Through a series of white papers and open forums, guided by a faculty-selected task force, we clarified what our theme and commitments might be, and began the challenging task of bringing together the many voices into our school's theme, so that it might be "sung" in many voices harmony. The effect was electrifying, and the many rich ideas brought forth quickly catalyzed other ideas and avenues of exploration. We became pleased and excited. And we began to slowly recognize that part of the impact of this process was actually embedded in the timeliness and inherent vigor of our focus: healing.

This process was occurring simultaneously with my writing and eventual publication of a book entitled *Negotiating at an Uneven Table: Developing Moral Courage in Resolving Our Conflicts*. I was interested in an issue within the field of conflict resolution that had a nagging impact on me. Every conflict resolution author had suggested that we should always set an even table. All the people that trained us gave this idea the same emphasis. Yet, I knew as a nurse and a woman that I was always at an uneven table, and generally, no one was committed to evenness emerging. I had worked with people of color and knew that they continuously had the same experience, as did the gay community, friends who were disabled, and others chronically disenfranchised in our society. I also began to notice that as a white woman, I seemed to have my feet in two worlds: one where I was clearly privileged and one where I was not.

Urged on by several national leaders in conflict resolution who had trained me and knew the importance of the issue, I wrote the book, opening by stating that it is "about negotiating conflicts in situations where some participants are at a disadvantage that others do not acknowledge" (Kritek, 1994). Here fairness and justice are unlikely to occur, and persons at the table, often unconsciously and sometimes consciously, proceed, accepting the social stratification, bias, active prejudice and cultural assumptions as givens which should be maintained. It is a worrisome issue, and one that has been both invigorating and frustrating to address. One dimension of this problem are the sustainers of the status quo who have privileges. Equally troublesome are the sustainers of the status quo who do not have privileges but who manipulate to get what they want and do not want this pattern jeopardized. In both cases, addressing the issue evokes conflict.

A year after the publication of this book, I contributed to one written by Leonard Marcus called *Renegotiating Healthcare: Resolving Conflict to Build Collaboration* (Marcus, Dorn, Kritek, Miller, & Wyatt, 1995). This book has had a rapid and significant impact, receiving several awards from both the conflict resolution and healthcare communities, including the *American Journal of Nursing*. In it, Lenny, along with our other colleagues at the program at Harvard, tells the story of the use of conflict resolution in healthcare, including the nature of our conflicts, the negotiation options we have available, the varied perspectives of healthcare practitioners, and the possibilities and promise of integrating constructive conflict resolution options into healthcare conflicts and negotiations.

My interests in conflict resolution and healing processes in nursing were increasingly converging for me. They were, at their core, stories with the same value assumptions and essence. They were indeed obverses, two sides of a coin, inherently related. In this chapter I record some of these linkages, and hopefully unveil for the reader the potentials and possibilities of scrutinizing both sides of the coin and beginning to understand the congruence that exists between the two enterprises. My intent is to be more exemplitive than comprehensive, drawing a sketch of possibilities knowing that readers will understand through their worldview and create a variety of options in the worlds where they live and work. Thus I see this chapter as more a catalyst than a guide, opening a window on a new and promising vista.

THE HEALER CONFRONTS CONFLICT

Very few healthcare providers in the United States introduce themselves as healers, preferring to be known as competent, scientifically trained professionals. Yet few in my experience would reject the label healer. We enter this field because we want to heal people, to give them access to a state of wholeness and integrity.

We have taken some quirky turns on our collective path of interpreting the nature of the healer's work, however, so that we are at our best under conditions I term *"in extremis"*: the dramatic life-threatening event, particularly one where the physical dimension of a person is at risk of not surviving. *In extremis* conditions are important to us: we admire these more, reward them more, and take greater pride in them. As a result, we are more likely to be healers of the severely physically damaged or dysfunctional, the person at extreme biological risk. In that sense, we are primarily healers of excessive physical fragmentation, giving illness care to persons by focusing on their physicality, often while minimally attending to either their minds or their spirits, and even less emphatically to the social, moral, or emotional challenges they incur while experiencing such health events.

And we have learned to call the dramatic medical intervention the healing event. Rarely, however, is a patient healed through this event. The risk is merely removed or diminished, the threat warded off. For the patient, of course, the damages of both the risk and the event purdure. Clearly it is only after the medical intervention that the sometimes tedious and frustrating process of mending, of becoming whole once more, of being able to "return to life," of healing begins. This distinction is critical, and the process acknowledged by almost no one, including many nurses is one where expert nurses make a central and compelling contribution.

Nonetheless, it is rarely admired, rewarded, or pridefully acknowledged more often being assumed to be a birthright that should be given, a healing presence in the patient's life that provides the path back to normal. It is the archetypal female role, and we presume upon it, as we do much of women's work and roles, as an expectation noteworthy only when done poorly or not at all.

It is nurses who are present for the fear, the embarrassing questions, the shame of the failure of a person's body to function properly. It is nurses who encounter the rage, the demand for changing a lifestyle and the subsequent despair and conviction that one will never fully heal. It is nurses who, in response, craft the healing web of hope and redirection, who unveil the possibilities, who walk the path with the person in search of healing. It is a vulnerable and tender role, one often sadly neglected by those nurses who have become convinced that healing is not their role because it is not accounted for in our timetables and scheduling, because it is not recorded as significant, because its impact is not acknowledged, because there are no rewards. Indeed, healing is often a process of risk, especially the risk of censure if you follow your inner convictions and intuitions about how to facilitate the healing process for this unique patient.

As a new graduate nurse, one of my first harsh lessons was how difficult it was to chose the healing act or role in the existing healthcare environment. What I knew was best for the patient was not permitted or rewarded by the environment because it was both outside the bureaucratic lexicon of rules and beyond the scope of my authority as judged by most other healthcare providers. I have a whole pack of these stories.

I once cared for a patient who was suffering from intractable insomnia, and thus was unable to heal from an incision. Everyone was worried and upset about him, and a variety of sleep medications had been prescribed, tried, and found problematic. The medications tended to make him groggy but anxious or simply agitated. I sat with him, we talked, and I asked him if he had any idea what would make him sleep better. He said his bed was in the wrong place in the room, and that at home he had it in a specific location that allowed him to sleep. I asked him where it needed to be, and I moved the bed where he indicated. He thanked me profusely and I left the room to announce the beginning of a new, creative intervention. At once I was told to move the bed back. When I asked why, I was told it was too far from the wall oxygen outlet. I noted that he was not on oxygen nor likely to be on oxygen. This intensified the debate and disapproval, and I was remonstrated for my unprofessional behavior with a patient. The head nurse went to the room and moved the bed back to its original location. I began to fear that I worked for a system that kept the hospital intact at the expense of the patient's well being. Since that fateful day, I have had numerous opportunities to validate this fear.

This simple story is for me a wonderful example of the intersection between conflict and healing. The effort to provide a healing experience has the potential of creating an institutional conflict that is usually resolved with the intervention of a "higher authority" who decides what is "right and wrong," and implements the "right" way to do things. I am continuously haunted by the insight of Warren Bennis, a favorite theoretician on leadership. In distinguishing leaders from managers, he notes that "the manager does things right; the leader does the right thing" (Bennis, 1989, p. 45). I had done the right thing, I thought, but I had failed to do things right. The outcome was conflict.

ON THE NATURE OF CONFLICT

Sometimes my nurse colleagues tease me that I have gotten myself embroiled in something as "negative" as conflict. I have learned to smile and proceed, since I have become more and more aware that the interpretation of "negative" says more about them than it does about me. Thomas Schelling (1960) noted that an individual can view conflict as either a problem or an opportunity. For me it has become an opportunity; for many others it is a problem. Why?

When I try to understand why someone posits the connotation a word should have, I go to the dictionary. In mine, conflict is variously described as competitive or opposing action of incompatibles, an antagonistic state or action, a mental struggle, a hostile encounter, a collision, and an opposition of persons. No where do I get the sense of an opportunity. This is not a chance to learn and grow; this is a really big problem and it doesn't look all that attractive. It is not difficult to understand where the negative connotation came from. It has always seemed to me that this definition was written by someone who needed to dominate and win more than they needed to connect or create.

But what if one were eager to connect or create. What better place than that nexus where the divergent viewpoint stands off in contrast to my own, notifying me that another has a perspective quite different from my own and in all likelihood, one I neither understand nor chose to honor. When everyone agrees with me, I have little need to either hone or enhance my worldview. It is difference and diversity of viewpoints that have always evoked the reflective reconsideration and the imaginative option in me.

Conflict asks me if I am capable of seeing the other side or if I am locked in a need to sustain my view. It unveils my blind spots and my prejudices. It serves notice that I do not know or understand everything, that my window on the truth is only one window. It also evokes moral consideration, when I discover that some of my beliefs and values are not negotiable, and while I may hold tenaciously to my moral convictions, I may indeed be contributing my energy, gifts, and time to an enterprise I cannot honestly support. This too is learning of another kind, and strengthens my commitment to an inner consistency that I cherish. It clarifies the choices I can and sometimes must make, including leaving an environment. Somewhere, at the beginning of this process, however, I must enter the dialog of the conflict in order for the opportunity presented to me to be realized.

CURRENT REALITIES AND PRACTICES OF CONFLICT MANAGEMENT IN HEALTHCARE

Marcus et al. (1995) identifies several forces that characterize the conflicts activated in the healthcare environment: ambiguity, requisite decisions and actions, complexity, stakes, competition, evaluation, hierarchical predicaments, obligatory cooperation, stress, pressure, consequences, and rapid change (pp. 12–16). Over the years, what we have learned in working with conflict in healthcare is that we start the conflict within the context of life and death issues, high human vulnerability, the need to not err or fail. This intensifies the dilemmas and the outcomes; few conflicts are as simple as they seem.

In addition, we have developed habits of conflict management that have become as ingrained and institutionalized as our clinical practices, and therefore seem unchallengeable and unchangeable. One popular model is appeal to a higher authority. This is how a nurse who questions a physician's decision can suddenly find the outcome is unemployment; for many physicians the solution to a disagreement with an "uppity" or "insolent" nurse is to simply to go to the hospital administrator and demand that the nurse be fired. The administrator directs the nurse administrator to take such action, and too often, the nurse administrator does as told. Everyone quickly learns that the higher power model involves power negotiations that do not even include the powerless party to the conflict, and the process continues.

This is also why it is so easy to ignore or deny the wishes of a patient or the patient's family members, why hierarchical dominance is so rigorously sustained in hospitals in particular, why neither racism nor sexism are confronted in healthcare environments, and why inappropriate ego inflation practices are directed at persons in power in healthcare. It is one of the reasons that it has proven so difficult for physicians to deal with the dramatic decrease in control and power they have experienced in hospitals over the past several years.

We all sustain the "higher power" model, either by exercising authority or accepting others' exercise of authority, even inappropriate authority, over us. Those of us without power have in particular learned the secondary gains of leaving accountability to others and then criticizing, even ridiculing their decisions. If others will not give us voice, we argue, then they can just suffer for it, and reap the fruit of their evil ways. We can also then excuse ourselves from the call to courage that exercising voice requires. *Negotiating at an Uneven Table* (Kritek, 1994) describes some of these traditional ways of negotiating with "higher powers," and calls them, quite aptly I believe, the "masks of manipulation" (pp. 93–113).

Another seemingly opposite response is conflict avoidance. Vulnerable parties, those chronically seated at uneven tables, simply avoid the occasion of conflict much as I was taught as a child to avoid the occasion of sin. If you're not really there, don't choose to understand, waffle on an issue, or simply stay silent, you can avoid conflict. As any healthcare practitioner can tell you, this eventually leads to a situation where harm is done to one or more patients.

As a young nurse working in the operating room, I once scrubbed for a physician who was obviously unskilled and who chose surgery to make tasteless remarks about his patients' sex lives while they were under anesthesia. I was deeply disturbed and was told by my nurse colleagues that he always did this and I had to get used to it. I then told my supervisor that I would not consent to scrub for him again. I was a popular scrub nurse, and he asked for me with his next case and my supervisor told him I refused to scrub for him. He was furious and complained loudly, so that soon everyone who worked in the OR knew of my decision. The outcomes taught me a great deal. For a week, my nurse colleagues who I knew agreed with my appraisal would not speak to me, noting sometimes quite vociferously that it wasn't fair that I did not have to scrub for him and they had to. Finally I simply asked the "ringleader" why she thought she had to scrub for him.

She was startled; then she "got it." She talked to the others and everyone refused to scrub for him.

Sequelae were interesting. My supervisor thanked me for my actions. She was a courageous and honest woman and stood her ground. When everyone refused to scrub for him, she had the support she needed to confront the fact that we had all been in collusion with his unprofessional actions. Happily, the hospital administrator backed her, an event that happens too rarely. The physician took his small number of cases to another hospital.

A week later I was scrubbing for one of the best of our surgical teams, the chief of staff and the chief of surgery. We were lined up at the sinks scrubbing when one of them, then the other, in a whisper thanked me for helping get rid of the offending physician. I was startled. "You knew!?!" "Of course" they replied, "everyone knew." In the intemperance of youth, I threw down my scrub brush, turned to them, and in a voice of poorly controlled rage confronted them with the fact that if they knew, they should have acted on this knowledge and not left it to the nurses to do so, saying, "We have plenty to do maintaining standards in our own discipline; we should not have to do it for yours also!" They both looked sheepish, and having not broken scrub as I had, they proceeded into the operating room, leaving me to start all over with my scrub. We never discussed this again, but on my last day on that job, these same doctors, walked me out to the parking lot and gave me gifts of farewell. I never could figure out if I was dealing with guilt or appreciation, but I understood better the nature of conflict avoidance.

It has seemed to me that these two approaches to conflict characterize much of what we consider to be conflict management in our healthcare environments. The one with the most power and/or highest in authority always gets to "win"; if you don't like the consequences of entering a conflict or perceive yourself as powerless or at risk, then avoid conflict at any cost. We do not resolve conflict. We actually thereby exacerbate it. Predictably, it will return and create another crisis. It is just a matter of time. We can even create relationships where the habit has become repeated so often that vendettas, machinations, and dirty deals to get even or redistribute power, and passive aggressive manipulations become the central character of working relationships.

Everyone may "pretend" their way through these rough waters, but nothing gets resolved. Conflict simply re-emerges and creates havoc later, only to be shunted aside again to return again. It is neither creative nor productive, costs a great deal, and harms the participants and usually the patients either directly or indirectly. There are few things scarier to a vulnerable patient trusting one's life to relative strangers than watching two health-care providers fight over what is best for oneself. We like to think that patients don't know this; this is an illusion.

THE SMOOTHING OVER MODEL: THE NURSES' SPECIALTY

It has seemed to me, watching nurses attend to conflict, that we too have a preferred mode, one I have tested on several groups of nurses either in training or in consultations in hospitals. They have all validated it without exception. Some even take an intense pride in this skill. I call it the "Smoothing Over Model of Conflict Management."

Among the many unacknowledged roles of nurses, one is the conflict manager. It is usually internally described as a patient advocacy activity. The many conflicts that emerge in healthcare frequently are delivered to the nurse, usually the one in charge of a given unit or service. The details of an unconscionable problem that the complainant knows is one of great importance to a given patient or patient's well-being are shared with the nurse. A second person is defined as the key deterrent to assuming this well-being. Most often there are at least two complainants reporting their different worldviews, ones that differ sometimes to the point of requiring the expression of hostile and destructive emotions.

It is the nurse's job to take in these complaints and make the problem go away. The nurse, exercising a secretive model of "shuttle diplomacy" figures out a potential solution to the problem and then goes about selling the solution to all germane parties, one by one. This can include such diverse skills as deception, cajoling, flattery, appearing to take the side of every party of the issue when it is discussed one on one, threatening, punitive measures, reassignment or removal, hazing, coyness, and withholding. This process proceeds until the conflict is "smoothed over."

The goal in this process is not conflict resolution but conflict removal or suppression. If we can just keep everything on an even keel, the patient will benefit. We consider these efforts necessary and appropriate to protect the patient from the potential untoward consequences of a given conflict. We feel successful when we smooth over the incident, and congratulate ourselves on our skill. We even tend to take pleasure in the secretiveness of our tactics, as if this secret gives us some sort of power. The only problem is that the conflict is not resolved and hence will re-emerge; the "tactics" used are often either unprofessional or dishonest, and the outcome gives the illusion of fixing something when it has merely prolonged the conflict and confused the participants. Everyone thinks he or she won, and no one did. In the end, it does not benefit the patient. It is costly in time and energy and creates a climate of conflict suppression and avoidance. It teaches nurses that the best way to deal with conflict is to avoid it or to make it go or stay out of sight and out of mind. It does harm.

What is perhaps even more sobering is that this model is used exclusively for others' conflicts. Many of the conflicts the nurse personally has go unattended, and rear their ugly heads in all manner of raging, blaming, projection, depression, and other tragic consequences. We are so busy fixing everyone else's conflict as good patient advocates that we fail to feel, know, address, and resolve our own. In training groups of health professionals, it fascinates me how often nurses, invited to learn about conflict, start from the position that they already know all about it and have wonderful skills. I ask them why they think this. They recite to me all the conflicts they have solved for others. When asked how they solve their own conflicts, it is clear that this is not part of the agenda. In addition, when asked if they have conflicts, they laugh at me. Of course they do, but that is not where they are to be doing their conflict resolution by their wisdoms. And besides, most of theirs can't be resolved anyway. This unique perspective troubles me. Why do nurses choose to ignore and sustain their own personal and professional conflicts while intercepting everyone elses? Those who claim our primary dynamic as a discipline is the enabling role of the codependent may be on to something here. What do we gain by solving others' dilemmas while enduring our own without any hope or intervention?

If nurses are busy smoothing over the conflicts of others, they are in essence absolving the involved parties from confronting and resolving their own conflicts, an infantilization of the conflicting parties. It reminds me of two kids in a sandbox with an overinvolved mother who solves the conflict for the children rather than teaching them the skills of resolving their own conflicts, a skill we will all need all of our lives. It also discounts the nurse's personal conflicts as irrelevant and reinforces an imperiled self-esteem. It creates an illusion of resolution while completely avoiding the essential conflict and never even attempting to resolve it. It sustains the nurses' conflict aversion. It festers the wounds of competing parties rather than creating a healing event.

Unacknowledged Dimensions of Conflict

As I noted earlier, for me conflict is always an opportunity. There are several reasons for this. The first and most noteworthy is that conflict is always first of all an inner event for the person involved in a conflict. I may hear many viewpoints and find them interesting, have several new experiences that activate my curiosity, create many relationships that enrich my life. In some of these, however, I will suddenly sense conflict stirring in me: I do not agree with that viewpoint and I don't like it or suddenly, the person who voiced it; I think this experience is awful and the persons who created it are bad, evil, or harmful to me; I don't like this person and I want out of the relationship. The first event in a conflict is my sudden realization that I am in an antagonistic stance. The other party may have no interest in a conflict, but once I am triggered, they don't have a choice. I disagree, and they are going to know it, one way or another. I can also elect to feed this inner struggle until it becomes quite intense and explodes all over innocent bystanders like some terrorist bomb.

Another curious thing about conflicts is that when triggered in me, they are not really so much about ideas as they are about emotions. We love to pretend that our differences are logical, rational, substantive, well-analyzed phenomena. If that were true, we would rarely pay the price we pay for conflict. We would sit down and logically, rationally, substantively analyze our way to some solution. But it is rarely the presence of differing ideas that give force to a conflict. It is emotion that undergirds and sustains the conflict: shame, fury, powerlessness, wounded pride, envy, fear, vanity, revenge, hatred, disdain to name just a few. If we were dealing merely with substance, a conflict would be hard to sustain. It is emotion that feeds a conflict and it frequently involves emotions we are loathe to acknowledge as part of our make up, especially in a healthcare environment where we self-present to ourselves and others as caring, competent, and compassionate professionals. We don't tend to open our discussion of a conflict by stating, "You've wounded my pride and evoked strong jealousy in me so I am enraged with you and want to get even!" Just saying an honest sentence like this would make most of us weak-kneed.

Another obvious but rarely noted characteristic about conflict is that it is always relational. I can't have a conflict until I have another party to engage with me in the conflict. If I'm disturbed about a hospital policy, I won't leave it in the abstract. I will find or assume the source of the policy, and announce to anyone willing to listen that the CEO or my supervisor or whoever else I judge to be the offending party is wrong. I may even tell the "bad guy" so, or, if I am a conflict avoider, I will tell everyone but this person but still actively engage in and feed the conflict, perhaps even requiring others to take sides. I may try to undermine or decrease trust in the offending party. One of my favorite examples of this is conflict with authority figures. When I served as a Dean of Nursing, some of the faculty I worked with had never met me but had discovered some traits of mine that were identical to the traits of one of their parents, usually their mother's, about which they still harbored some unresolved conflict. Sometimes the response was so incongruous with who I perceived myself to be that I would ask a second party to sit through a negotiation to provide me with some feedback. It is difficult at best to unwillingly be related to as someone's unknown parent, and the resolution of conflicts in this context is difficult without a third-party intervention. Once locked into a role that you do not choose to assume, negotiations take a crooked turn and can only be righted with great difficulty.

Conflicts can be sustained; we have the choice to keep a conflict going. It may stem from an unconscious malice, a desire to shame another or seek revenge, an unwitting effort to shift power differentials in the relationship, or unresolved frustration. The decision to sustain a conflict is a real one and it is foolish to pretend that someone who has elected to sustain a conflict will suddenly make a new choice. Resolution has to be in the self-interest of the parties involved, or the options presented have to be more compelling than the reason for sustaining the conflict. If that shift is not achieved, then the conflict may not yield to resolution. This is a valid and important discovery. One of the clearest cases of this is the conflict where one or both parties have included vengeance as a desired outcome, or retain the right to sustain envy or jealousy toward the other party. If that's the case, it is a waste of time and energy to try to create a meaningful resolution, and alternatives such as lawsuits or wars find their voice.

This is particularly poignant in healthcare. By way of example, some malpractice lawsuits stem from avarice or the desire for revenge. No meaningful mediation can bring these to a positive outcome for all parties unless those motives shift and they may not. Perhaps more interesting is the tendency among healthcare providers to assume that some powerful other is constructing policy. Such persons may then decide that having voice in this is either hopeless, a political practice of deceit, or a waste of time. Having absented themselves from the process, they then become enraged at the emergent policy, wasting substantially more time opposing or berating others about the policy than they might have spent participating in its crafting. This always seems to me like a strange expression of an inability to understand a democracy.

One of the most subtle dimensions of the power of the hidden emotion or intention surrounds the issues of power and control, winning and losing as a struggle for dominance. Our culture puts a very high priority on power and control, and much of our energy is invested in power negotiations posing as issue exploration. In a crazy quilt image of conflict, we seem devoted to continuously either maximizing our dominance over others, making sure that they fail to maximize theirs over us, or simply maintaining a power status quo.

Power is very important to us, and a particular type of power is our focus. We do not perceive power as an opportunity for self-agency or a responsible dimension of self-actualization or a resource we can use to support the fullness of life and self-agency of others. We are simpler than that: power is the opportunity to control others and their outcomes. It is a crude and unimaginative model, but one that we are nonetheless deeply attached to, and often unable to imagine replacing with some alternative viewpoint of power. It is a central commitment in our healthcare environments, and often the one type of conflict that we believe cannot be resolved, is one where a substantial redistribution of power would be required.

We tend to not give up our dominance power without a fight, and we fight to win. The need for physicians to have control of nurse practitioners by legally mandating supervision that often reduces itself to mere protocol signing or fee splitting is a good example. One of the amusing observations about this power struggle is that nurse practitioners are supported for indigent care, rural communities, disenfranchised populations such as migrants, where physicians do not chose to practice. They are, however, actively opposed if they attempt to give care to populations physicians view as their care populations. This introduces the strange realization that apparently nurse practitioners are good primary care providers in some geographical locations and not so in others. Clearly this is a conflict that has nothing to do with competency.

After my medical-surgical stint and my OR stint as a young nurse, I began practice in my personal passion and subsequent specialization: psychiatric nursing. My first job was at a state hospital in a large metropolitan center in the Midwest. We were considered the dregs of the state system, and I worked on a unit labeled pre-adolescent that actually provided long-term care for children aged 8 to 18. They were mostly street kids, often referred to us from the juvenile detention center, and often rootless and without any support. They had learned violence as a life solution, and invoked it as needed. The physician assigned to our unit was frightened of the children, and had actually never met any of them. Her job was a "political plum" appointment and gave her the opportunity to earn a second substantial full-time salary, larger than any of the nurses on the unit. She however only came to the unit once a month.

It was quite a ceremony. We nurses were required to corral the children in some area away from the medicine room so she could safely walk from our front door to the medicine room without encountering any child. Our next job was to have prepared a list of the medication changes we knew were needed. We were then to sit with her and tactfully get her to sign off on our recommendations so our children could get what they needed. She had a very volatile personality, in part I believe because she knew what she was doing was indefensible, so we had to work very hard at not disagreeing with her in any way, yet getting the medications we needed ordered. She would feign knowledge and decision-making behaviors, and if we didn't participate in this noxious charade, she would stomp out and leave us with no orders for medication for the children. The children, of course, knew what was transpiring and were alternately antagonistic and disdainful of her, us, and the process, looking for ways to scare her even more.

Each month we would go through this bizarre ritual, and I would ponder the realization that this was clearly not covered in any textbook on nursing management that I had studied. This was an early and compelling lesson in political power, hierarchies, and dominance in healthcare. It is perhaps the most pervasive and unyielding characteristic of our healthcare institutions that they sustain existing power structures to the point of irrationality, and the conflicts that challenge these structures are often doomed to nonresolution. The overall caste system often seems intractably locked in, impervious to even the discussion of potential change, and is fueled daily by unacknowledged fear, vanity, and insecurity. It does not benefit patients.

I take time to comment on these characteristics of conflict because I believe that they are critical in honestly analyzing our conflicts. They also become the driving forces in the process of conflict resolution and are too often given short shrift by the theorists of conflict resolution, most of whom are men and hence reflect men's comfort with and interest in content, objective data, and functional interventions that honor some culturally accepted norms of logic and reason. James Laue, one of the founders of the field of conflict resolution, put it best for me when he once encouraged me to write the book I wrote, "Yes, Phyllis, it's a white guys' field and reflects our style and beliefs and ways of seeing and doing things. We know that this is a weakness, but the only way it will get fixed is if people like you provide the balancing voice. Write that book already!" I knew he was right, and I also knew better than he how hard it would be to "sell" this alternate viewpoint, what I call the unheard voice or the silent voice, an idea crystallized for me by Belenky, Clinchy, Goldberger and Tarule in their analysis of women's ways of knowing (1986).

THE OTHER VOICE IN CONFLICT RESOLUTION

The patterns of conflict-related behaviors that I describe above can evoke a variety of responses. If I am an unreflective person, I will fail to notice that conflict is first of all inner. I will assume it is outside of me, and I will approach its resolution quite differently. If I am only minimally in touch with my feelings, I will not even notice that the fuel that feeds my role in a conflict is not conviction but emotion. This too will lead me to approach the resolution quite differently. If I am unskilled about the nature and demands of effective relationship building and maintaining, I will not focus on the relational dimensions of the conflict, but turn more comfortably to the content of the conflict, which may or may not have anything to do with the real substance of the conflict. And if I do all of these things, I will be ill-equipped to differentiate the conflict that has the potential to be resolved from the one where my energies will simply be wasted. I mediate differently, I negotiate differently, and the outcomes will often be quite different.

Indeed, I may discover that both I and other parties will leave the mediation or negotiation with the same inner conflicts intact, only to be reactivated when the next stimulus arises with the same party or another. The opportunity to learn about myself and my inner conflicts from the negotiation will be lost. I will also never learn about the nature of my emotions, how I engage in conflict, what unacknowledged and very probably projected emotions I have failed to discover, confront, express, or resolve. I will have learned little new about relationships and I will still be unable to know the resolvable from the unresolvable conflict. This may say more about why we consider conflict a problem rather than an opportunity than we realize.

What is this other voice about? It seems to be interested in the inner conflict as a key ingredient in the externalized conflict, one that can be discovered so that conscious choices can be made. It seems to acknowledge and attend to emotion and relatedness. It seems to know that some conflicts won't be solved because intentions prevent that resolution. These things are often easier to see from a position of powerlessness and are easier to study because one has less to protect or preserve in terms of dominance over others. As a powerless player in the conflict, it is also very much in my self-interest to know and understand the unacknowledged dimensions of a conflict. Indeed, it may be the key to my safety from those interested in dominating me. There are also embedded in these traits of conflict some initially covert issues that have both personal and moral repercussions, and ignoring them can leave me engaged in actions and choices I do not support or condone. They can leave me a passive pawn in a conflict I have failed to understand.

There is a bit of caution in introducing this alternate voice. The reason is quite simple. This voice is the silenced voice, the one not heard or heeded. It posits a different set of beliefs, values, convictions and skills than the ones that currently prevail in our culture. These beliefs, values, convictions and skills are absent for a reason; they are not desired or preferred. It is for me the other side of human, the one currently undervalued in our culture. It is my belief that the absence of this voice explains to a disturbing degree why our culture is so painfully out of balance in so many dimensions.

In my book, I image these two voices as two strands in a DNA like molecule, where each is distinct but both are needed to create the molecule and both are bonded together creating a balance. Dimensions of each voice are identified, and called the dimensions of the dominant and the emerging paradigm. I support the bonding and the balance as essential to wholeness, integrity and harmony within and among persons.

The dominant paradigm is characteristically analytic, hierarchic, compartmentalized, aimed at controlling, containing and predicting, linear, and in pursuit of scientific knowledge. The emergent paradigm is characteristically synthetic, interactive, embedded and contexted, likely to explore possibilities, aimed at connecting and expanding, and pursues multiple ways of knowing (Kritek, 1994, p. 179). They are called dominant and emerging because one is currently the worldview of choice and the other introduces an alternate voice. For many, these two voices are not complementary obverses of human capacity, but competitive voices where one must win and one must lose.

For many, these two paradigms also are images of socially nurtured traits of men (dominant) and women (emerging). Dealing with this issue is a bit tricky. They seem to me to be human capacities. They are certainly more socialized into one gender, and indeed we are quite imbalanced in our culture because one voice tends to dominate dialog, but nonetheless they seem to me to be human traits, albeit ones largely associated with the essential nature of one gender or the other. What does seem real to me is that men are often more skilled at the dominant voice and women at the emerging voice, but it is also true that many men excel in the latter and many women excel in the former. It is rare to meet a nice balanced bilingual. As I often comment, in my professional life, I speak fluent male but it is not my native tongue. I often wonder why I have been encouraged, sometimes even required to maintain this fluency in male while so few men even recognize that there is an alternate voice or seek to learn of it. The fact is, both voices are human voices, and the more bilingual we all are, the better.

A more subtle observation involves the nature of masculine energy and feminine energy, or masculine strength and feminine strength. Here the discussion can become more challenging. There is an intensity of emotion on this topic of gender energy or strength in our culture, and few people seem indifferent. It seems clear to me that while men and women are all humans, we do seem generally speaking, to come in two different versions of gender, with each having some traits and capacities that are stronger than these same traits and capacities manifest in the other. For most women, one good pregnancy makes this pretty clear. I find the Chinese Yin/Yang symbol useful, because it notes that each side of contrasting sides of this image also has an aspect of the other embedded in it, and together, the two sides create a harmonious circle, yet retain their individual natures.

We often view the contrast between genders as an invitation to a competition. Indeed, it is a wonderful exemplar of emotion-laden conflict. We even casually refer to the "war" of the sexes, as if it were an inborn trait. It seems equally valid to note the complementarity of the sexes. This, of course, puts me squarely in the world of the emerging paradigm, no doubt a "typical woman."

Educated by discriminating Jesuits and committed logical positivist scientists, I know the dominant paradigm well enough to know I do not want to live on this planet without its strengths and its clear voice. I want a conversation where both this voice and the emergent voice are strong and articulate and can have a meaningful and enriching dialog. To achieve that, and to give the planet the balance such a dialog would engender would seem to me some ultimate step toward conflict resolution and world peace. Neither voice need or should prevail in my worldview. The reality is that the silent voice has often been the voice of women. When the voice is clear and articulate, it is often the voice of women both because of the nature of being a woman and the social reinforcement of the understandings of this voice in our culture. Feminine energy is not weak; it is capable of great strength. It is merely different. We are not, in the main in this culture, adapted to this kind of strength and often find it disturbing, even frightening. This strong women's voice is often the alternate voice of choice that can give us access to greater balance.

In healthcare that has often been the voice of nurses, 96 percent women and the largest provider group in the nation. And it is nurses who have honed the skills of the emerging paradigm. Some nurses have clearly abandoned this voice, giving up on it and consenting to speaking only in dominant paradigm terms. It is equally noteworthy that other healthcare providers such as women who are physicians have contributed to the alternate voice in healthcare. It seems to me, however, that the highest potential for manifesting this voice resides in nursing.

I recently participated in an animated discussion at a national conference on conflict resolution. The discussion focused on a question that persistently emerges: Is conflict resolution a form of therapy? The strong and even strident answer of most group members was "absolutely not!" I felt their response expressed a good deal of unacknowledged intensity and emotion. Substantiating this was a chorus of voices who noted that we are not experts in nor are we prepared to do therapy; we do not want to alienate the world's therapists by implying we are horning in on their turf; we use a process of analysis and logic, not emotion, and we do not try to fix the participants or deal with emotional problems.

The image of therapy presented was one of a complex process designed for chronically ill persons with schizophrenia or a history of long term use of illegal narcotics. Many people, however, seek therapy for inner or relationship conflicts. These conflicts manifest in the process of conflict resolution and if we deal with them well, there can be a therapeutic outcome. Perhaps in every good resolution of a conflict, something therapeutic happens to the disputants. We may not set out to do therapy, but we may often have therapeutic outcomes. I shared my views, and no one really contested or explored them with me, though many of the earlier voices seemed discomforted by this idea. They then continued the exploration, sustaining a commitment to being positional about their beliefs. I reflected then, and have since reflected often on this discussion. I sensed I was introducing the other voice. It was not comfortably received. It was also not explored or addressed.

The Alternate Voice as the Healing Voice

For me, this experience helped to clarify the relationship between conflict resolution and healing processes. All that I have said thus far is merely prolog, a description of a set of realities that warrant our attention and begin to unveil a series of insights. It is however a necessary prolog, since it begins to point arrows to the common ground of the healer and the resolver of conflicts.

The editors of *Healers on Healing,* Carlson and Shield (1989 observe that many healers view their role "as guiding those who have fallen out of balance to reestablish harmony and wholeness in their lives" (Carlson & Shield, 1989, p. 33). Several authors (Hay, 1989, pp. 22-25; King, 1989, pp. 26-30; Simonton, 1989, pp. 48-52) focus on the search for harmony while others (Krieger, 1989, pp. 124-126; Kübler-Ross, 1989, pp. 127-130), focus on the theme of balance. Most authors, citing the origins of the word "healing," posit that the process of healing is one of moving toward wholeness.

These ideas of harmony, balance, and wholeness have a powerful meaning for the individual seeking to heal from an illness or injury experience. They have an equally powerful meaning for the individual seeking resolution of a conflict that will restore balance and harmony, making the parties involved whole again. We humans innately strive to once more become whole. We want to be in harmony, to feel a sense of balance both within ourselves and with our environment. These ideas seem virtually self-evident. But what if we analyze lack of harmony, imbalance, and wholeness when it is disrupted within relationships, either between two or more persons, families, groups, institutions, communities, or nations. We do not tend to call this illness except in a metaphorical sense. We tend to call it conflict.

Nurses have historically claimed that they provide nursing care to individuals, families, groups, and communities. This is a sincere claim, and we educate our students accordingly. The reality is, however, that until very recently, most nurses practiced in institutions where they worked primarily with individuals, somewhat with families, occasionally with groups, and rarely with whole communities. Depending on the statistics of choice, 60 percent to 75 percent of the nurses in the United States practiced nursing in hospitals until very recently. We were in the main acute care providers, experts in the individual course of a treatment program, its sequelae, and its final outcomes. Our focus was primarily on the ill individual, no matter how often we protested that we were really interested in wellness. We got paid for doing illness care, with due consideration given to families dealing with the impact of the patient's experience on their lives and fears.

The recent publication of the revised nursing's social policy statement by the American Nurses' Association (1995) exemplifies this tendency. In reviewing a range of potential definitions of nursing which start with Nightingale's "charge of the personal health of somebody . . ." (p. 5), they conclude that there are four essential features of contemporary nursing practice. Only one of these refers to practice with groups, and while all are worded so they might apply to more than the individual, each sounds more like a focus on the individual. Indeed, it is often hard to address nursing care in a model that goes beyond the focus on the individual, and even when we try to deal with numbers of patients, we can easily drift to a one-by-one model. Our traditions are more individual-focused than group-focused. Exceptions of community health or world health policy delineation are present, but of a different order, one thing you can do but not the most common thing.

Our one-by-one propensity leads to an understanding of healing that focuses on a single person, usually the patient, and sometimes individual family members. This, coupled with our focus on physical illness, tends to prepare us for a fairly narrow range of understandings of healing. What does healing look like as we move beyond this one-by-one focus? What are the healing activities appropriate to the nurse when the client is a family, or a group, or a community, or a nation? What is the treatment of choice, the nature of the healing process, the indicators of a desired outcome when the diagnosis is conflict? When a relationship experiences a disruption through conflict, how does it again become whole, in harmony, balanced? When a community is fragmented, engaged in passionate disputes about desired healthcare services, unable to find common ground to assure a healthy community living in harmony, what do we healthcare providers offer as the service of choice? We increasingly choose to describe as societal illnesses the damages incurred not only by the individual but indeed by a whole nation because of an escalating incidence of problems such as domestic violence, dysfunctional families devoid of skills that promote harmony and balance, chemical dependencies that fragment and destroy whole communities, and abusive behaviors toward children that create long-term imbalances in the child and the abuser. How do we heal these societal wounds? Who will heal them? What healers are needed for the task?

Quinn speaks to the relationship dimension of healing in her contribution to the discussion on *Healers on Healing* (Carlson & Shield, 1989). Noting that healing and health concerns tend to focus on "harmony of body-mind-spirit," she continues, exploring the meaning of harmony:

> *The word harmony can be found in a thesaurus as a synonym for* connection. *Other synonyms for connection are relationship, congruity, and unification; synonyms for harmony include unity, order, peace, and reconciliation. If we consider and reconsider these words, allowing them to gently wash over us and settle into our consciousness, they begin to weave themselves into a rich and meaningful tapestry. The image that emerges suggests that when we talk about*

wholeness, we are talking about relationship. This relatedness is the opposite of alienation, isolation, estrangement, and fragmentation ... We can be alienated from our bodies, from our own deepest self, from our closest friends, or from society. No matter at what level, when we are alienated or isolated, we are not whole; we are diseased. When true healing occurs, relationship is reestablished. (pp. 139-140)

Her understanding of healing thus emerges from an understanding of relationship, what she calls right relationship. There is a harmony that can only be achieved through reconnecting. The disharmony is one of alienation, of disconnecting.

Quinn's suggestion to reflect on these ideas was one I acted on, and in the process began to uncover a better understanding of my deep interest in conflict resolution and its potential, my sense that it was a way of healing alienation and disconnection at the relationship level, and that this understanding was deeply congruent with our wisest understandings of nursing. It also brought to mind my interest in the other voice, the one of the emerging paradigm, with its emphasis on interaction, connection, context, and a commitment to diversity. It was clear to me that effective conflict resolution assures the exploration of possibilities and the expansion implied by this paradigm, and was one congruent with the highest levels of excellence in nursing practice. The first and most interesting conflict that became apparent to me was the one involved in the silencing and discounting of this alternate voice, and the willingness of the silenced and discounted to sustain this state of affairs or intensify the problem through alienating countermaneuvers. There is perhaps no better example of this than the persisting, destructive, often venomous, and frequently personalized "wars" between and among our professional organizations. Not much healing going on there!

There is an intrinsic irrationality in presenting ourselves as healers and yet manifesting so many behaviors and attitudes that exemplify the continuation and intensification of conflict. Hay (Carlson & Shield, 1989, pp. 22-25) observes, as do others, that the healer must first attend to healing oneself. Harner (Carlson & Shield, 1989, pp. 135-138) notes that the healer, through assisting others to seek healing, also heals oneself. If indeed we intend to be authentic in our practices of healing, attention to self-healing is not an option; it is intrinsic to our role of healer. I noted earlier in this paper that nurses do not attend to their own conflicts, preferring to attend to smoothing over the conflicts of others. Their own go repressed or unconsciously acted out on others. In like manner, a nurse who does not attend to his or her own healing processes is ill equipped to become an effective healer.

If indeed the preferred response to conflict is one of avoidance or smoothing over, then we are approaching the activity of healing relationships from a disturbingly superficial stance, one we are ill-equipped to defend. One can only imagine noting an infected wound or a severe drug reaction and viewing it as too uncomfortable to address, hence either avoiding or denying its presence. We would readily concur that such a nurse was dangerous and incompetent, not to be trusted with patient care, certainly not capable of being a healer. In like manner, the nurse who ignores or denies conflict, its alienation and isolation, its steady erosion of connection, and its disturbing sequelae for all parties could equally be called a dangerous and incompetent nurse, one not to be trusted with patient care, certainly not capable of being a healer.

We might lightly tinker on occasion with a family conflict, but beyond that we tend to absent ourselves, attempt to stay unaware of issues, avoid, and deny. Yet conflict is the manifestation of the illnesses of relationships. If we are not skilled in addressing these illnesses constructively, we at least need to reevaluate our commitment to families, groups, and communities. And we need to examine our relationships among ourselves and with other healthcare providers and those who administer the systems of care where we work. All of these are complex and challenging relationships. We may work intensely to assist a patient recovering from heart disease, yet try to block out the implications of the disease worsening due to an ongoing and unresolved marital conflict with his wife that we have been observing daily. We are too often willing to leave that to "them" and claim that this is beyond our scope of practice, that they need a therapist or psychiatrist, that they are disturbed or hopeless, or that this is actually none of our business. We do cardiac function, not the conflict of a heart relationship. We know our place.

Part of our claim to the role of healer is our personal willingness to model health promoting behaviors. It is hard to imagine that our patients view the internecine wars of healthcare, sustained over decades, as useful models of how to weave new tapestries of harmony, peace, or wholeness. Bear (Carlson and Shield, 1989) posits that "in order to become totally healed, a person has to throw out hatred, envy, jealousy, and other destructive attitudes and feelings" (p. 150). He summarizes his observation by noting that "all genuine healing addresses the problem of unblocking negatives in one way or another" (p. 150). The editors state that the healer serves as a "reflective mirror, yet as a role model at the same time" (p. 117). These observations give one pause about the behaviors and attitudes we model. Are they perceived by our patients as healing?

Over time a lurking question has grown clearer to me. Can a person who lays claim to the role of healer in nursing do so without demonstrating competencies in conflict resolution? I think not, and I think our failure to address this issue raises troublesome questions about our ability to participate in the healing process within a relationship. As the conflicts in healthcare today become increasingly costly and deep-rooted through neglect, as the forces of change activate substantive conflict in most persons experiencing these changes, as we move into community-based practice and notice increasingly that communities lack harmony, balance, and wholeness because of substantive conflicts, we will discover that avoiding conflict, or entering into it in a positional or prescriptive fashion will become more and more dysfunctional for everyone.

As the demographics in our society steadily shift, the potential conflicts inherent in difference and diversity will intensify, and we are collectively ill-equipped to address these conflicts. Not the least of our problems will then be our inability to personally address the fact that the healthcare delivery systems we have created practice healthcare on the terms of European-Americans and the patients, families, groups, and communities we serve may increasingly find this worldview dissonant with their own, and therefore a source of conflict. When I ponder Quinn's observations on healing as right relationship, I wonder how we will address the challenges of these new relationships.

HEALING AS CONNECTING

Complex new communications and information technologies have increased the awareness among all peoples on earth that we are indeed connected, that what happens to one of us in some sense happens to us all. The ecological movements have heightened our sensitivity to the fact that harms suffered in one location on our planet will eventually affect the whole. We are beginning to notice we are connected in a complex network of relationships. We often describe this as if we are creating connections. The more realistic image is one of discovering and unveiling our relatedness. We start out connected: we just seem to not notice it until there is a disruption or dislocation of the connection. We wait for harms to show us the nature of the connection.

It is much like how we experience our own health status. Until very recently, we felt that we were integrated and whole and that this was a natural state that should take care of itself. More recently we have realized that the diverse dimensions, powers, and capacities of the human person are all connected, and that we can choose to strengthen and enhance these relationships. This tends to involve both avoiding harmful behaviors and committing to constructive and creative behaviors. We are learning to enhance our connectedness within ourselves and with all other forces and creatures on planet earth by starting from a premise that these connections can be either strengthened or damaged, and that our behaviors determine which. At the personal level, that may involve something as simple as balancing exercise and rest. At any level beyond this, it will inevitably involve recognizing our connections and investing in behaviors that enhance these connections. When the connections are disturbed or damaged, we need to know what to do. While there are no doubt other useful tools, an obvious one that is gaining more and more credibility and utility is conflict resolution. It is the tool of choice for addressing complex international relationships and tensions. It can keep our connections intact, and thereby benefit us all. It can help to heal the wounds of a fragmented planet, nation, community, group, family, or individual.

Validation from the Conflict Resolution Community

The actual process of conflict resolution focuses on mending a fractured relationship. As Christopher Moore (1986) notes in his excellent and balanced analysis of the mediation process, this process emerges when two parties determine that they cannot handle their conflict on their own and need the assistance of an impartial third party. He observes that in such a case, a prior attempt at negotiation has proven unable to resolve the conflict, so the parties move on to mediation. He notes that parties lose a degree of control when they move on to the introduction of a third-party neutral. Mediation is actually a midpoint, however, since the parties can then go on to arbitration where a neutral third party makes a binding decision for the disputants.

Negotiation, the first stage of resolving a conflict is however, for me the most interesting, promising, and rich in potential. In this, parties create a "bargaining relationship" because they have an actual or perceived conflict of interest (Moore, 1986, p. 6) Moore further notes that "the participants voluntarily join in a temporary relationship designed to educate each other about their needs and interests, to exchange specific resources, or to resolve one or more intangible issues such as the form their relationship will take in the future or the procedure by which problems are to be solved" (p. 6). Moore is a practicing mediator and arbitrator. As a student of Moore's, I have had the opportunity to watch him actually model the skills of the negotiator and have admired these skills for their grace, clarity and creative possibility. He has always seemed a healer to me.

There is an inherent pragmatic sanity in Moore's description, a more promising response in healthcare than the one's we are currently using. It is noteworthy to me that Moore describes this process as a relationship and the outcome as one of crafting ways to sustain the relationship. One can only imagine what would happen in healthcare if all nurses, focusing consciously on their role as healers, used negotiation skills and competencies to resolve the conflicts directed at them for solution, their own conflicts with others in their environment, including nurses, and the diverse wounds of the patients they serve. It would seem we would see a good deal more healing and good deal less smoothing over.

The basic primer on conflict resolution is the small introductory book by Fisher and Ury called *Getting to Yes: Negotiating Agreement Without Giving In* (1981; second edition, 1991). It is the one book on conflict that I find some nurses have read and studied. This book gave a strong impetus to the developing field of conflict resolution and introduced many of its fundamental tenets and possibilities.

Fisher, the lead author, was at the time the book was published, teaching negotiation at Harvard Law School and was himself a lawyer. Ury, the second author then served as an Associate Director and Co-founder of the Harvard Negotiation Project, a vital laboratory exploring conflict and its resolution.

In 1988, Fisher wrote a sequel coauthored by the new Associate Director of the Harvard Negotiation Project, Scott Brown. The new focus caught my eye immediately. The book was titled *Getting Together: Building Relationships as We Negotiate*. In this second book, emphasis was placed on the concept of relationship. The goal discussed was "a relationship that can deal well with differences"; the primary strategy was to "be unconditionally constructive"; and the basic elements of a working relationship, which must be put all together for congruence, were listed as rationality, understanding, communication, reliability, persuasion, and acceptance (pp. ix–x). The book is a composite of practical suggestions for building relationships. Once more, the centrality of relationships emerges, and the assumption of enduring relationships is given particular attention. These leaders in conflict theory were addressing connections as they explored conflict.

In 1994, Jeffrey Kottler, a practitioner of counseling and educational psychology, wrote a book titled *Beyond Blame: A New Way of Resolving Conflicts in Relationships*. His primary message is that in order to resolve relationship conflicts, one must abandon blame as a response and looking inward to identify one's own patterns of conflict and taking responsibility for these. He posits that a person can change only one party in a dispute: oneself. He provides tools for assessing and making decisions of choice about the inner triggers, primarily fears, that arouse conflicts in our relationships. Once more, the theme of relationship is central and the inner nature of conflict is confronted. Solutions that address emotions are identified. The book includes an analysis of the positive functions of conflict.

That same year, Bush and Folger (1994), established experts in the field of conflict resolution, startled many of their colleagues by publishing a book called *The Promise of Mediation: Responding to Conflict Through Empowerment and Recognition*. In this book, they provide a critique of the current practice of mediation, where reaching agreement has become the central concern of the mediator. They wrote the book, they state, because they experienced the most exciting part of mediation to be not the agreement reached but the potential for personal transformation of the disputants, one they perceived as having an impact well beyond the confines of the simple conflict mediated. They set out to describe an alternative approach to mediation, one focused on its transformative potential to empower and strengthen people. They include in their analysis the worldview undergirding their approach, which they describe as one that is relational in contrast to the individualistic one that currently dominates the field (Bush & Folger, 1994, pp. 248-256). They also sound a note of caution concerning an organic worldview that focuses on harmony. They observe that this worldview is dangerous if it leads to the suppression of conflict rather than its resolution (pp. 239-241). They posit that the individualistic worldview focuses on the satisfaction of the disputants while the authors' relational process focuses on the transformation of the disputants through empowerment and recognition. They do not discard the strengths of either the individualistic or the organic worldview, but subsume them under the more compelling focus of transformation. In the end, they argue for a relational worldview because it is more robust, it values the personal strength of the disputants, it includes the capacity for compassion, and enables people to grow and learn. Transformative mediation, they posit, changes people. This occurs because through mediation, disputants find ways to avoid succumbing to conflict's most destructive pressures; they avoid acting from their weakness but rather act from their strength; and they no longer choose to dehumanize the other, but rather elect to acknowledge one other. They go on to observe that "overcoming these pressures involves making difficult moral choices, and making these choices transforms people—changes them for the better. They discover within themselves capacities for good that they did not know existed. And they learn how to draw on these positive capacities in dealing with life's problems and relating to others" (p. xv).

While these are merely examples of a much larger collection of written resources on conflict, available to anyone with the interest and commitment to access and read them, they all share a theme of relationship. They also uncover some of the same salient features of the healing process, and search for some of the same outcomes. They demonstrate the conceptual relationship between activities that are directed at assisting others to heal and activities that are directed at assisting others to resolve their conflicts. We may indeed be singing out of the same hymnal at some level, even if we are not aware of it.

OPTIONS FOR THE PRACTICING NURSE

If one decides that the relationship between healing processes and conflict resolution is real, meaningful, and substantive, how does one go about acquiring the necessary competencies? Since so little has been done thus far to bring together the fields of conflict resolution and healthcare, and the primary impetus has been the program at Harvard School of Public Health, my responses are likely to sound like a marketing ploy. The fact is, however, that the training sponsored by that program is an ideal way of developing competency since they focus specifically on the heathcare context and its realities. There are both one-day introductory training sessions and a one-week certificate program, some geared to specific audiences and offered to groups throughout the United States. Other programs specifically designed for healthcare professionals are beginning and may also be available in a given region.

Books abound, and one can wisely start with the ones I reference here, particularly the book by Marcus which focuses specifically on healthcare negotiation. The others require some translation since they do not include a focus on healthcare, but can be very useful. Journals such as the *International Journal of Conflict Management* and the *Negotiation Journal* provide a regular link to developing theories, practices, and research. Local mediation centers often have newsletters or training programs in the basics of conflict resolution.

There are two national organizations that meet regularly: the Society for Professionals in Dispute Resolution (SPIDR) and the National Conference on Peace and Conflict Resolution (NCPCR), one of James Laue's contributions to the field of conflict resolution. The former is located in Washington, DC, and the latter is headquartered at George Mason University in Fairfax, Virginia. Attendance at these national programs is another useful option for learning.

A first phase of this developmental process, however, might be taking the steps recommended by Marcus et al. (1995, pp. 28-43) as ways one can move beyond conflict:

1. Accept conflict as a given.

2. Recognize the consequences of conflict, what price is exacted for ignoring a shared problem.

3. Formalize motive, to communicate a willingness to settle disputes in which we are participants, a step many are reluctant to take when confronted with this decision, yet nonetheless essential to this process.

4. Begin the learning process of how to settle a dispute. Like all learning, one must endure the stages of ineptness, confusion, and stupid errors. It gets better over time.

5. Find the logic, begin to look beyond the polarization and simplification of issues that tend to characterize conflict. One must conduct a balanced assessment of the concerns of all parties and collect all information that may better inform one about the actual nature of a given conflict.

6. Check your choices. This is a lot more interesting and fun than it sounds. Since we drift toward a win/lose worldview, imaging three or seven or twenty other outcomes to a conflict is often the most engaging and creative part of the process.

7. Imagine the possibilities. What could be if our disputes were creatively resolved; how would it benefit you and others?

8. Search, with another party or other parties in a dispute, to identify common purposes, shared goals, and intents. In the process, we also unveil common responsibilities, values, and desired outcomes; our inherent interdependence. In learning these steps, we begin to understand the places where conflict is likely to occur.

9. Because we both recognize the harms of unresolved conflict and the potential in conflict resolution, we learn to anticipate and

prevent conflict, or expeditiously introduce negotiations that address the conflict in its initial stages.

10. Move beyond conflict. We become skillful at seeing the whole picture in a situation, to widening our lens on reality and to imaging a more constructive and creative way to deal with difference and diversity.

The steps are neither easy nor simple, but they are a wonderful pathway to new options, all of which feel a good deal better and work a good deal more constructively than the practices we currently engage in when confronted by a conflict. While some conflicts cannot be resolved, those that can be give us access to new opportunities for synergistic and constructive outcomes. In the process, we may also discover that effective conflict resolution is indeed transformative, an opportunity to learn a good deal more about ourselves and others.

COMING FULL CIRCLE

At the beginning of this chapter, I stated that I hoped it would serve as a catalyst, one that enabled others to see and understand the possibilities and potentials in linking the worlds of conflict resolution and healthcare. I see my work in conflict resolution as healing work. It brings the pleasure and deep satisfaction of all other healing activities I embrace. I recognize that in resolving the conflicts in which I am a negotiating party or the ones where I mediate, I am enabling myself and others to activate and benefit from the intrinsic capacity we humans possess to heal fractured relationships, restoring balance to these relationships in ways that can not only heal wounds but open up new vistas of opportunity, growth, and collaboration. Conflict resolution is a useful tool for the healer, indeed increasingly a necessary tool. And healing processes, with the desired outcome of wholeness, balance, and integrity, are improved with the contribution of the knowledge and skills of the resolver of conflicts. The call to the connectivity, the expansion, and the synergy available in the interaction between these two worlds is a call not only to heal what is fragmented and to resolve what is conflictual. It is also a call to create options and possibilities for us all that can lead to a more whole and healthy planet, and to the health and wholeness of each person on the planet. My single contribution is modest, but joined with others, has the potential for transformation, not only at the individual level but in our common practices, values, creations, and dreams.

References

American Nurses Association (1995). *Nursing's social policy statement.* Kansas City, MO: Author.

Bear, S. (1989). *Healing attitudes.* In R. Carlson & B. Shield (Eds.), *Healers on Healing* (pp. 149–153). New York: Putnam.

Belenky, M. F., Clinchy, B. M., Goldberger, N. R., & Tarule, J. M. (1986). *Women's ways of knowing: The development of self, voice, and mind.* New York: Basic Books.

Bennis, W. (1989). *On becoming a leader.* New York: Addison-Wesley.

Bush, R. A. B., & Folger, J. P. (1994). *The promise of mediation: Responding to conflict through empowerment and recognition.* San Francisco, CA: Jossey-Bass.

Carlson, R., & Shield, B. (1989). *Healers on healing.* New York: Putnam.

Fisher, R., & Brown, S. (1988). *Getting together: Building relationships as we negotiate.* New York: Penguin Books.

Fisher, R., & Ury, R. (1981). *Getting to yes: Negotiating agreement without giving in.* New York: Penguin Books.

Fisher, R., Ury, W., & Patton, B. (1991). *Getting to yes: Negotiating agreement without giving in.* New York: Penguin Books.

Harner, M. (1989). The hidden universe of the healer. In R. Carlson & B. Shield (Eds.), *Healers on healing* (pp. 135–138). New York: Putnam.

Hay, L. L. (1989). Healer, heal thyself. In R. Carlson & B. Shield (Eds.), *Healers on healing* (pp. 22–25). New York: Putnam.

King, S. K. (1989). Removing distress to reveal health. In R. Carlson & B. Shield (Eds.), *Healers on healing* (pp. 26–30). New York: Putnam.

Kottler, J. A. (1994). *Beyond blame: A new way of resolving conflicts in relationships.* San Francisco, CA: Jossey-Bass.

Krieger, D. (1989). The timeless concept of healing. In R. Carlson & B. Shield (Eds.), *Healers on healing* (pp. 124–126). New York: Penguin.

Kritek, P. B. (1994). *Negotiating at an uneven table: Developing moral courage in resolving our conflicts.* San Francisco, CA: Jossey-Bass.

Kübler-Ross, E. (1989). The four pillars of healing. In R. Carlson & B. Shield (Eds.), *Healers on healing* (pp. 127–130). New York: Putnam.

Marcus, L. J., Dorn, B. C., Kritek, P. B., Miller, V. G., & Wyatt, J. B. (1995). *Renegotiating health care: Resolving conflict to build collaboration.* San Francisco, CA: Jossey-Bass.

Moore, C. W. (1986). *The mediation process: Practical strategies for resolving conflicts.* San Francisco, CA: Jossey-Bass.

Quinn, J. F. (1989). Healing: The emergence of right relationship. In R. Carlson & B. Shield (Eds.), *Healers on healing* (pp. 139–143). New York: Putnam.

Schelling, T. (1960). *The strategy of conflict.* London: Oxford University Press.

Simonton, O. C. (1989). The harmony of health. In R. Carlson & B. Shield (Eds.), *Healers on healing* (pp. 48–52). New York: Putnam.

CHAPTER 39

Reciprocity in the Healing Relationship between Nurse and Patient

ELNORA (NONIE) P. MENDIAS, RN, CSFNP, PHD

We all have an idea about what reciprocity is, in the social sense. You do something nice for me, and I do something nice for you. Someone has helped you, or me, or someone we care about, when we were in need, so you and I help someone else in need. A negative form of reciprocity is revenge or getting even.

Reciprocity is also an important component of healthy nurse-patient relationships. It is essential to the satisfaction nurses and patients feel about nurse-patient relationships. The importance of reciprocity in nurse-patient relationships is reinforced by the literature, my own research, and my personal experiences, as a nurse, as a patient, and as the family member of a patient.

Within this chapter, I will explore the concept of reciprocity in relationships between nurses and their patients/clients, including families and communities. Although reciprocity may be positive (involving rewards) or negative (involving penalties or costs), it is the positive form which is a desirable component of professional-client relationships.

OVERVIEW OF RECIPROCITY

There are many sociopsychological definitions of reciprocity in the literature. In general, reciprocity is characterized as an interpersonal exchange, customarily expected to be symmetrical or equivalent in quality, involving the giving or receipt of some thing or commodity (Chadwick-Jones, 1976; Van Baal, 1975). The thing/commodity we exchange may be tangible or intangible, intrinsic or extrinsic (Dowd,

1975, 1978). For instance, we may exchange something tangible, such as food or assistance, or something intangible, such as love, appreciation, or information. Other terms used to describe exchanges include gifts, obligations, rewards, costs, and benefits.

The Norm of Reciprocity

Reciprocity is a norm of interpersonal behavior (Blau, 1964; Chadwick-Jones, 1976; Gouldner, 1960; Homans, 1974; Mauss, 1925/1967; Nye, 1982; Van Baal, 1975). Although we know of no society in which total, balanced reciprocity prevails, reciprocity is thought to be a universal phenomenon, occurring in some form in every society (Befu, 1980). The concept of reciprocity is so ingrained in human societies that we generally assume it occurs and may view its absence or imbalance as a wrongdoing or offense. It is a universal standard of social behavior, apparently proscribed for social life (Nye, 1982).

The notion of reciprocity has existed for a long time. Writings of Seneca (as cited in Greenberg, 1980), in the 8th century BC, and Democritus (as cited in Greenberg, 1980), in the 4th century BC, imply a cultural more of giving and receiving, with attendant expectations of equality or equivalence in exchanges.

Theoretical Review

Reciprocity is an important concept in its own right and in social exchange, social support, caring, and other theories. Study of the phenomenon of reciprocity appears in the anthropological works of Westermarck and Rivers in the early 20th century, followed by Malinowski's work shortly thereafter. Malinowski (1922) reports his work with Trobriand Islanders and describes a complex and prescribed system of reciprocal relationships in gift-giving, payments, and business interactions. Mauss (1925/1967) reviews his own work and that of other anthropologists regarding gift exchange in primitive societies. Mauss describes the three obligations of reciprocity: to give, to receive, and to pay back. Mauss also warns that violation of the expected (reciprocal) protocol resulted in open or private warfare!

In contrast to Mauss, Gouldner (1960) lists only two conditions for reciprocity: helping those who help you, and not hurting those who have helped you. Gouldner's concept of reciprocity addresses only repayment, not giving and receiving (Befu, 1980).

Social Exchange Theory and Reciprocity

Social exchange theory both supports reciprocity as a key concept in interpersonal relationships and allows for reciprocal interactions between patients and clients. Only social exchanges, and not economic exchanges, Blau (1964) says, "engender feelings of personal obligation, gratitude, and trust" (p. 94). Further, economic transactions involving service are closer usually to social exchanges than are pure forms of economic exchanges involving service products or commodities.

Chadwick-Jones (1976), exploring social exchanges occurring in "professional services" (p. 321), notes that, while normative standards could prohibit reciprocal social exchanges in client-professional exchanges, social exchange rewards, nonetheless, may be given or received. These rewards may be offered by colleagues, society, or in direct exchange transactions between clients and professionals.

Kazan (1978), discussing Meyeroff's concept of caring, describes caring as a "process or a way of relating to someone or something which involves development" (p. 6). Kazan describes the reciprocal evolution occurring in a caring interaction: "in caring for the other, . . . I myself grow. . . . As the other needs me to grow, so do I need the other to be myself" (p. 6).

Nursing Theories

Many nursing theories also emphasize reciprocity in nurse-patient relationships. Peplau's concept of mutuality has been described as referring to a reciprocal process, legitimizing growth in both clients and nurses in specific circumstances (Beeber, Anderson, & Sills, 1990). Peplau has provided an example of reciprocal exchange between nurses and clients: nurses offer information, and, in exchange, patients offer their identities and needs (Greenberg-Edelstein, 1986). Leininger (1977) has written of care-giving and care-receiving as reciprocal behaviors that satisfy participants in interactive caring processes.

Watson's concept of caring has been interpreted as being a dynamic and reciprocal interaction between nurses and patients (Cooper, 1989). Watson (1988) has described a reciprocal transaction between nurses and patients when a model of Transpersonal Caring is used by nurses: "What is learned from others is self-knowledge" (p. 180).

Using caring theory, Gadow (1985) proposes that caring as intersubjectivity between nurses and patients is the ideal, with the alternative being, "not simply reduction of the patient to an object, but reduction of the nurse to that level as well" (p. 39). Gadow believes that nurses and patients have valuable gifts to exchange. Patients often and routinely are asked to give healthcare professionals a priceless commodity—their trust.

Marck (1990) has described "therapeutic reciprocity" (pp. 49–58) between nurses and patients. Marck defines therapeutic reciprocity as mutual, instructive, empowering, collaborative exchanges of thought, feelings, and behaviors, with the purpose of "enhancing the human outcomes of the relationship for all parties concerned" (p. 57).

Rawnsley (1990) has described "instrumental friendship" (pp. 46–47) as a metaphor appropriate for the special human bonding that occurs in nursing. Rawnsley suggests that nurses, through acknowledging patients as being lovable or worthy of love, actualize mutual goals or expectations established with patients, thus fulfilling their own professional or personal goals.

Writing about nurturance, Greenberg-Edelstein (1986) describes nursing as professional nurturance "par excellence" (p. 9). She notes that the giver, in giving, sometimes receives, and also describes reciprocity as a norm in nurturance. Greenberg-Edelstein describes five levels of reciprocity: (1) nonreciprocity—where the professional nurtures a mostly passive client; (2) elementary reciprocity—where there is some minimal response from the client; (3) social reciprocity—where there is some socially acceptable mutual response, such as listening, clarifying, reflecting, or sharing; (4) therapeutic reciprocity—where professionals and clients are equals, with personalized exchanges; and (5) in-depth reciprocity—which involves transcendence. Greenberg-Edelstein's model describes the spectrum of reciprocity that nurses experience with their patients. Although nurses can participate at any of the five levels, it is the last three which both patients and nurses find the most rewarding.

Types of Reciprocity

Two basic types of reciprocity have been identified: restricted exchanges and generalized exchanges. Restricted exchanges occur between two persons (Ekeh, 1974; Gillmore, 1987; Levi-Strauss, 1969). Generalized exchanges are complex and involve exchanges in a cycle or chain of persons. Restricted exchanges attempt to maintain equality, and reduce indebtedness, for the two persons involved (Roloff, 1981). Generalized exchanges operate more from a mode of faith or trust, with the expectation that those who help others will be helped in return, although perhaps by different persons.

Reciprocity appears to be a fluid and dynamic concept. It is not required in all relationships, nor is it perfectly balanced. We all know those patients with whom we have "clicked" and those with whom we have not, patients who glow in our memories and reaffirm our career choice, and patients who make us question that choice. This spectrum of rewards and costs reflects the five levels of reciprocity described previously. However, viewed from a "global" or overall perspective, exchanges will balance out over time. Both in social life and in "professional" life, what one gives and what one receives should be roughly even, unless there is some other condition that modifies the expectation. Although some patient interactions may be truly "peak experiences," it is the overall balance that I believe affects nurses' general satisfaction with their relationships with their clients and their career choice.

FACTORS AFFECTING RECIPROCITY

The idea that some conditions may modify the norm of reciprocity, so that reciprocal behavior is neither expected nor required, has been explored by several theorists. For instance, Gouldner's work is significant for recognizing a causal imbalance in reciprocity. Although Gouldner (1960) believes that reciprocity is a universal phenomenon, he also believes that it may be conditional, depending, for instance, on the status of exchange participants and the interpretation of equivalence in the exchange.

Reciprocity Based on Social Distance

Van Baal (1975), citing Sahlins, has identified three kinds of reciprocity, based upon "social distance" (p. 37): generalized, balanced, and negative. (This generalized reciprocity is not to be confused with the type previously described.) Generalized reciprocity refers to altruistic transactions, such as those occurring in families (Pryor & Graburn, 1980). Examples of this type of reciprocity include generosity and payment of tributes and kinship gifts, and generalized reciprocity frequently benefits the indigent or sick (Van Baal, 1975). Such transactions carry only a weak expectation of symmetrical exchange. In families, the obligation to give persists, but the obligation to receive or repay is diminished, and sustained beneficence may appear to be one-way for a long time (Pryor &

Graburn, 1980). However, Leach (cited in Pryor & Graburn) asserts that the beneficence is balanced by intangible returns.

An example of generalized reciprocity occurring within a family is when Relative A financially assists Relative B through college, without expectation of repayment. Despite the lack of expectation of repayment, Relative A, the giver, may be rewarded by the gratitude or success of Relative B, the receiver. To the giver this reward may be as valuable as, or more valuable than, financial reimbursement would be. Another example of generalized reciprocity might be parents who provide emotional, physical, and financial support to their children. The parents may receive as rewards intangible returns such as the children's love. Yet another example is the adult child who provides care for an aging or ill parent, out of feelings of past obligation or moral responsibility. Knowing that one is doing one's duty may be the reward in this instance.

Balanced reciprocity is "intratribal" (Van Baal, 1975, p. 37) and is more like trading or gift-giving, usually implying commensurate exchanges. Sahlins (cited in Pryor & Graburn, 1980) asserts that these exchanges may be unequal at times but tend to balance eventually. An example of balanced reciprocity is the car pool. People in the car pool take turns in providing transportation to members of the pool, and it is generally expected that each person "fairly" participate. Another example of balanced reciprocity is the neighborly exchange of courtesies, such as accepting packages, taking turns mowing certain pieces of property, exchanging child care, and so forth.

Negative reciprocity is "intertribal" (Van Baal, 1975, p. 37). Sahlins (cited in Pryor & Graburn, 1980) asserts that negative reciprocity exchanges tend to occur among enemies or strangers and are malicious or evil. Negative reciprocity is typified by chicanery, theft, or other mean-intentioned activities. Examples of negative reciprocity include things such as warlike exchanges between countries (strike and counterstrike) or cutting off another car on the freeway if the driver has somehow offended you.

Reciprocity Based on Motivation to Reduce Indebtedness

From another perspective, Greenberg (1980) has described three categories of reciprocity, based upon motivation to reduce indebtedness: utilitarian, attraction-mediated, and normative. In utilitarian reciprocity, the recipient is motivated by hope that a benefactor will give future (external) rewards, presuming that a benefactor can indeed provide other rewards. As an example of utilitarian reciprocity, an employee may give an employer a gift, in hopes of attracting positive attention and, ultimately, a promotion or salary increase.

In attraction-mediated reciprocity, the recipient is motivated by attraction to the benefactor, increasing the recipient's positive regard or concern for the benefactor and enhancing the recipient's enjoyment of the exchange. An example of attraction-mediated reciprocity is giving flowers, a special gift, or candy to those dear to us. We both hope the recipients appreciate our carefully chosen gift—and us, for giving it—and we enjoy their pleasure in the gift.

In normative reciprocity, the recipient is motivated by an internal force to comply with the reciprocity norm, based upon a felt obligation rather than external rewards. Examples of normative reciprocity include giving a gift to someone who has given you a gift, doing a favor for someone who has done you a favor, or paying a compliment to someone who always compliments you. The goal in this type of giving is to "match" or "pay back" someone else.

The Significance of Reciprocity in Professional-Patient Relationships

Reciprocity, Status, and Power

In most cases, reciprocity is a "given" in social life. However, in reciprocity, much more is involved than a superficial analysis of who gives and who receives. For instance, we know that reciprocity is an important determinant of major social issues such as status and power balance (Gouldner, 1960). In general, the giver has more status and power than the receiver, and it is the reciprocal interaction that provides the leveling of power/status.

Van Baal (1975) notes that members of some cultures have used gifts as weapons of status, with the "power to humiliate" (p. 26), derived from the proposition that superiors give more than inferiors. The one who gives the most is perceived to have the highest status, leading Van Baal to conclude, "Unequal status generates unbalanced reciprocity, and balanced reciprocity suggests social equality" (p. 16).

Using exchange theory, Dowd (1975) discusses reciprocity in exchanges between the elderly and other younger cohorts. Dowd posits that the majority of elderly in our society are less powerful than younger members of society. He further describes the lack of power as synonymous with dependence, generated by the inability of one exchange partner to reciprocate. The less dependent participant is seen to have a "power advantage" (p. 587), which then can be used to bring about compliance or approval from the more dependent exchange partner.

Dowd (1975) presents the elderly as usually having fewer or limited power resources (examples of power resources include such things as knowledge, money, social position, or power of persuasion). He makes a critical point: the elderly, having limited or few power resources or rewards to offer in an exchange, are often forced to offer a "generally available response which is universally experienced as rewarding—money, approval, esteem or respect, and compliance" (p. 590). Dowd believes that the elderly offer first esteem, then compliance. The value of esteem is pictured as decreasing quickly with further exchanges, until esteem loses its value as a reward and compliance, perceived as a very expensive commodity, must then be offered. Significantly, Dowd believes that the elderly, because of scarce power sources, may choose to disengage from relationships, because "the costs of remaining engaged—that is, the costs in compliance and self-respect—steadily increase" (p. 591).

The idea of reciprocity does not sit well with all health professionals. There is something about the idea of mutual gain in nurse-patient interactions which some nurses find odd, inappropriate, or even unprofessional. After all, most of us have been strictly socialized in professional ethics and behavior to think of ourselves as benevolent givers, too professional to allow a return. However, even altruism is "at least an indirect kind of reciprocity" (Chadwick-Jones, 1986, p. 51), and Homans (1974) also argues that altruistic persons help themselves as they help others.

Less noble reasons may also play a part in nonallowance of reciprocal exchanges between nurses and patients. Haug (1988) notes that some nurses, doctors, and dentists find it difficult to share information with clients because of a diminishment of the "power gained from their expert knowledge and, thus, their authority and influence" (p. 231).

Reciprocity is also important in status and the power balance within professional-patient relationships. It easily could be argued that many, if not all, our patients come to us in a "one-down" position. They may be sick, even helpless; they may need assistance, information, aid. They may be economically, physically, psychologically, emotionally, spiritually, or educationally disadvantaged by their health status, life circumstances, or the healthcare environment.

I can think of significant questions about relationships with those who find it difficult to reciprocate for any reason, including poverty, ill health or disability, illiteracy, a very young or very old age, other social disadvantages—or healthcare professionals who do not "allow" reciprocation. In nurse-patient relationships, if nurses are doing all the giving, and patients are doing all the receiving (without being able to reciprocate), then who has the higher power and status? Will patients unable to reciprocate feel angry, inadequate, or indebted? Will they feel embarrassed or diminished by their experience? Will they withdraw? Perhaps most significantly, will they feel themselves to be, and will nurses feel them to be, equal partners in their healthcare?

Further, if nurses are doing all the giving, without receiving, will nurses feel angry, used, abused? Will nurses "burn out?" Will they withdraw from the patient? Or will nurses become the "powerful" partner in the relationship—with all that potential for misuse/abuse or just plain inequity in the relationship?

If we are to discuss healthcare "partnerships" with patients, we must discuss interactions between equals. It is this that drives me to examine the reciprocal interactions that I know do occur.

Review of Reciprocity in the Nursing Literature

Nursing literature contains theory that provides a basis for understanding the importance of reciprocity in nurse-patient relationships, as well as examples that further enlighten us about the presence and significance of reciprocity. A brief review of some of these follow.

Rempusheski, Chamberlain, Picard, Ruzanski, and Collier (1988), studying patient/family satisfaction with nursing care provided in an inpatient primary nursing setting, find a consistent desire in patients and families to reciprocate or acknowledge nursing caregivers. They interpret this attempt to equalize relationships with caregivers, a "symbolic 'payback'" (p. 49) for care received or not received.

Thorne and Robinson (1988a, 1988b) studied relationships between chronically ill patients and their families and health professionals. They describe patients' and families' attempts to "humanize" (1988a, p. 298) relationships with healthcare providers, fostering "reciprocal trust" (1988b, p. 786), through methods such as joking, asking about professionals' health or families, acknowledging the difficulties of working with sick persons, giving gifts, and rationalizing healthworkers' mistakes as human error. Development of reciprocal trust is said to facilitate patient satisfaction with care received and patients' feelings of competence by promoting self-esteem and confidence.

Morse (1991) studied 44 Canadian nurses willing to discuss incidents when patients or their families had given them gifts. Morse identifies five categories of gifts: those meant to reciprocate a particular nurse; those given because a patient perceived an obligation to do so; those meant to manipulate or change relationships with nurses or quality of care; those given to an institution by a patient-benefactor desiring to acknowledge excellent care; and serendipitous gifts. Morse writes that nurses found it most rewarding to receive gifts from patients with whom they had felt a profound professional relationship. She suggests that gifts offered with a manipulative purpose not be accepted, but recommends that gifts offered because patients felt an obligation or felt gratitude be accepted as a "normative courtesy" (p. 613) or "an essential part of the patient's recovery process" (p. 613).

Geissler (1990a, 1990b) interviewed a total of 36 nurses about the two-way stream of nurturance flowing between nurses and patients. Reciprocal interactions benefit both nurses and clients.

Gilbert (1993) discusses a particular pattern of reciprocity in nurse-client interactions: reciprocal "involvement activities" (p. 764), occurring during interpersonal interventions involving listening. She concludes that "reciprocity is a pattern found with regularity in nurses' behavior during a specified interaction" (p. 684).

Schroder and Maeve (1992) studied "nursing care partnerships" (p. 25). One nurse in the study comments on her reason for liking this term: "It means we both struggle through what happens in the course of the disease" (p. 36). Another nurse, describing her works with AIDS patients and their families, says, "the rewards for all of us are worth it" (p. 37).

Nolan and Grant (1993) studied a concept they called "rust out" in healthcare workers for elderly clients in long-term settings. Rust-out is described as similar to the concept we know as burn-out, but occurs because of the boredom resulting from a lack of stimulation. They found that workers most appreciated "meaningful interpersonal relationships" (p. 1308) with their clients, which added to workers' job satisfaction.

Sherlin (1990) describes receiving a plant and a thank you note from a patient "who nurtured me during a time when I most needed it" (p. 18). Mallinson (1990) writes about "how long nurturance from certain patients sustains us" (p. 7) and describes three instances in which patients nurtured their nurses: a dying prisoner who wrote a thank you note to his nurse; patients who nurtured by serving as nurses' teachers; and a Vietnamese refugee using "his precious bucket of clean water to wash the nurse's feet and sandals" (p. 7).

Hall (1990) describes flowers given to intensive care nurses by the father of a baby who had died. Frank (1993) describes the profound significance of receiving Christmas cards from HIV/AIDS clients in a nursing home setting. White (1993) describes the rewarding but difficult job of caring for AIDS patients on readmissions: rewarding, because of the "strong sense of trust" (p. 2) between herself and these patients; difficult, because of witnessing patients' increasing debilitation and illness. White also discusses the reward of helping patients "die with dignity," and adds, "A simple 'thank you' from a patient, family member or lover is enough to make the day a success" (p. 2).

Mitch (1991), a psychiatric aide and freelance writer, discusses nurses she knows who talk about "throwing in the towel, none of them ever did" (p. 108). She speculates, "Maybe it's because the satisfaction of their successes outweighs the moments of despair" (p. 108). Or, maybe, she adds, "it has something to do with a sense of devotion and responsibility . . . . Or maybe they're just plain crazy for taking on a job like this" (p. 108).

Paternostro (1994) says that, despite the discouragement of limited resources and hard work, "the impact nursing has on the lives of others keeps me holding on" (p. 12). However, she adds, "it's nice to have someone notice . . . . You make a difference—you're a nurse" (pp. 12–13).

Brady (1994) discusses being present with friends when a family member was admitted to critical care. As she explained what was happening and interpreted care being given, family and patient were relieved and thankful. "Suddenly I felt wonderful. I was the American Embassy in a foreign land, Superman swooping down to save Lois Lane from the balcony of a burning building" (p. 54).

Stefanko (1994) describes the "ecstatic" feelings she experienced when a head injury patient in her care was able to speak again. She describes the "surge of joy and wonder" (p. 80) she feels when severely neurologically impaired patients awaken. "Though my work can be difficult and sometimes discouraging, there's always a patient . . . to spur me along and strengthen my pride in nursing" (Stefanko, p. 80).

Chapman (1994) describes working with a patient with breast cancer. She tells the patient, " I want you to know that you have touched me in ways I can never describe to you. Through your strength and endurance, you have made me become stronger" (p. 57).

Miller, Haber, and Byrne (1992), discussing the experience of both patients and nurses in caring interactions, note reciprocal positive outcomes for both nurses and patients. Patients report increased trust, self-esteem, feelings of happiness, being comfortable, and feeling relaxed. Nurses feel "a 'magical' feeling of deep satisfaction that prompts them to love nursing . . . everything else falls right into place; indeed, both nurses and patients feel better" (p. 146).

In a slightly different approach, Stockton (1994) writes that the "genuine care and professional attitude" of nurses taking care of her terminally ill father motivated her to enter nursing. "I am finally able to give back the gift given to me" (p. 4). Somewhat similarly, Phillips (1994) writes that, in becoming a nurse, she "will have accomplished my goal in life—to do for others what I could not do for my mother" (p. 5), who was dying of cancer.

Personal Experiences of Reciprocity in Nurse-Patient Relationships

Each nurse is an individual, and, while some rewards are fairly generalizeable, what each of us values is different. I am one who values "connectedness" with my clients. Kazan (1978) has words which describe this connectedness I value: "I feel that I belong or that I have found my place" (p. 7). This feeling of connection is what keeps me in this career.

Reciprocal interactions with patients permeate my nursing career. There is the severely depressed, elderly man with rheumatoid arthritis, in severe chronic pain, with hands terribly gnarled and twisted, who made me a pink "paper clip holder" that looked like a miniature bedpan. Later, this same man made me a ceramic angel with my name hand-lettered on it. The institution where I worked did not allow nurses to accept any form of gifts from patients or their families. But, it was such an important "normative courtesy" (Morse, 1991, p. 613) to accept, that I instinctively knew that I simply could not decline these gifts of affection and appreciation.

There is the note from the withdrawn young man with severe psychosis: "Dear No-Knee, I like U. Love, Marty." It's been more than twenty years, and I remember the note perfectly. I am still entranced by the way he spelled my name (Nonie), and what I perceive this spelling to mean: that I was someone he could trust to do him no harm—no small gift from someone who usually trusted no one.

There is the 94-year-old woman who taught me that you can still dance, no matter how old you are. What fun she was! Every time I saw her, I thought, "Now, this is the way I want to age!" She was heartening and a joy.

There is the family who taught me so much about enduring disability with grace and meeting death with dignity. Their faith and their love and devotion to each other were awe-inspiring.

These are just a few of the patients over the years who have taught me so much about life and living, death and dying, health and illness, healing, coping, humility, hope, and acceptance. How many times, when I have been on the verge of throwing in my own nursing towel, has a patient reminded me why I chose my career and what I love about it? I have not kept a count, but the number is great.

I also have experienced reciprocity as a patient and as a family member. I will never forget the delivery room nurse who came to my room to tell me she had baptized my baby, who had died. I cannot put into words how much I value the kindness of this nurse, of how much it meant to me and to my family. When I went home, I wrote a note to the hospital, telling them how special this nurse was, to think about my spiritual needs, when I was too distressed to think of them. That was "total patient care."

As the daughter of a critically ill parent in intensive care, I will not forget the nurses who bent hospital rules so that all ten of my brothers and sisters and I and our significant others could quietly, two-by-two, stand at Dad's bedside for a few minutes three times a day. I wanted to write a letter to hospital administration, praising this wonderful sensitivity—but I was afraid I would get the nurses in trouble for breaking the rules! So, I thanked them profusely and gratefully (and very quietly), proud of this demonstration of the real meaning of caring and nursing professionalism.

Selected Factors Affecting Nurse-Patient Relationships

I have studied reciprocity in relationships between public health nurses and their clients/patients (Mendias, 1995). Prior to the study, I interviewed, formally and informally, many nurses, and I also talked with many nurses in the recruitment phase and as the study progressed. I immediately noticed one very important thing: nurses liked this concept of reciprocity, and they saw my study as valid and important. Nurses were quick to tell me about the rewards which kept them in nursing—straight-from-the-heart stories about the rewards they had received over the years from many patient encounters. They were interested in this study, they wanted to participate, and they wanted to know the results. I was not surprised to find statistically significant relationships between nurse-perceived reciprocity and a number of variables in my study: career satisfaction, case management, satisfaction with nurse-patient relationships, years with current employer, work satisfaction, the "other" category of nursing care delivery systems (this answer refers to a type of nursing care delivery system, typically selected when nurses either did not practice in just one particular form of nursing care delivery or when their mode of care delivery did not fit the responses given), satisfaction with workload, the "functional" type of nursing care delivery system, and primary nursing.

CONCLUSION

Roach (1991), discussing the creation of "communities of caring" (p. 123), describes nursing as a "personal service to persons in need" (p. 128). Caring, she says, is a

> *total way of being, of relating, of acting; a quality of investment and engagement in the other—person, idea, project or self as "other"—in which one expresses the self fully, and through which one touches most intimately and authentically what it means to be human.* (pp. 130-131)

Caring consists of caring both for ourselves and for others, which sometimes requires us to "allow others to enter our personal space to share our vulnerability and to heal our woundedness" (Roach, 1991, p. 132). Nurses are not very good at this, but must get better, if we are to bring into being the caring environments needed to "set us all free" (p. 132).

Many nurses have told me that the patient is the reason why they love nursing. Many nurses already know that the rewards we feel in our profession are often interpersonal and that these are critical to our work satisfaction and, perhaps, to our life satisfaction. The concept of reciprocity is not new to nurses, although it may be one of those things we know intuitively, rather than something we are taught professionally. The point of this paper is that we need to consider reciprocal interactions between nurses and patients as empowering, and thus, normal, necessary, healing, desirable, and useful—good for patients and nurses alike.

In this time of change of healthcare delivery, our systems of care, nursing roles, and expectations of clients/patients are metamorphosing. With change comes opportunity. We can choose how we practice our profession. We have an opportunity to develop a healing milieu, with nursing practices, care delivery systems, and care environments in which patients are allowed and encouraged to participate in therapeutic reciprocity—and wherein they are acknowledged for their roles as equals, as partners in their healthcare. This would indeed be healing for nurses and patients alike.

REFERENCES

Beeber, L., Anderson, C. A., & Sills, G. M. (1990). Peplau's theory in practice. *Nursing Science Quarterly, 3*, 6-8.

Befu, H. (1980). Structural and motivational approach to social exchange. In K. J. Gergen, M. S. Greenberg, & R. H. Willis (Eds.), *Social exchange: Advances in theory and research* (pp. 197-214). New York: Plenum.

Blau, P. M. (1964). *Exchange and power in social life.* New York: John Wiley.

Brady, J. (1994). Being there. *American Journal of Nursing, 94*(5), 54.

Chadwick-Jones, J. K. (1976). *Social exchange theory: Its structure & influence in social psychology.* London: Academic Press.

Chapman, K. (1994). When the prognosis isn't as good. *RN, 57*(7), 55-57.

Cooper, M. C. (1989). Gilligan's different voice: A perspective for nursing. *Journal of Professional Nursing, 5*, 10-16.

Dowd, J. J. (1975). Aging as exchange: A preface to theory. *Journal of Gerontology, 30*, 584-594.

Dowd, J. J. (1978). Aging as exchange: A test of the distributive justice proposition. *Pacific Sociological Review, 21*, 351-375.

Ekeh, P. (1974). *Social exchange: The two traditions.* Cambridge: Harvard University Press.

Frank, S. K. (1993). Long-term AIDS care given from the heart. *The American Nurse, 25*(2), 2.

Gadow, S. A. (1985). Nurse and patient: The caring relationship. In A. H. Bishop & J. R. Scudder, Jr. (Eds.), *Caring, curing, coping* (pp. 31-43). Birmingham, AL: The University of Alabama Press.

Geissler, E. M. (1990a). Nurturance flows two ways. *American Journal of Nursing, 90*, 72-74.

Geissler, E. M. (1990b). An exploratory study of selected female registered nurses: Meaning and expression of nurturance. *Journal of Advanced Nursing, 15*, 524-530.

Gilbert, D. A. (1993). Reciprocity of involvement activities in client-nurse interactions. *Western Journal of Nursing Research, 15*, 674-689.

Gillmore, M. R. (1987). Implications of general versus restricted exchange. In K. S. Cook (Ed.), *Social exchange theory* (pp. 170-189). Newbury Park, CA: Sage.

Gouldner, A. W. (1960). The norm of reciprocity: A preliminary statement. *American Sociological Review, 25*, 161-178.

Greenberg, M. S. (1980). A theory of indebtedness. In K. J. Gergen, M. S. Greenberg, & R. H. Willis (Eds.), *Social exchange: Advances in theory and research* (pp. 3-26). New York: Plenum.

Greenberg-Edelstein, R. R. (1986). *The nurturance phenomenon: Roots of group psychotherapy.* Norwalk, CT: Appleton-Century-Crofts.

Hall, M. D. (1990). The way it is. *American Journal of Nursing, 90*, 86.

Haug, M. R. (1988). Professional client relationships and the older patient. In S. K. Steinmetz (Ed.), *Family & support systems across the life span* (pp. 225-242). New York: Plenum.

Homans, G. C. (1974). *Social behavior: Its elementary forms*. New York: Harcourt Brace Jovanovich.

Kazan, S. (1978). Adler's gemeinschaftsgefuehl and Meyeroff's caring. *Journal of Individual Psychology, 34*(1), 3-11.

Leininger, M. (1977). The phenomenon of caring, part V. *Nursing Research Report, 12*(1), 2-3.

Levi-Strauss, C. (1969). *The elementary structures of kinship*. Boston: Beacon.

Malinowski, B. (1922). *Argonauts of the Western Pacific: An account of native enterprise and adventure in the archipelagoes of Melanesian New Guinea*. New York: E. P. Dutton.

Mallinson, M. B. (1990). How about an "interdependence day"? *American Journal of Nursing, 90*(7), 7.

Marck, P. (1990). Therapeutic reciprocity: A caring phenomenon. *Advances in Nursing Science, 13,* 49-59.

Mauss, M. (1967). *The gift: Forms and function of exchange in archaic societies* (I. Cunnison, Trans.). New York: W. W. Norton. (Original work published 1925)

Mendias, E. P. (1995). *Selected factors affecting nurse-perceived reciprocity in nurse-patient relationships*. Unpublished doctoral dissertation, The University of Texas at Austin.

Miller, B. K., Haber, J., & Byrne, M. W. (1992). The experience of caring in the acute care setting: Patient and nurse perspectives. In D. A. Gaut (Ed.), *The presence of caring in nursing,* (NLN Pub. No. 15-2465) (pp. 137-156). New York: NLN Press.

Mitch, C. (1991). Thank heavens for crazy people. *American Journal of Nursing, 91*(1), 108.

Morse, J. M. (1991). The structure and function of gift giving in the patient-nurse relationship. *Western Journal of Nursing Research, 13,* 597-615.

Nolan, M., & Grant, G. (1993). Rust out and therapeutic reciprocity: Concepts to advance the nursing care of older people. *Journal of Advanced Nursing, 18,* 1305-1314.

Nye, F. I. (1982). The basic theory. In F. I. Nye (Ed.), *Family relationships: Rewards & costs* (pp. 13-31). Beverly Hills: Sage.

Paternostro, J. M. (1994). Recognition: A little bit goes a long way. *RN, 57*(4), 11-12.

Phillips, K. (1994). Forum. *The American Nurse, 26*(9), 4-5.

Pryor, F. L., & Graburn, N. H. H. (1980). The myth of reciprocity. In K. J. Gergen, M. S. Greenberg, & R. H. Willis (Eds.), *Social exchange: Advances in theory & research* (pp. 215-237). New York: Plenum.

Rawnsley, M. (1990). Of human bonding: The context of nursing as caring. *Advances in Nursing Science, 13*(1), 40-48.

Rempusheshki, V. F., Chamberlain, S. L., Picard, H. B., Ruzanski, J., & Collier, M. (1988). Expected and received care: Patient expectations. *Nursing Administration Quarterly, 12*(3), 42-50.

Roach, M. S. (1991). Creating communities of caring. *Curriculum Revolution: Community Building and Activism* (NLN Pub. No. 152398) (pp. 123-138). New York: NLN Press.

Roloff, M. E. (1981). *Interpersonal communication: The social exchange approach.* Beverly Hills: Sage.

Schroder, C., & Maeve, M. K. (1992). Nursing care partnerships at the Denver Nursing Project in Human Caring: An application and extension of caring theory in practice. *Advances in Nursing Science, 15*(2), 25-38.

Sherlin, M. M. (1990). On nurturance [Letter to the editor]. *American Journal of Nursing, 90*(12), 18.

Stefanko, T. (1994). Awakenings: Still a thrill. *American Journal of Nursing, 94*(7), 80.

Stockton, S. (1994). Forum. *The American Nurse, 26*(9), 5.

Thorne, S. E., & Robinson, C. A. (1988a). Health care relationships: The chronic illness perspective. *Research in Nursing & Health, 11,* 293-300.

Thorne, S. E., & Robinson, C. A. (1988b). Reciprocal trust in health care relationships. *Journal of Advanced Nursing, 13,* 782-789.

Van Baal, J. (1975). *Reciprocity & the position of women.* Amsterdam: Van Gorcum, Assen.

Watson, M. J. (1988). New dimensions of human caring theory. *Nursing Science Quarterly, 11,* 175-181.

White, S. (1993). Patients challenge RN to learn more. *The American Nurse, 25*(2), 2.

CHAPTER 40

Project Hope Alliance

GERALDINE A. DORSEY-TURNER, RN, MS, PNA, CS

Healing can be defined as the act of overcoming an undesirable condition. This chapter describes a project called Project Hope Alliance that was designed to provide an opportunity for a group of high-risk students to experience healing and to overcome an undesirable condition. They were able to do this by having the opportunity to enter a nursing program. Project Hope Alliance refers to "Having Opportunities Produces Excellence."

Project Hope Alliance provided an avenue for healing the learner with marginal academic achievement. This project was instituted to assist minority students whose grade point average (GPA) did not reflect criteria of achievement. These students were given an opportunity to complete the academic requirement for a Bachelor of Science in Nursing. This article will describe the initial project and strategies used to facilitate the students' academic healing process. In Project Hope Alliance, students empowered themselves and found freedom to embark on the road to success, fulfilling their dream of becoming a professional nurse.

GRADE POINT AVERAGE AND ALTERNATIVE MEASURES

Grade Point Average is a quality point average that educational institutions use as a predictor for success. In our society, there are students who do not measure up to the standard of quality grades. However, these students may have other qualities, such as motivation, leadership, commitment, and past personal achievements that can be considered in the admission process. This article addresses our experience with students who did not have the quality grades to compete with high academic achievers, but who had other personal qualities which we believed worthy of consideration for admission to our BSN Program.

Often students arrive at our academic door in need of healing. Are we equipped to heal the potential healers so that they can in turn facilitate the healing process in their practice? The backgrounds of our students are very diverse. Some come with rich resources obtained from their home environments and the educational institutions that they attended. Success has been their roadmap; their futures look bright and positive. Other students may not be supported by their families and their past experiences with higher education are less than optimal. These students' transcripts do not necessarily reflect their personal attributes and abilities. These may need to be uncovered and polished, like diamonds in the rough.

These students come from environments and academic institutions that may have crippled the students' sense of self-worth as well as their aspirations for success. Will they come into an educational institution that provides a caring environment, where healing can begin, or will they arrive at our doorstep broken and dejected without realizing that someone cares enough to assist them in the healing of old wounds? Can mending and healing be accomplished, so that these individuals can enter the professional ranks of nursing with a wholeness of mind and spirit that adds to our growth as a profession, or will our professional ranks be encumbered with individuals who are unable to contribute to the growth of our profession? Avenues are immediately closed to many potential nurses if all that is seen is their GPA. Precious resources may never be uncovered when seeds are not even given the opportunity to grow.

Perhaps some of these students have been allowed to enter the Halls of Ivy, but the hostility of the environment is neither nurturing, nor therapeutic, nor does it foster growth. These students fall by the wayside, never having been given a chance nor having been met halfway, so that their resources and potential have not been uncovered. However, this bleak picture can be brightened if faculty have the foresight and insight to infuse their program of study with a caring model. An environment can be created that fosters hope and caring. Within this environment, the student can be provided the opportunity to grow, by using institutional resources that support avenues for success and excellence.

CREATING A CLIMATE FOR HEALING

Much has been written about the recruitment and retention of minorities, but much remains to be done. Barriers to education can be lifted. One of the initial barriers that can be altered are inflexible admission criteria that focus only on the applicants' GPA. Other barriers that we need to consider include the requirement for full-time study, lack of adequate financial aid, and insufficient academic support services.

What is needed for the learner to be successful? Not all of the answers are known, but some are quite obvious, and include peer tutorials, opportunities for remediation, academic counseling, personal counseling, financial support, committed faculty, and most especially, administrative support. The students also need to contribute to their own learning through motivation, a commitment to study, realization of strengths and weaknesses, ability to seek assistance when needed, and most importantly, a sense of self and hope that is necessary to attain goals. It is also important that the students have a good support system. Faculty members and administrators can play a key role in the healing process through personal involvement in the students' activities and recognition of their personal achievements and worth.

Faculty may question why they have to assume so much responsibility with these students. "I don't have the time," "I didn't decide to teach in a professional school to remediate learners." These philosophical issues need to be addressed prior to initiating a program of caring for high-risk minority students. After all, time is a key element for both students and faculty. Commitment by all is essential to the program's success. Not everyone on the faculty has to become personally involved, however, caring should be the keystone of all faculty members. A model of caring and healing that is subscribed to by the faculty can be transmitted from the faculty to the students and from the students and faculty to the patients and clients. Implementation of such a model will allow healing to be a continuous process.

PROJECT HOPE ALLIANCE

The philosophy of Project Hope Alliance was to institute a program for high-risk minority students that would fulfill a twofold objective: (1) increase the number of minority students in our program, and (2) provide students who might not have been admitted under the competitive GPA model, an opportunity for success in a baccalaureate nursing program. Our initial group consisted of six students who were admitted after a telephone interview and two personal interviews with selected faculty members and an administrator. The interviews focused on assessment of the students' motivation and commitment as well as providing information about the project requirements.

One of the admission requirements was that the students complete necessary remedial work during the summer term prior to beginning the nursing courses in the fall semester. The remedial work was individualized, based on assessment of need, and was provided by a local community college at no cost to the students. For example, students whose reading level was not at the twelfth grade level participated in activities that increased their reading skills. All students were at the twelfth grade level or above for reading and math skills prior to the fall semester. Seminars in motivation, leadership, impromptu speaking, test taking, and writing skills were also provided during the summer term. These activities were considered as requirements rather than optional and this was clearly understood by students prior to their admission. Students were allowed to audit the Pathophysiology course that would be one of the required courses in the fall term.

Although our usual curriculum sequence set forth a prescribed course of study for two years (five academic terms), one of the provisions of Project Hope Alliance was that students would complete the course of study in three years instead of two. They began with a reduced workload during the first year, which provided time for adjustment to the requirements of a professional school and to further strengthen their academic skills. They gradually progressed to a full-time course load during the second and third years. This schedule change was instituted with the belief that although the students' GPA was below 3.0, given support and more time to learn, these students could be successful. Faculty presented the students with a certificate of commendation for successfully completing the summer sequence at a luncheon to which family members were invited. This activity was meant to actively recognize the students' achievement and to further encourage the students.

During the fall semester, along with the regular courses, students were required to attend monthly meetings to address any issues that arose and to use this time for reflecting on and assessing their own progress. Events such as birthdays and good examination grades were celebrated. Peer tutorials were available, as were materials from the Learning Resources Center, to enhance learning. Academic and personal counseling were provided through the counseling center on campus on an "as needed" basis.

Financial resources were a problem for most of the students to varying degrees. As the project director, I worked closely with the University's student financial aid office to ensure that the students were aware of all potential sources of assistance. Several scholarship opportunities available only to minority nursing students were identified and several of the students benefited. The University has a "Work Study" program that students could apply for, and several students worked in various capacities at the University, including work in the Nursing Skills Lab and the Office of Student Affairs.

At the end of the second summer, one of the original six students left the program due to personal problems. Prior to the student leaving, career counseling was provided along with personal counseling. Communication with this student has continued and she is now successful as a social worker. The five remaining students gained confidence and grew in leadership skills as they progressed through the program. Leadership opportunities, such as assisting with student recruitment activities and volunteering within the community, resulted in leaders emerging within the group.

Five students graduated in 1993. Four successfully passed the NCLEX examination the first time, and the fifth student passed the examination on the first repeated attempt. Each of the original six has achieved a Bachelor of Science Degree. Providing an opportunity to hope, and a healing environment to succeed helped heal old wounds. These students were provided a chance to heal, to succeed, and to realize their dreams. A dream is a goal put into action.

The students' efforts and the therapeutic and healing environment opened a beginning pathway toward success and allowed these students to become contributing members of our honored profession.

ROLE OF DIRECTOR

It is very rewarding to have a dream realized. I had a dream that I hoped would come to fruition. Past experiences as a student and faculty member made me aware that some barriers to achievement could be eliminated. My goal was to be a positive part in the link of helping students in their quest for achievement. Standardized testing, and often GPAs, do not reflect the true potential of most minorities. As a member of an underrepresented group, this has been my personal experience. Experiences like these can cause frustration and discouragement when striving to reach personal goals. Many opportunities are not available to individuals who may not have outstanding academic achievements, so that their potential talents may not be observed or nurtured. Educational opportunities vary depending on the community and the educational system attended. Everyone has a different learning style and rate to process information. Some individuals, like flowers, may need more nutrients for growth, such as more water, sun exposure, and care. People vary in their needs and in reaching full growth.

Nurses, as a vital part of the health team, focus on healing of the patient/client. Caring historically has been a concept instilled and inspired within the profession. It is my personal belief that environments can alter behavior, so what better way to start than with beginning students in a nursing program? We are what we repeatedly do. "Excellence then, is not an act, but a habit"—Aristotle (cited by Covey, 1990, p. 46).

As project director of Project Hope Alliance, my role was to help motivate and provide support and encouragement to the students. It was also important to present opportunities for personal growth attainment and excellence. It is very important to offer a positive therapeutic environment, so healing through the realization of dreams and aspirations can bring about desired outcomes. Internal healing for the student is necessary, so they as healers, can continue the process. Although faculty are not academic dream makers, as a faculty member I represent a vital part in helping the student realize a life goal and also have the responsibility to aid in the direction that goal will take.

Project Hope Alliance was my dream, and my goal was to empower a group of students helping them make their dream a reality, the dream of becoming a professional nurse. If a student meets the qualifications of a program, is committed to learning, is working toward striving to attain that goal, I believe faculty and the institution have an obligation to help them succeed. This was the philosophy behind Project Hope Alliance. This can be accomplished if some educational barriers are lifted and a healing therapeutic environment is in place.

"What lies behind us and what lies before us are tiny matters compared to what lies within us"—Oliver Wendwell Holmes (cited by Covey, 1990, p. 96). The focus of Project Hope Alliance was to recall the past, not dwell on it, reflect on the future, strive for it, win the race and attain the goal. All this was accomplished because of something strong and powerful within these students. Their potential was made evident as barriers to their education were lifted, opportunities for growth were opened and finally realization of dreams was made attainable through healing, the cornerstone of care. We found that our project HOPE (Having Opportunities Produces Excellence) was an example of what can be achieved in a healing environment.

REFERENCE

Covey, S. R. (1990). *The 7 habits of highly effective people.* New York: Simon & Schuster.

CHAPTER 41

Soul Image: A Healing Metaphor

PHYLLIS BECK KRITEK, RN, PHD, FAAN

this house
has many wings, mirror shapes that
    curve
both private and full public;
stairwells known only to me;
beds for loving, rooms for living.

this house
is under reconstruction: some
expansion, mild refurbishing,
colors brightened, textures hewed,
woods of every tree i ever loved.

this house
is mine for breathing, music pulses
broken by my bracing silences, my
secret songs and my cleansing tears:
intimations of a soaring symphony.

this house
has doors and locks on it, open as air
and welcome as sunlight or moonlight
in rhythm; closes completely like
the morning glory, spreads like a rose.

this house
touches everything with simple awe
for only that it is and will perdure,
for frenzy turned to peace, and this,
a gift for all the turns of pain.

this house
is nothing special, nothing new, not
flashy or serene: rock bands play here
on holidays, fuses blow, the toilet
overflows and with it all else.

this house
was constructed eons ago; was framed
    in
homicides, crushed and caked with
    mud
and seaweed from prior storms, broken
completely in unnamed hurricanes.

this house
rests on a sure earth i trust as i trust
water and air, fire in winter, spring
breezes and tomato plants, rocks
and the moon that speaks clearly to
    me.

this house
sits by ageless seas cycling the wet
wonders in tempos like my own
    wizened heart;
keeps me honest in wild weather,
    mimics
my rages and my quiescent states.

this house
has no basement and two stories and
stories too numerous to tell or write;
has mysteries in every space,
    whimsies
in every moment, has history to
    shape.

this house
has trees and trees and trees to
    comfort
and protect the land, embraceable and
strong, deep rooted and old, tall

and firm and full blooded with tree
    juices.

this house
has grassland for ambling carpet and
    love
making and sky dreaming, has space
for running for the play of it, has play
for the space and time of it, has grass.

this house
is more window that wall, more rag
    rug
than tile, more trickster than sage,
more mother than friend, more
    laughter
than sighs, more loving than life.

this house
was never up for sale, never on the
market, never priced or overpriced,
never assessed, never mortgaged,
never sold, and never owned.

this house
has lofts for the lofty, overnight
guests, dream makers and dream
    weavers
and dream catchers; beds them all
for the interim, serves notice.

this house
has rules, tough stuff requirements:
dress codes and honor codes and
    places
to hang the towels and store the
    boots;
restrictions that stick, and stricken.

this house
is staffed by volunteers: spirit waifs
who tidy up, note damages, do repairs,
mend fractures, heal tissue splits,
conjur among themselves bemused.

this house
has lush places, rooms sensuous as
pomegranates and summer rain, scarlet
spaces where entry is a stirring
celebration, where love explodes.

this house
has rooms as dark as night, light free
space where works are tunnels and
victories are fires and rainbows
form from ebony and flame.

this house
has lots of toys and trinkets;
frolics splashing games that never end
because the laughter and the giggling
light the rainbow, spark the love.

this house
is word riddled, swelling, libraries of
reflection and despair, paradox and
    hope:
piping thought through the heating
    system,
piping language through the doors.

this house
looks outward, lightly pensive and
    perturbed,
now peaceful, now amused, now
    saddened,
now assured, now silent, now
    concerned,
now certain of the outer warp and
    woof.

this house
has housed some miracles, some
    loving of
this life, some birthings and some
    dyings,
and some silent struggling wars, and
this house has been beloved, every
    inch.

CHAPTER 42

Psychosynthesis: A Perspective for Growth and Healing of Self

PATRICIA ROMICK, RN, MS, RNCS

This chapter introduces the theory of psychosynthesis as envisioned and developed by Roberto Assagioli, M.D., a contemporary of Freud and Jung. By sharing my own experiences with psychosynthesis as a consumer, student, and practicing provider/guide, the implications of psychosynthesis as a healing modality are highlighted.

I was introduced to psychosynthesis in the late 1970s when I attended two workshops led by directors of the Kentucky Center of Psychosynthesis. I had completed my Masters Degree in Psychiatric/Mental Health Nursing and had previously been interested in transactional analysis and gestalt therapy. However, I had been reluctant to enter a formal training program in either. My initial workshop exposure to psychosynthesis represented what I, as a nurse therapist, understood to be true about people and change, health and illness, growth and healing. Thus, I made a three-and-a-half-year commitment to the training program for professionals at the Kentucky Center of Psychosynthesis.

What was it about psychosynthesis that had such a profound impact on my personal and professional "being?" There are many answers to this question: Some are within my awareness and some still remain unconscious. Those I do recognize, however, start with my attraction to the holistic nature of this combination of psychology, philosophy, and spirituality. This was a way of helping and working with people as whole beings: body, mind, and spirit—with the recognition that what affects one part also affects the other parts. Psychosynthesis reflected not only a perspective on the personality, but also a perspective on humankind—a worldview. The perspective of psychosynthesis also allowed for the incorporation of other modalities, schools of thought, and effective methods for psychological work and growth. Assagioli was always open to new hypotheses in relation to Psychosynthesis theory, methods, and areas of use. Psychosynthesis methods themselves allowed for in depth work, providing for the possibility of healing and transforming an individual's inner pain. Further, Assagioli realized that any healing or transformation took place from "inside out," not from the "outside in." According to Assogioli, the psychosynthesis therapist, or guide simply guides and does not fix. The client, or traveler, heals him or herself with the assistance of the traveler's Higher Self inner wisdom.

Laura Huxley, in her Foreword to Ferrucci's book, *What We May Be,* reported a conversation she once had with Roberto Assagioli, during which he asked her what she did with people. She replied, "Well, I don't do anything really; I just help them get rid of their garbage. And, what do you do?" Without hesitation, he replied, "I do just the same thing you do" (Ferrucci, 1982, p. 1).

What I believe Dr. Assagioli was saying is that, in using the psychosynthesis approach, he stayed out of the way of his client's internal process and allowed the person's Higher Self to be the "director." He simply helped and guided the process of therapy, using his knowledge of psychiatry, personality, counseling methods, and techniques of his contemporaries as well as his own "psychological laws," and his commitment to self-awareness and self-understanding.

Psychosynthesis: A Journey toward Healing

No one method of working with people is right or best for everyone. However, for me, psychosynthesis has provided an approach to healing our inner children, our internalized critics, and some core issues such as anxiety, phobias, and depression. There is more healing to take place; healing is a life-long journey and process. However, I have personally experienced and seen in others a depth of healing and growth that I have not witnessed in other work. These observations have led to an integration and some synthesis of how I would define self-healing, which includes the following:

- Knowing, accepting, and affirming who I am: my light and dark sides, my strengths and limitations, my feminine and masculine qualities, my purpose, and my human condition.
- Having the full range of my emotions present and available to me and having a willingness to express my emotions as well as my thoughts.
- Acknowledging that within me resides a "Higher Self" who is guiding my process, thus, what is happening at any moment and time in

my life has a higher purpose for my soul's development within this lifetime.

- Recognizing, although they are a part of me, that I am more than my body, drives, sensations, thoughts, and emotions.
- Being fully conscious when I am identified with one set of feelings, thoughts, and behaviors and being able to disidentify from that pattern, thus reconnecting with my "self" and, thus providing the opportunity to connect with my "Higher Self."
- Having my work and career reflect and be congruent with my recognition and acknowledgment of my life purpose.
- Trusting that the individual, with whom I am guiding/counseling, has the Higher Self inner strength and knowledge that is needed to resolve issues and become more integrated and whole without my interference or fixing; but rather, with my presence to the individual's process and self-identified intention, goals, and purpose.
- Continuing to work toward bringing more harmony, balance, and integration into my personality; my body, mind, and spirit; and my professional, personal, and spiritual life so that I can continue to strive toward my highest potential and greater good.

These statements flow from Assagioli's philosophy about healing and human beings, which has been well-summarized by Whitmore (1991) in her book, *Psychosynthesis Counseling in Action* (p. 5). Assagioli proposed that the purpose of psychological healing was to contact a deeper center of identity, the self; to nurture the self's unfoldment while removing obstacles to the self's actualization. He articulated an optimistic vision of human nature. This premise led to several others. He emphasized the soul, man's spiritual being, by positing that the soul was the source of psychological health. He recognized that meaning and purpose were fundamental to human existence and well-being. He perceived life as an evolutionary journey of development and differentiation; he saw problems as opportunities to further develop the evolutionary journey. He viewed the human being both as a unique individual as well as a universal entity interconnected with others and the environment. He maintained that evoking human potential was necessary in treating pathology. He noticed that, along with the repression of negative aspects of oneself, the repressed individual also represses intuition, altruism, creativity, love, and joy.

I, as a nurse therapist, was attracted to this philosophy regarding people and change, health and illness, growth and healing. I found the congruence with my own discipline, nursing, striking. Florence Nightingale stated, "Nursing is an art; and if it is to be made an art, it requires as exclusive a devotion, as hard a preparation, as any painter's or sculptor's work; for what is having to do with dead canvas or cold marble, compared with having to do with the living spirit? It is one of the Fine Arts; I had almost said, the finest of art" (Letter to the Editor, Macmillan's Magazine, 1867). Nursing has always considered the spiritual aspects of health and healing. Nursing has always viewed individuals as whole beings both in health and illness. Virginia Henderson, an internationally known nursing educator and writer, in describing the nature of nursing stated that, "the unique function of the nurse is to assist the individual, sick or well, in the performance of those activities contributing to health or its recovery (or to peaceful death) that he [sic] would perform unaided if he had the necessary strength, will, or knowledge. And to do this in such a way as to help him gain independence as rapidly as possible" (Henderson at the International Council of Nurses, 1958).

Schlotfeldt (1972) stated about nursing: "the goal of nursing as a field of professional endeavor is to help people attain, retain, and regain health. . . . The knowledge base for nursing is man's [sic] behavioral mechanisms . . . The intellectual concern of nurses is thus man's voluntary and involuntary, conscious and pre- or subconscious, behavior through which he is motivated to seek health, to avoid threats to health, and to cope with life's crises, as well as with diagnostic procedures and therapeutic modalities, during illness, injury, infirmity, and decline" (pp. 245–246). The congruence between psychosynthesis perspectives and these three nurse leader exemplars is striking as you will see.

Descriptions of Psychosynthesis

Psychosynthesis is first and foremost a dynamic, even a dramatic conception of our psychological life, which it portrays as a constant interplay and conflict among many different and contrasting forces and a unifying center which ever tends to control, harmonize and use them (Assagioli, 1976, p. 30). Psychosynthesis brings the matter to a point of extreme simplicity, seeing the self as the most elementary and distinctive part of our being, its core. This core is entirely different from all the elements (body, sensations, feelings, thoughts, etc.) that make up our personality. As a consequence, it can act as a unifying center, directing those elements and bringing them into the unity of an organic wholeness (Ferrucci, 1982, p. 16).

These descriptions refer to the theoretical basis of personality structure, integration and development. The following speak more of the application of psychosynthesis in clinical practice.

Psychosynthesis is a synonym for human growth, the ongoing process of integrating all the parts, aspects, and energies of the individual into a harmonious, powerful whole. Like most "natural" processes, this one can be enhanced and facilitated by awareness, understanding, and specific techniques (Brown, 1983, p. 3). Anne Yeomans states, "Psychosynthesis is self-care; it is both learning to care for yourself and allowing your self to care for you" (Weiser & Yeomans, 1984, p. 65). Psychosynthesis conceives of the human being as an element or cell of a human group. This group forms associations with larger and more complex groups (family, social classes, national groups), and these larger groups form the entire human family. Thus, psychosynthesis conceives of the universe as one cosmic energy (Assagioli, 1976, p. 31). Each description hypothesizes that all humans have a basic drive toward maturity, freedom, and creative self-expression. Psychosynthesis practice is rooted in the effort to support this drive, work through whatever blocks it, and affirm and strengthen the expression of who we are (our true selves). Thus Thomas Yeomans asserts, "This is the touchstone for healing and for growth." (Weiser & Yeomans, 1985)

Viewed as a composite, these descriptions provide a useful overview of the world of psychosynthesis. It is my intent to show you the depth and breadth of this energetic healing modality called Psychosynthesis. I have chosen to share with you the ones that have had meaning for me and my work.

STAGES OF PSYCHOSYNTHESIS

There are two stages of psychosynthesis: personal and transpersonal. Personal psychosynthesis has the goals of integrating the personality around the personal self and assisting individuals to reach their highest potential within their chosen life work and within their relationships with others. Transpersonal psychosynthesis has the goal of aligning the self of the personality with the Higher Self (residing in our superconsciousness), thus allowing for the expression of Higher Self energies. This results in the manifestation of transpersonal (Higher Self) qualities such as compassion, cooperation, courage, creativity, generosity, goodwill, gratitude, inclusiveness, joy, love, responsibility, serenity, service, trust, truth, understanding, and wisdom. Both of these stages overlap one another creating movement between the stages of work.

ASSAGIOLI'S IMAGES OF HUMAN PERSONALITY

Assagioli developed several images as ways to view human personality: the "Egg Diagram," the "Star Diagram," the "Will," the "Subpersonalities," and "Body, Feelings, and Thinking Mind." Each is briefly discussed below.

The Egg Diagram

In the Egg Diagram (Figure 42.1), the area within the small circle is the field of consciousness. This contains sensations, thoughts, feelings, desires, impulses, and images, of which we are aware. At a conscious level, these can be observed, analyzed, and criticized. At the center is the "I" or "self."

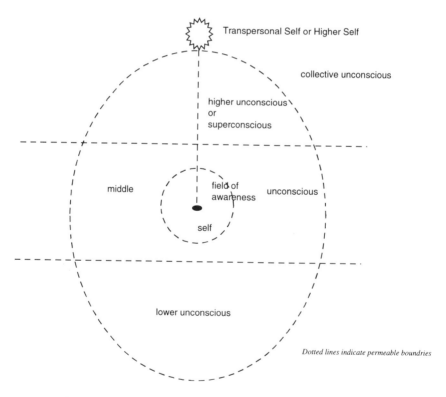

FIGURE 42.1.

This is the center of pure awareness and will, and serves as the integrating center of the personality. The "I" is permanent, unchanging, and self-accepting of faults and limitations. The "I" is self-conscious; it can observe itself. The Higher Self is also a center of consciousness and will; it is the center around which spiritual/transpersonal integration takes place. The area within the oval egg is the personal unconscious and relates specifically to the individual's life experience and inner qualities. Outside of the oval egg is the collective unconscious referring to Jung's term for the psychic environment beyond the individual.

The personal unconscious is divided into three levels: lower, middle, and superconscious. The lower unconscious is what Freud called the unconscious; it holds repressed desires and traumatic experiences, basic drives, and basic psychological activities which direct body functions. The middle unconscious is one's normal waking state of consciousness and can be remembered and experienced at any time by choice. The superconscious is the source of the higher human functions and activities: the drive for purpose and meaning in life, authentic values, superior intuitions, and altruism.

The Star Diagram

A second way to view the personality is to see it as a set of psychological functions. The functions include: sensation, emotion/feeling, impulse/desire, imagination, thought, intuition, will, and the central point (the "I" or personal self). "Through the Will, the "I" acts on the other psychological functions, regulating and directing them" (Assagioli, 1974, pp. 12-13). The Star Diagram, shown in Figure 42.2, displays these dimensions of psychological function as Assagioli depicted them.

The Will

The Will is a third way to view the personality. The Will is the function closest to the self; the energy employed by the self to regulate and direct all the other functions. To train the Will, an individual must first recognize that a Will exists; then that he or she has a Will; and lastly, that he or she is a Will. When Assagioli spoke of Will, he was not referring to "will-power." Will power is something wanted by one of our parts, which is usually in opposition to one or more of our other parts. Assagioli was speaking of being born as a Will, part of the self. When we clarify our intentions and align

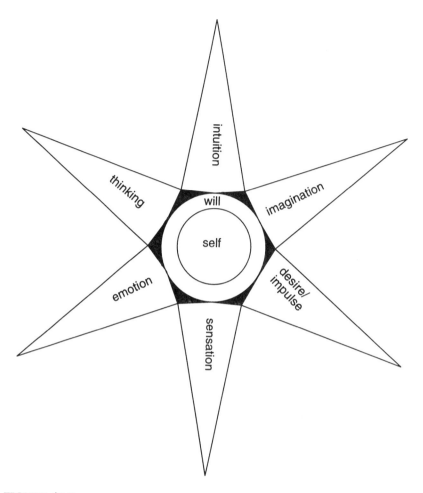

FIGURE 42.2.

them with the strength, skill and goodness of our Will, we can reach our goals and purpose.

I once had a client who had every reason to not come into therapy: financial reasons because she earned very little and although she had insurance, it only paid a small amount; a family system that was unsupportive of her making literally any changes in her life; a terror of talking with people she did not know; a traumatic childhood and adulthood that might have left most individuals stuck and unable to recognize a need for change, let alone seek out help to change. For the first year we worked together, each session was spent sitting in silence much of the hour. I experienced a terrified child sitting across from me. As we sat, she clearly had the intent to talk with me and wanted help in making some changes in her life. Most of the time she sat with her head down and, at first infrequently, later more frequently, looking up at me visibly trembling and attempting to speak. Sometimes her mouth would move without any sound. This was the major obstacle she had to overcome before we could continue our work.

I intended to remain fully present to her until she connected her intention to talk with her Will. Very slowly she began to check out the safety of talking with me. I also worked out a payment plan with her in order to remove one of her obstacles to therapy. No matter how painful and difficult it is to change, with help from an intentional and willful guide, a traveler can gather: intention, connection with the qualities of her Will, and courage from her Higher Self energies. Over a lengthy period, this young woman demonstrated courage, determination, patience, and discipline and although change was slow for her, some of the changes she wanted to make in her life happened. As a guide, I had to utilize the qualities of my Will in order to remain consistently present and to remain connected with my purpose in sitting across from this traveler.

The Will has three levels: personal, transpersonal, and universal and six stages: purpose, deliberation, decision, affirmation, planning, and implementation.

The Will, when in action, includes a wide range of qualities: (1) Energy-dynamic power-intensity; (2) mastery-control and discipline; (3) concentration, one-pointed-attention-focus; (4) determination-decisiveness-resoluteness-promptness; (5) persistence-endurance-patience; (6) initiative-courage-daring; and (7) organization-integration-synthesis (Assagioli, 1974).

The Will also has three major aspects of strength, skill, and goodness. The qualities of a strong will are courage, determination, and decisiveness. The qualities of a skillful will are discipline, organization, and mastery. And the qualities of a good will are patience, faithfulness, and right action. It is important to bring balance between the aspects of the Will and to integrate those aspects. When there is a major imbalance, the result is destructiveness in the world, such as ethnic cleansing and man's inhumanity against humankind and the planet.

Subpersonalities

Subpersonalities are psychological satellites, coexisting as a multitude of lives within our personality. Each subpersonality has a style and motivation of its own (Ferrucci, 1982, p. 47). Subpersonalities are learned responses to legitimate needs: survival needs, needs for love and acceptance, needs for self-actualization and transcendence. A subpersonality is a distorted expression of a valuable quality and a valid need (Brown, 1981, p. 32). The sources from which subpersonalities develop include: roles, internal conflicts, fantasy images, the personal unconscious, the cultural unconscious, and the collective unconscious (Rowan, pp. 22–23).

Subpersonality Work

I have learned to value psychosynthesis doing my own subpersonality work and doing subpersonality work with my clients. What I have noticed most is that although we each have numerous parts that make up who we are, there are two primary groups of subpersonalities (introjected critics and inner children) which, if not integrated, create most of our inner stressors. Life brings to us many external stressors; and, it seems that as soon as one is removed, there is always one or more to replace it. Therefore, our work on stress needs to attend to our inner stressors, which are caused by the battles that go on inside our heart and mind. These occur between the child subpersonalities (our inner children) and the critical subpersonalities (our introjected critics that often resemble one or more of our parents or other adults in authority, who were critical of us when we were young). I believe that, if we resolve these "battles" by integrating these parts and bringing balance between these parts, that we have done a major healing of self during our lifetime.

The phases of subpersonality work were delineated by Vargue in the early 1970s. They include: recognition of the subpersonality by both the guide and the traveler; acceptance of the subpersonality by the self of the traveler; coordination of the subpersonality's needs and wants, positive attributes, and irrational attitudes; and integration of the subpersonality's positive attributes into all aspects of life: intrapersonal, interpersonal, life work and purpose, and spiritual. The final phase of synthesis is a continually evolving work. This phase is commensurate with Maslow's "self-actualization," described within his hierarchy of needs model (Maslow, 1970). Each phase of subpersonality work must be grounded before moving on to the next one. Grounding means putting into practice, in concrete terms of daily life, the insights that have been acquired in each phase of subpersonality work. This fosters the client's potential for significant behavioral and attitudinal change as an outcome of insight and self-awareness.

In subpersonality work, it is important that the traveler be aware that the purpose is not to get rid of any part of him or herself; but, rather, to integrate that part of the personality into the whole being; this results in the individual knowing more clearly who he/she is; the result of subpersonality work is to better know the "self." It is important also, that the client understand that there are no "good" or "bad" subpersonalities and that no matter how negative they may appear initially, all subpersonalities have positive and important attributes. The goal is to transform the negative aspects in order to identify and use the positive attributes. In order to transform the negative aspects, the individual must update the subpersonality's information bank, determine the needs and wants of the subpersonality, discover ways to meet those needs and wants, and heal the subpersonality's past traumas.

I remember working with a therapist who was attending a series I was presenting on psychosynthesis. We had just covered subpersonalities and he volunteered to be a traveler while I guided him using some of the principles of subpersonality work. I asked him what he wanted to work on in order to be clear of his intent and purpose. He said that, although he had worked in therapy on the subject of feeling insecure, this problem continued. To deepen his intent, I asked him what benefit would come from this work. He was able to determine benefit and we continued the process. I asked if he were willing to do some imagery work around this issue. The purpose of using the word "willing" in this question was to engage his Will. If this is accomplished, the traveler becomes more committed to the process. After establishing if he was a visual or mental imager (establishing the type of imager is of importance because that assists the guide to choose the correct words to use during the imagery experience), I guided him into a state of relaxation and connection with his quiet space within. From that place within, I asked him to allow an image to form which would represent that part of himself that felt insecure. His image revealed a small little boy around five years old. I asked him to fully describe this little boy in as much detail as possible. Asking him to do this assists the traveler to more fully connect with the image and gives the guide clarity. At this point, there is recognition of the subpersonality by both the guide and the traveler.

I then asked him to check out if the little boy in the image knew who he was. Often, I have found, our inner children (particularly the younger ones) do not realize that they have grown up to be who we are. It is important for the inner child to have his information bank updated in this regard. Incidently, it is important to update the child's information bank in many areas as the subpersonality work continues. I then asked him to check out his feeling toward his little boy and the little boy's feelings toward him. This is the stage of acceptance of the subpersonality by the self of the traveler. If acceptance is not occurring, then the guide has to work with the subpersonality or subpersonalities that are hampering this process. Those are usually critical subpersonalities getting in the way. The next step was to work toward coordination, and because this was a demonstration, I only made several interventions. Through a series of interactions, using imagery and gestalt work, between the traveler and his little boy, the traveler was able to: ascertain some information regarding the source of the little boy's insecurities; ascertain some of the little boy's wants and needs regarding his feelings; and begin the process of healing himself and the inner child. To ground this experience, I asked the traveler if he was willing to make an intentional statement in order to get to know his inner child more. He committed to making contact with his little boy daily for the next month, through the creative use of his imagination.

Body, Feelings, Thinking Mind

A fifth way of viewing the personality is to consider it as a three-part structure of body, feelings, and thinking mind, with an integrating center, the self. Splits in our society are found primarily between mind and body and mind and feelings. Most individuals identify with one of the personality aspects more than the other two. Working with the personality from this perspective requires recognition that what affects one part of the structure has an impact on the others.

As an example of this, consider the traveler who presents highly identified with his or her feelings but is unable to think of options to current problems or would like to be more intellectually stimulated but is fearful of failing. This person needs guidance in disidentifying from feelings and becoming more identified with thoughts and the thinking process. The process of disidentification begins with an awareness of the identification. So, a traveler may be asked by the guide to allow an image to form which would depict the feeling. The image/feeling can be explored in the same way one might work with a subpersonality. When travelers disidentify from a feeling state, there is a realization that they are not their feelings and that they can think, make decisions, and be successfully intellectual. This disidentification with feelings and identification with mind requires many grounding experiences over time. An example of grounding might be to ask the traveler to become an observer of his or her feelings regarding different situations. At the time of each situation, the traveler is asked to disidentify from the feelings by becoming an Observer (disidentification occurs when in the Observer). The traveler, at this time, can choose to observe his or her thoughts about the situation and becomes conscious of both thoughts and feelings. Conversely, when a traveler presents totally disidentified from feelings and highly identified with mind, guiding assists the traveler to disidentify from mind and identify with feelings and their expression. What we are looking for is a balance between feeling mind and thinking mind. This same process is true when working with a mind/body split.

Other Major Principles of Psychosynthesis

There are several other concepts used in psychosynthesis that it would be helpful to understand because they are the foundation upon which psychosynthesis practice occurs in each therapeutic encounter. They include presence, intention, purpose, identification and disidentification, intuition, and grounding. I will describe each, briefly.

Presence.   For the clinician, presence is the inclusion of the whole person of the guide including body, mind, feelings, imagination and intuition. Presence includes concentration so that there is full attending to the process of the traveler, guide, and the therapeutic encounter. It includes the guide's willingness to let go of the outcome of the session, nonattachment, and the conscious choice by the guide of his/her perceptions, models, and beliefs related to the guide's ability to be with another's reality. Thus presence includes wisdom and intuition, the guide's inner knowing. It means the guide is willing to open to his or her highest qualities and highest good. Finally, presence requires trust, empathy, acceptance, honesty, intention, and practice (Brown, 1983, p. 49).

Intention.   Intention usually refers to what a person means or plans to get or do. In his book, *Love and Will,* May stated: "Intentionality is the structure which gives meaning to experience. It is our imaginative participation . . . to form, to mold, to change ourselves, and the day in relation to each other" (May, 1969, p. 80). In psychosynthesis, intention is the Will in action; intention is a willingness to work toward a goal or purpose. Intention must be evoked and strengthened during a therapeutic encounter. This allows for the possibility of the traveler's "self" to connect with purpose and choice.

Purpose. Purpose is greater than goal. A goal has an outcome whereas purpose has a direction. Purpose is as vital to a session as it is to life; it provides meaning and direction, a context within which to make choices and experience oneself (Brown, 1983, p. 71). Ferrucci states that purpose is present within us. At each stage of our life, there are subordinate purposes. This is a process of unfoldment which is marked by joy (Ferrucci, 1982). Qualities of purpose, Assagioli pointed out, include presence, connectedness, broad vision, understanding, experience of uniqueness and wholeness, unaltered sense of inner knowing, dedication, serenity, and ability to be practical as well as spiritual. Assagioli viewed purpose as the beginning and essential stage of the act of Will.

Identification/Disidentification. The concepts of identification and disidentification are primary to psychosynthesis. The processes of disidentification from subpersonalities and identification with the self and the Higher Self are central to psychosynthesis and subpersonality work. When one is identified with a part, one believes that he/she is that part because that part is acting out its thoughts, feelings, and behaviors so convincingly that the other parts are hidden. Thus, when one disidentifies from a part, he/she can reconnect with centeredness and can identify with self: who "I" am. The "self" has the freedom of choice to be who we are, know what we want, and know where we are going. The process of disidentification and self-identification is developmental and occurs throughout the therapy, regardless of what techniques are being used (Whitmore, 1991, p. 93).

Intuition. Intuition is defined as the immediate perception or understanding of truths, facts, or events, without reasoning. As Ferrucci states, the importance of this deeper kind of understanding is almost universally neglected (Ferrucci, 1982). In psychosynthesis, the nurturing and further development of the awakening of intuition is considered necessary and useful for the traveler and the guide. Ferrucci states that intuition can be fully assimilated when it is also coordinated at the mental level; thus, providing for correct interpretation, connection with everyday reality, and clarity in communication of the knowledge gained from the intuition. Intuitions have a synthetic character because they have a spontaneous ramification in several dimensions of one's life. A single intuition may often throw light on previously unrelated issues, showing the existence of the same pattern in all of them (p. 224). Intuition, therefore, provides for a wholeness of knowing not only who we are, but how to heal ourselves.

Grounding. Grounding is defined as "to fix firmly; establish." For the clinician, grounding reflects "the need for significant behavioral and attitudinal change as an outcome of increased self-awareness" (Weiser & Yeomans, 1984). Psychosynthesis views change as active rather than reactive. Therefore, at the end of psychosynthesis sessions, homework is suggested that aims at grounding the therapeutic insights.

Psychosynthesis Tools

When the guide is clear on purpose and intent and remains present to the traveler's process and when the traveler is clear on purpose and intent and remains present to his/her inner and outer process, remarkable growth and healing occurs. This worldview accommodates incorporation, by the guide and the traveler, of the rich array of tools available to assist a person in this journey. These tools are drawn from depth psychology and psychoanalysis, gestalt methods, Jungian methods of dream work and free association; mental imagery methods, spontaneous movement and drawing; psychodrama; body work; and meditative and inner dialogue techniques. In addition, flexibility, silence, focusing on an issue, affirmations, journal keeping and homework are also utilized.

Psychosynthesis Applications to Nursing

Psychosynthesis processes and ideas have been applied to psychotherapy, counseling, medicine, education, religion, and management. Its application to therapy and counseling has been in individual and group work with varied presenting issues: existential and spiritual issues, anxiety and depression, childhood abuse, relationship issues, stress-related issues and illness, to name a few. In medicine, there has been an increasing number of physicians who have brought a spiritual and holistic dimension into their practice. Clergy have been trained in the principles and methods of psychosynthesis and many psychosynthesis trained teachers have incorporated their training into working with primary school children. In the field of management, psychosynthesis has contributed to enhancing organizational and staff development, creative problem solving, and conflict resolution. This is the list one usually finds cited.

I would like to see nursing added to this list since there are many links between nursing and psychosynthesis. Newman, an acknowledged nursing theorist of our time, states that health is the expansion of consciousness.

"The meaning of life and health . . . will be found in the evolving process of expanding consciousness" (Newman, 1986, pp. 2–3). "Within the new paradigm, pattern recognition is the essence of practice. Pattern recognition is the heart of human interaction. It is basic to responding to the individuality of another person and therefore basic to the health professional's effective use of self in therapeutic interaction. What we sense in terms of pattern is a function of our own level of awareness, sensitivity to self, and point of view" (Newman, 1986, p. 18).

Psychosynthesis offers a conceptual framework and a set of clinical skills that enables the nurse to recognize client patterns and assist the client in conscious repatterning. Assagioli's image of subpersonalities is, in fact, a constellation of interrelated energy patterns. The knowledge and use of psychosynthesis helps the nurse guide to help his or her client recognize conditioned patterns, disidentify from those patterns, and integrate those patterns into a more whole self.

In 1980, the American Nurses' Association published: "Nursing: A Social Policy Statement." In that statement, the nursing definition was "intended to maintain the historical orientation of the Nightingale and Henderson definitions, as well as reflecting the influence of nursing theory that is a part of nursing's evolution: *Nursing is the diagnosis and treatment of human responses to actual or potential health problems.*" Examples given of these human responses include . . . "pain and discomfort; emotional problems; deficiencies in decision-making and the ability to make personal choices" (American Nurses Association, 1980). In 1995, a revised document, "Nursing's Social Policy Statement" was published which references the 1980 document reiterating this definition focused on diagnosis and treatment.

Psychosynthesis offers a variety of ways to determine a nursing diagnosis. The nurse psychosynthesist can assist the client in exploring the presenting issue: how it is now manifesting in the client's life; the client's perception of how it is affecting relationships; and the sensations, emotions, attitudes and belief systems which contribute to the presenting issue. Treatment, from a psychosynthesis perspective, would mean guiding the client, based on a hypothesis from the above exploration, toward options, choices, self-awareness, and integration. "Nursing diagnosis is the title given to the stage of identifying the problem" (Roy, 1975, p. 91).

Psychosynthesis practice exemplifies holistic nursing practice and the characteristics of a nurse healer as described by Barbara Dossey (1995). The nurse psychosynthesist is aware that self-healing is a continual process, has familiarity with the terrain of self-development, recognizes his or her weaknesses and strengths, is open to self-discovery, continues to develop clarity about life's purpose, is aware of present and future steps in personal growth, models self-work, is aware of the importance of presence, respects and loves clients, is willing to offer methods for working on life issues, guides the client in discovering creative options, presumes that the client knows the best life choices, actively listens, helps client to empower self, shares insights without imposing values and beliefs, accepts what clients say without judgment, and perceives time spent with clients as service and sharing of self. (Dossey et al., 1995, pp. 63–64)

For the psychiatric/mental health clinical specialist, psychosynthesis training can provide an opportunity for self growth and healing. In addition, as Linda Tuyn pointed out: ". . . many of the psychological theories and frameworks commonly used in psychiatric nursing practice offer little or no recognition of the spiritual dimension of human experience, and virtually no guidance on how to incorporate this dimension in treatment strategies. Psychoanalytic, behavioral, and interpersonal frameworks, while offering many valuable pieces to the puzzle of understanding human beings, fall short of adequately addressing spiritual needs of clients" (p. 260). One of the attributes of psychosynthesis is that the therapist/guide *does not* have to throw out previous knowledge or methods; but, can simply incorporate these into the perspective of a holistic model.

For the nurse educator, psychosynthesis training can provide an opportunity to employ different teaching/learning methods as well as discover more effective methods of relating to students and other teachers. In regard to the use of psychosynthesis in education, Assagioli stated, "It is axiomatic that the prevention of any disorder is better than the cure . . . What, we wonder, are the implications of such a statement? Examine the kind of education in the Western World from a viewpoint of: First producing a human being who functions harmoniously, radiantly and productively in relation to his [sic] own capacity. And second, establishing the conditions in which such an ideal could be realized" (Whitmore, 1986, p. 22). Would it not be professionally sound to provide our nursing students with a learning environment that not only provides a strong scientific nursing curriculum, but also those learning experiences which enhance the students' growth and development as harmonious, radiant, and productive "professional nurse" human beings? One might say at this point: What an idealist! After 33 years as a professional nurse, a part of me is still idealistic. But, a part of me is also a realist. And my experience teaches me that if each of us does our own inner work, we can help our students be open to explore their own process and become healthier professionals and individuals on this planet.

And, for nursing managers, psychosynthesis can provide conflict resolution skills, new ways of dealing with communication problems, creative problem solving, staff growth and development skills to address transition issues occurring as a result of healthcare reform, and the managerial modeling of self-growth and development. Kritek (1994) describes "constructive ways of being at an uneven table": find and inhabit the deepest and surest human space that your capabilities permit; be a truth teller, honor your integrity, even at great cost; find a place for compassion at the table; draw a line in the sand without cruelty; expand and explicate the context; innovate; know what you do and do not know; stay in the dialogue; and know when and how to leave the table. (pp. 187–316) Although these ways of being are difficult to achieve in our culture, they would be easier to attain by individuals who were familiar with Assagioli's philosophy about healing and human potential, meaning and purpose, and viewing the human being as both a unique individual and universal entity that is interconnected with others and the environment.

For all professional nurses, psychosynthesis offers the opportunity for change, growth, the healing of personal and professional issues, and empowerment.

SUMMARY

Persons interested in holistic healthcare and healing practices would greatly benefit from the use of psychosynthesis in clinical practice. Nurses will find this approach to working with a human being highly congruent with nursing both as a science and an art. Its flexibility, adaptability, and humanism make it a useful and valuable approach to nursing.

REFERENCES

American Nurses Association (1980). *Nursing: A social policy statement*. Kansas City, MO: Author.
American Nurses Association (1995). *Nursing's social policy statement*. Kansas City, MO: Author.
Assagioli, R. (1976). *Psychosynthesis*. New York: Penguin.
Assagioli, R. (1974, 1992). *The act of will*. New York: Penguin.

Assagioli, R. (1991). *Transpersonal development.* Great Britain: The Aquarian Press.

Brown, M. Y. (1981). Discovering the self. *Psychosynthesis Digest, 1*(1), 20–38.

Brown, M. Y. (1983). *The unfolding self.* Los Angeles, CA: Psychosynthesis Press.

Brown, M. Y. (1993). *Growing whole: Self-realization on an endangered planet.* New York: Harper-Collins.

Dossey, B., Keegan, L., Guzzetta, C. E., & Kolkmeier, L. G. (1995). *Holistic nursing,* 2nd ed., Gaithersburg, MD: Aspex Publishers.

Ferrucci, P. (1982). *What we may be.* Los Angeles, CA: J.P. Tarcher.

Ferrucci, P. (1990). *Inevitable grace.* Los Angeles, CA: J.P. Tarcher.

Henderson, V. (1958). *International council of nurses.* Paper presented

Kritek, P. B. (1994). *Negotiating at an uneven table.* San Francisco, CA: Jossey-Bass.

Macmillan's Magazine (1867, April). *Letter to the editor.*

Maslow, A. H. (1970). *Motivation and personality.* New York: Harper & Row.

May, R. (1969). *Love and will.* New York: Norton.

Newman, M. A. (1986). *Health as expanding consciousness.* St. Louis, C.V. Mosby.

Rainwater, J. (1979). *You're in charge.* Culver City, CA: Peace Press, Inc.

Remen, N. (1980). *The human patient.* Garden City, NY: Anchor Press/Doubleday.

Rowan, J. (1990). *Subpersonalities.* London/New York: Routledge.

Roy, C. (1975). A diagnostic classification system for nursing. *Nursing Outlook, (Feb),* 23:91.

Schlotfeldt, R. M. (1972). This, I believe . . . . nursing is health care. *Nursing Outlook, 20*(4), 245–246.

Stauffer, E. (1987). *Unconditional love and forgiveness.* Burbank, CA: Triangle Publishers.

Tuyn, L. K. (1988). Psychosynthesis: Evolutionary framework for psychosynthesis. *Archives of Psychiatric Nursing, 11*(3), 260–266.

Weiser, J., & Yeomans, T. (1984). *Psychosynthesis in the helping professions: Now and in the future.* Canada: The Department of Applied Psychology/The Ontario Institute for the Studies in Education.

Weiser, J., & Yeomans, T. (1985). *Readings in psychosynthesis: Theory, process and practice.* Canada: The Department of Applied Psychology/The Ontario Institute for the Studies in Education.

Whitmore, D. (1986). *Psychosynthesis in education.* Rochester, VT: Destiny Books.

Whitmore, D. (1991). *Psychosynthesis counseling in action.* London: Sage.

PART SIX

HEALING AS A FOCUS OF NURSING SCHOLARSHIP

PHYLLIS BECK KRITEK, RN, PHD, FAAN

The final part of this book points to the future, the implicit outcomes of an effort to reflect on healing processes in nursing. It is in the act of reflecting that we set our course of scholarship, learn to take note of the salient features and challenges of the land our path leads us through. Too often we nurses, given to imitating when we might better trust our own instincts and create, have designed paths of scholarship characterized more by what others thought we might best study, or worse still, thought we must study if we wanted to earn credibility in the academic community. We have not cut our own path, but followed paths prescribed by others. The antidote to this tendency is reflection. As we reflect, we discover avenues of discovery that make sense to us, that capture our imagination and our attention, that compel us forward toward goals worthy of the profound nature of nursing. In this closing section of the book, we provide some examples of the kind of scholarship that emerges when we apply our reflections on the nature of healing to the scholarly activities we elect to engage in. We find new vistas in the process.

The first of these contributions, by Rita Cascio, highlights the opportunities community health nurses have to promote wholeness, and therefore healing, in the communities they serve. Rita notes that community health nurses have a unique set of competencies that make them a central resource in a community's effort to heal, to find health. She focuses specifically on assessment and planning founded on principles of mutuality, cohesion, and holism. She describes a specific model and process used to implement a community-based assessment and planning process focused on women's health within a specified community.

Rita describes in detail the assessment process itself, initiated with the creation of a community advisory board. She posits that the community health nurse serves not as an impartial or detached observer, but as an engaged participant if indeed healing of communities is sought. She details the assessment and statistical outcomes, the subsequent planning, and the implementation of a health promotion program for women. She concludes with the observation that such a process can empower communities toward "the ultimate goal of healing."

Doris Rosenow, in the next chapter, demonstrates the potential of theory development that emerges in the analysis of healing as a central construct in nursing. Her interest is in the process of self-reintegration as a dimension of the process of healing from an illness. She sees this as bringing together parts of a whole, bringing about a balance from a prior state of illness or disturbance. Her theory emerges from the philosophical foundations provided by Marcel, Erikson, and Erickson and includes constructs of adjustment, self-responsibility, returning to a normal life, affirmation of attitudes, and obtaining a high quality of life/well-being. The core of her theory concerns resources available to the individual to assist in the healing process.

Having crafted a careful description of her theory, Doris then sets out to apply this theory to nursing practice using a case study, demonstrating the utility of the theory in assisting the nurse in understanding and deciding appropriate goals, grounded in coherent principles and aimed toward specific outcomes. This theory development exemplar demonstrates the type of useful middle-range theories that can reasonably be expected to emerge in the careful and reflective study of healing processes in nursing.

In the next chapter, Karen Brykczynski and Phylicia Lewis focus on the research process, providing another useful exemplar. They were interested in studying the role of nurse practitioners using Benner's descriptions of practical knowledge and clinical competencies as a basis of understanding. The data-rich examples provided by Karen and Phylicia, which they generated through interpretive phenomenological research, help reveal the healing activities of these nurses, and help us better begin to understand the nature of such activities.

Karen and Phylicia posit that research such as theirs is valuable in bringing "to open discourse" aspects of nursing care such as healing practices that have been largely covered over and not acknowledged explicitly. At a time when the simple removal of nursing care has become acceptable, this observation has particular relevance. Their report also provides a useful model for identifying other healing practices in nursing, and explaining their role in the healing processes of patients.

Donna Morris provides a thoughtful analysis of healing from yet another perspective: she grapples with the question of healing processes when the patient is a community. Assuming the questioning posture of the scholar, she examines the assumptions of traditional approaches to community health planning, programming, and research, and offers a constructive appraisal of the limits of these approaches. She demonstrates how an honest exploration of the concept of healing leads inevitably to new approaches, where the traditional "control" agenda of the external healthcare provider is supplanted by a model of community control.

Having analyzed the limits of the traditional model, she then describes a "new" model where the community determines who, when, and how healthcare professionals provide service in their community. Donna's description of LaFrontera, a community committed to controlling its own fate, is a powerful example of the healing impulse from within a community. She identifies the many adjustments that healthcare providers will need to make if they intend to facilitate healing in communities of this nature.

Bobbie Lee summarizes several years of research in the epidemiology of violence and violent injury, and provides a model of healing that demonstrates the array of issues and problems that emerge when this topic is explored from a healing perspective. She focuses specifically on victims of violence, and identifies the complexities of violence research. Her data summary provides a sobering glimpse into a major national problem, one with powerful implications for nurses and nursing. The role of the nurse who wishes to facilitate healing in victims of violence is amplified in the process, since the complexity of the data undergirding the role is revealed.

Her analysis of this complexity concludes with recommendations for nursing research, political action, research support, and attitude awareness. She notes the congruence between nursing's commitments to healing practices and its commitments to addressing the problems of violence and victimization. She serves notice that to support healing processes without a systematic and responsible appraisal of factors that contribute to violence is to deal only with superficial factors and ignore causal phenomena. As such, she demonstrates the impact that understanding healing in all its complexity can have for the nurse scholar.

The final chapter in this final part of the book is aptly provided by the dean of the school, Mary Fenton. Mary tackles an issue that runs like an undercurrent throughout this book, the existence of what she calls "underground nursing." This underground nursing occurs, she posits, as a "behind-the-scenes process," one that is healing at the physiological, psychological, social, spiritual, and cultural levels. It includes the use of listening, presencing, comforting, and touching skills. She notes that nurses often serve as patient advocates attempting to force the healthcare system and other agencies to respond. The focus of this work is one of "guiding and assisting the person, the family and friends to cope, adapt, accept, and come to terms with the illness, problems and prognosis." Often nurses use alternative therapies in these efforts. In most cases no one but the nurses and the patients know about these activities and efforts.

Mary goes on to ask the obvious question of why these are secretive activities and provides the perhaps equally obvious answer that nurses fear reprisal or suppression. As a result the practices most essential to the promotion of healing are not named, described, studied, documented, acknowledged, or owned. Yet it is clear that healing practices may be the highest possible level of nursing practice. She concludes: it is time for this "underground nursing" practice to become the "standard of professional nursing care and part of the mainstream of healthcare." She aptly summarizes the rationale for all the many choices that have led to the publication of this book.

CHAPTER 43

Opportunities to Promote Healing: Community-Based Assessment and Planning

RITA S. CASCIO, RN, PHD

The potential for healing a community can be found in the high-level, aggregate, and community-focused activities conducted by community health nurses. Healing is promoted and achieved within the community when professional community health nurses facilitate wholeness within their chosen communities. The important underpinnings of the healing process must include communication and substantive interaction with the community. Mutuality of intention between the community health nurse and her chosen community is central to the goal of healing in a community.

Community health nurses bring a unique and specialized repertoire of skills that have the potential to promote healing within their communities. They are armed with the expertise to facilitate and assist the process of healing through the activities of community-based assessment and planning.

The following description of community-based assessment and planning interventions in Southeast Texas highlights the translation of the concepts of mutuality, cohesion, and holism within the community with the ultimate goal of promoting healing.

The Women's Health Issues Project (WHIP) was funded by the Health Education Training Alliance of Texas (HETCAT). HETCAT is a consortium of Texas educational institutions and state agencies formed to improve the access to healthcare by residents of Texas counties within a 300-mile range of the border between Texas and Mexico. There are three HETCAT regional offices which promote and coordinate the development of community-oriented projects (Figure 43.1). One, the East Texas Area Health Education Center (ETAHEC) was developed to improve the supply, distribution, quality, utilization, and efficiency of health professionals in East

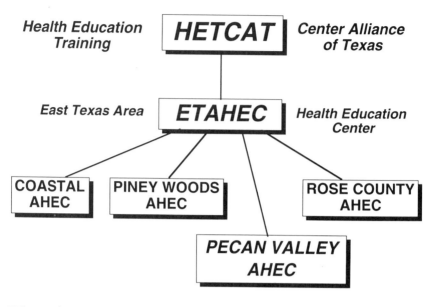

FIGURE 43.1.

Texas. In addition, ETAHEC addresses the informational needs of practicing health professionals in designated regions. The ETAHEC is divided into four regions: the Coastal AHEC, the Piney Woods AHEC, the Rose County AHEC, and the Pecan Valley AHEC. Each AHEC is the catalyst for developing partnerships between communities and educational institutions which offer health science/allied health programs. In conjunction with ETAHEC, this study focused on the assessment of and planning for community healthcare needs. Specifically, assessment was centered on the expressed healthcare needs and concerns of women aged 35 to 65 who reside in the Pecan Valley AHEC region. Through community assessment, the women of the region expressed their perceived needs and concerns. Healthcare needs and concerns were truly community-determined.

As women move from childbearing years to mid-age, they may participate less often in screening for reproductive cancers, sexually transmitted diseases (STDs), and HIV infection (Horton, 1992). Delayed identification and treatment of reproductive cancers and STDs, and exposure to HIV infection in females results in a tremendous cost to individual women, their communities, and to society as a whole. Furthermore, women may be less likely to engage in health-promoting and disease-preventing activities. Mutuality of concern regarding these specific areas of women's health was shared by our team at the University of Texas Medical Branch, the Director of the Area Health Education Center, the Regional Health Department Director and staff, as well as consumer-community representatives residing within the region.

The purpose of this research project was threefold: (1) to develop a local community advisory board; (2) to conduct a needs assessment relevant to reproductive cancers, STD/HIV infection, and health-promoting behaviors among women 35 to 65 years of age; and (3) to compile a resource roster of available health services for women in the target area.

As a logical first step to assure community acceptance and collaboration as well as community ownership, a Community Advisory Board (CAB) was established. The support and assistance of the medical director of the Regional Health Department were crucial to the successful interaction within the community, the target population, and the establishment of a Community Advisory Board. With her help and the assistance of her staff associates, key community representatives were identified. These included providers, traditional and nontraditional community leaders, as well as women consumers of healthcare services. Initial contact by the Project Team through independent visits with community representatives allowed further identification of other key individuals and interested consumers. A significant amount of time was spent cultivating interest in, support of, and formation of a Community Advisory Board. As potential members were visited, their support of the project and their participation on the Board was solicited. A CAB meeting was subsequently held. The meeting served several purposes:

1. To allow the exchange of ideas and concerns;
2. To inform the CAB membership of the project's overall purpose;
3. To reflect and incorporate ideas and concerns and integrate them into the goals of the project;
4. To solidify support for the project;
5. To create community involvement, enthusiasm, and ownership of the project; and,
6. To build the concept of the CAB as the infrastructure for future health planning and provision of healthcare resources for women in the region.

In addition, the CAB members provided vital background and historical information benefiting the process and outcome of the project. The community health nurse, as researcher and member of her community, cannot function as a detached observer, measurer, and estimator of the reality of women "out there" in the community. It is only through personal contact, skilled communication, and mutuality of concern and intent shared among the members of the CAB, the women of the community, and consumers and providers of healthcare that progress toward wholeness and, therefore, healing can occur.

HEALTH NEEDS ASSESSMENT

The next step in the project was to gather information relative to the perceived problems. Of prime interest was determining what the target population of women identified as health needs and concerns.

Instrument

A personal interview format was adapted from a previous project (Morris et al., 1990) and was validated by a panel of experts. The format was substantively expanded to include sections on HIV infection, self-care, and health promotion. The final format, *The Household Interview,* contained approximately 75 questions divided into five main sections: (1) demographic data, (2) breast cancer data, (3) cervical cancer data, (4) STD/HIV infection data, and (5) self-care/health protection/health promotion data (Cascio, Landis, & Morris, 1992). *The Household Interview* was translated into Spanish and was piloted by the interviewers during the scheduled Interviewer Training Session in order to assess the translation.

Data Collection and Methodology

Procedures for our target population began with a sampling plan. Household addresses for the county were obtained from the 911 listing provided by the county EMS and city addresses were obtained from the City Planning Commission. In consultation with a statistician in the Department of Psychiatry at the University of Texas Medical Branch, a systematic probability sampling with a cluster of five was developed for selecting a sample from the population of interest. For sampling purposes, the county and the city were treated as separate populations to ensure proportionate representation. The sample size for city and county women aged 35 to 65 was calculated based on the proportionate population and total number of households in the city and county. Next, cluster sampling was employed to facilitate interview completion. Cluster sampling allowed interviewers to complete several interviews in one location, reducing travel time and expense.

The sampling goal for city household interviews was 148. A 1:5 ratio of completed interviews was anticipated. Therefore, a total of 740 addresses were randomly selected through nine computer repetitions. The sampling goal for county household interviews was 52. Similarly, a 1:5 ratio of interview completions was projected, and 260 addresses were randomly selected from nine computer repetitions. Repetitions for both the city and county were sent to the Project Director for assignment to the interviewers.

Five criteria were established for recruiting project interviewers. They would be: (1) female, preferably 35 years of age or older; (2) residents of the target community; (3) preferably bilingual; (4) have their own transportation; and (5) be available throughout the data collection period. Eight interviewers were recruited through newspaper advertisements and by word of mouth. Half of these women were bilingual. The on-site Project Director was responsible for coordinating all of the activities of the interviewers.

An *Interviewer's Manual* (Landis & Cascio, 1992) was compiled and distributed to each interviewer. Mandatory training sessions were conducted to prepare interviewers for collecting the data. The *Interviewer's Manual* was essential as a guide in the group sessions. Sessions covered the purpose of the project and rationale for data collection methodology, issues of confidentiality, interview techniques, recording of data, and problem solving in the field. The interviewer group also role-played situations that could be encountered during data collection.

Data collection occurred during the summer of 1992. Additionally, the on-site Project Director contacted approximately every tenth interviewee by telephone to verify the accuracy of the information.

Data Analysis and Findings

A total of 212 household interviews were completed. Data were analyzed using descriptive and chi-square statistics. Over half of the sample were married Anglo women with an average age of 48 years. Most (81%) had completed high school and 40.4 percent were employed full time outside of the home. Almost 30 percent have household incomes of less than $16,000. A total of 35 women refused to give financial information.

Five potential barriers to healthcare were examined. Half of the women (50.5%) had responsibility for their own children, their grandchildren, or another person's children. Furthermore, 4 percent had responsibility for elder care. Approximately 17 percent had no health insurance. Travel time to access healthcare is another known barrier. Approximately 80 percent of the sample traveled 20 minutes or less to obtain healthcare. Gynecological healthcare was obtained through private physicians in 74 percent of the sample. Time since the last general healthcare visit was examined. It was found that 30 percent had not visited their healthcare provider or clinic in the past year. Of these women, 44 percent had not made a visit in the past two years. For gynecological healthcare, 32 percent made no visits within the past year and almost half of these had not received gynecological care in more than two years.

Findings related to breast cancer revealed that 15 percent are at increased risk for breast cancer because of a positive family history of the disease. Knowledge of breast self-exam (BSE) was assessed: 7 percent did not know how to check their breasts and 2 percent did not know of the need for self-examination or did not believe that BSE was necessary. Although a high percentage of the sample is aware of the need for monthly BSE, less than half actually performed BSE monthly. Knowledge of and education about BSE came from a variety of sources but 65 percent reported that nurses and physicians were the main sources of their current knowledge of BSE. More than one out of every three women (36%) has never had a mammogram. Further, of the women who *have* had a mammogram, 17 percent had the last one more than two years ago.

A chi-square analysis was performed to determine if income was a significant factor in determining if the women had obtained a mammogram in the past 12 months ($x^2 = 3.321$, df = 1, p = .06 before Yates correction). Although there was no significance at the .05 level, this variable of income warrants consideration as a potential factor affecting breast cancer screening.

Findings related to cervical cancer revealed that 20 percent of the sample was at increased risk because of a positive family history of the disease. Although 97 percent reported having a Pap test at least once in the past, 35 percent have not had one in the past year.

Race and income were significant factors in determining if women had obtained a Pap test in the past year. Significantly fewer lower income women and women of color obtained Pap tests in comparison to their

Anglo counterparts. Various sources encouraged these women to obtain reproductive cancer screening. Physicians and nurses were predominating encouragers (32%) with 59 percent reporting that no one encouraged them to obtain a Pap smear.

Findings relative to STD/HIV in the sample revealed that 80 percent were sexually active within the past year. However, only 15 percent of these women used some method of protection against sexually transmitted diseases. Forty-two percent reported that they use no protective measures because they have only one sexual partner. Five percent of the sample had been treated for a sexually transmitted disease (STD). Most of the sample (98%) denied use of IV drugs.

In the sample, one out of every five women has undergone HIV antibody testing. This high proportion of testing was discussed with the Medical Director of the Public Health Department in the community, the Director of the Coastal AHEC, and a biostatistician in the Department of Infectious Disease, Texas State Health Department. It was thought that an element of uncertainty and fear due to lack of knowledge regarding modes of transmission of the virus may be causing these high rates. However, in light of the findings from the women of this community, testing may be prudent given that only 15 percent of those sexually active protect themselves from STDs. Interestingly, all HIV testers obtained testing outside the community.

Findings related to health protection/promotion activities demonstrated that 68 percent are trying to control their weight, 59 percent use stress reduction techniques, and 51 percent exercise less than three times per week. Seventeen percent of the women smoke, and 43 percent of these wish to stop. When asked about their learning needs, the women expressed a need for more information primarily about weight control, stress management, exercise, and assertiveness training.

USE OF THE PRECEDE-PROCEED MODEL

Usefulness of a needs assessment can be enhanced when it is part of a conceptual framework which gives structure and form to relationships among important data and concepts. The PRECEDE-PROCEED Model proposed by Green and Kreuter (1991) is an effective tool for developing and evaluating a variety of health promotion programs and was selected as the organizing framework for this community project. Health promotion programs seek to provide interventions that short-circuit illness or enhance quality of life. These interventions usually involve some change or the development of health-related behavior and living conditions conducive to improved quality of life.

The PRECEDE-PROCEED Model (Figure 43.2) consists of two sequential frameworks that work together to provide a tool for health promotion planning. First, the PRECEDE framework identifies the multiple factors that shape health status and allows the planner to generate a highly focused set of target factors for intervention. The PRECEDE framework forces attention on outcomes rather than inputs. Therefore, the planner is encouraged to ask "why" before asking "how." One begins by defining the desired outcome and then by deciding on what must "precede" this outcome. The factors important to an outcome must first be identified. Only then can a successful intervention be planned.

Next, the PROCEED framework seeks to implement and evaluate the intervention. Based on the PRECEDE framework diagnoses, an effective intervention may be enacted. Similarly, evaluation in the PROCEED

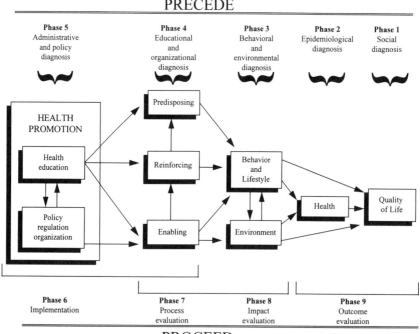

FIGURE 43.2.

framework is largely based on the information gathered in the PRECEDE framework.

In addition, the PRECEDE-PROCEED Model addresses comprehensive planning, a major need in health promotion and health education. The model is applicable in numerous situations. Specifically, it has been shown to be successful as a guide to the development of local health department programs (Green & Kreuter, 1991).

In order to demonstrate the utility of the model for the reader, selected findings from the assessment are placed within the PRECEDE-PROCEED framework. The following illustrates use of the model.

Phase I: Social Diagnosis

The following Quality of Life factor priorities were derived from *Healthy People 2000* (Public Health Service, 1991) and from concerns of local health officials in the target area:

1. Prevent, detect, control cancer.
2. Prevent, detect, control STD/HIV infection.
3. Increase health protecting/health-promoting behaviors.

Phase II: Epidemiological Diagnosis

The following health factors were derived from statistical reports and physiological risk factors identified in the sample population:

- *Breast cancer:* This type of cancer represents 28 percent of all female cancers and is the leading cause of cancer deaths among women. Risk factors for breast cancer include a positive family history and increasing age over 40 years. Mortality rate for breast cancer in our target area was high. Fourteen percent of the sample had a positive family history for breast cancer.
- *Cervical cancer:* There are interrelationships among cervical cancer, STDs, and HIV. STDs predispose women to cervical cancer and also increase the risk of HIV transmission. Likewise, HIV+ women have an increased prevalence and recurrence of cervical cancer. Risk factors for cervical cancer include a positive family history, a high fat diet (which predisposes to obesity), smoking, and STDs. Mortality from cervical cancer in our target area was not significantly high.

Twenty percent of the sample has a positive family history of cervical cancer.

- *STD/HIV:* Data on the incidence of these diseases are difficult to assess because of under reporting of STDs and confidentiality of HIV information. Nationally, about 14 percent of STDs occur among those 30 years and older. However, Texas ranks in the top five states in the number of reported AIDS cases. Risk factors for STD/HIV include multiple sex partners, unprotected sexual activity, IV drug use, and blood transfusion.
- *Health protecting/promoting behaviors:* These behaviors include those activities which decrease probability of illness by protecting the body against stressors or by early detection of disease and include BSE, mammography, PAP smears, and screening procedures. Health-promoting behaviors are continuing activities that are an integral part of one's lifestyle and include consistent use of condoms for protection against STD's/HIV, exercise, nutrition, and stress management.

Phase III: Behavioral and Environmental Diagnosis

In this phase, behavioral and environmental factors related to preventive actions, self-care, and utilization of healthcare services among the target population are identified and placed in the following subsections of Phase III. The following illustrates examples of the types of data that should be placed in each section.

Behavioral Factors

- *Breast cancer:* Percentages of the total sample of women who have never had a mammogram or do not practice BSE monthly, for example, would be indicated in this specific section.
- *Cervical cancer:* Similarly, the percentages of the total sample who have not had a PAP smear in the last year, for example, would be indicated here.
- *STD/HIV:* Reported here would be the percentage of the total sample who were sexually active, the percentage of those who utilized some form of protection against STD/HIV and those who do not, the ratio of HIV antibody testing in the sample population, the percentage of the sample reporting diagnosis of a STD, and receipt of blood transfusion, for example.

- *Health protecting/promoting behaviors:* Included in this section would be the percentages of the sample who are attempting to control their weight, use stress reduction techniques, are attempting to stop tobacco use, report exercise as a consistent healthy lifestyle choice, and indicate a need for further knowledge regarding selected health promotion topics.

Environmental Factors

- Education, employment, transportation, and family responsibilities are reported here. An example of this, again to illustrate from the community-based assessment findings, is the percentage of women with less than a high school education, who are unemployed or have incomes at or below poverty level.

Phase IV: Educational and Organizational Diagnosis

This phase includes factors that impact health status and health practices. Predisposing factors include knowledge, attitudes, and beliefs relevant to healthcare of women in the sample.

- *Breast cancer:* Beliefs regarding BSE, and knowledge about performance of BSE would be reported here from the findings, for example.
- *Cervical cancer:* Beliefs about the importance of PAP tests, percentage of the sample women who have a friend who has experienced cervical cancer, and their desire to obtain more knowledge about selected health promoting strategies related to the area of reproductive cancers would be indicated in this section.

Reinforcing factors include attitudes and behaviors of health professionals, spouses, and others that affect health behaviors of the sample population. One example from the findings is that nurse and physician support and encouragement is an important factor in the women's decision to obtain screening mammography.

Enabling factors include availability and accessibility of health resources, community assets, and health-related skills. Findings derived and analyzed as enabling factors would include the percentage of the sample that did not have health insurance, and received no general or gynecological healthcare in the past year. Required travel time to access care, presence of a smoking cessation clinic in the area, and the fact that

The following is an overview of interventions and strategies that we recommend to the CAB for their consideration. These as well as others suggested by board members can serve as components within the framework that provide direction for program planning and interventions.

Specific Interventions: Breast Cancer Screening, Diagnosis and Treatment in Women Aged 35–65.

1. Increase number of women receiving screening for breast cancer.
2. Increase and direct community and professional attention to the importance of healthy breast care behaviors in middle-aged and older women.
3. Provide health education specific to screening, diagnosis, and treatment of breast cancer.
4. Obtain additional information concerning barriers to mammography screening, clinical breast exam and breast self exam in this target group.
5. Initiate strategies which motivate breast care behaviors. An "Encouragement Campaign," for example, undertaken by health professionals and key community members in conjunction with healthcare agencies can serve to increase the number of women screened by mammography.
6. Develop plans for interagency collaborations among the Health Department, M.D. Anderson Cancer Center and UTMB Clinics.
7. Develop collaborative agreements between the Community College's Division of Nursing and the Health Department to promote and conduct a "Women's Health Fair."
8. Increase the number of professional and staff resources in the State/County Health Department for the specific purpose of implementing breast health promotion, education and screening programs.
9. Study the feasibility of developing a Breast Cancer Center within the Health Department.

Specific Interventions: Cervical Cancer Screening, Diagnosis and Treatment for Women Aged 35–65.

1. Increase number of women receiving cervical screenings.
2. Gather additional information concerning barriers to regularity of cervical screening.
3. Increase regularity of repeat cervical screening; monitor timely follow-up and treatment of abnormal findings.
4. Develop community-based outreach strategies specifically targeting low income women and women of color to combat issues related to access to initial screening and regularity of screening.
5. Increase professional awareness that the healthcare provider must play a greater role in referral process.

FIGURE 43.3.   Suggested Interventions and Strategies.

Specific Interventions: STD/HIV in Women Aged 35–65.

1. Increase community and professional attention to the high rate of HIV testing of women in this age group (1 out of 5).
2. Increase the provision of STD/HIV education, screening, diagnostic and treatment services county-wide to women in the target group; coordination and development to be conducted by the Health Department and HIV Case Manager, targeting women aged 35–65 who engage in high risk behaviors.
3. Obtain additional professional staff to assist in the implementation of HIV testing conducted within the Health Department.

Specific Interventions: Self-Care Practices and Expressed Needs of Women Aged 35–65.

1. Increase community and professional focus on expressed needs for increased knowledge on the topics of weight control, stress management, exercise and assertiveness in the target population.
2. Study the feasibility of developing a "Women's Wellness Center" for the specific purpose of providing program and behavioral support in the problem areas identified by women aged 35-65 in the community.
3. Increase awareness of existing programs that address the identified topics.

FIGURE 43.3. (Continued)

the women reported that they would use the public library for additional health-related information would be appropriately reported in this section of Phase IV.

Phase V: Health Promotion Planning

Recommendations (Figure 43.3) to the Community Advisory Board (CAB) were made, moving the Project into Phase V in which the intervention program is developed. The community health nurse researchers through small and large group formats and the development of and interaction with the CAB, challenged their abilities to enlighten, educate, and develop a broader awareness of the major forces, pressures, and trends that affect the health of women in the community. The members of the CAB did respond, demonstrating an increased sensitivity and motivation to complete the work ahead. Inherent here is the process of healing; it will be carried on through the continuing work of the CAB. The CAB must now prioritize and set objectives for appropriate programs that address the issues that were clearly communicated by the women of the community. The Board must assess the resources required to implement needed programs of intervention. Phase V assessment requires an in-depth knowledge of local policy and community organizations. Thus, the CAB must determine what resources are needed, what is available, and identify barriers to program implementation (Green & Kreuter, 1991). For example, a program to promote healthy breast behaviors was recommended to the CAB. Components of the health education program include direct communication to the public and women clients identifying healthy breast behaviors which would impact predisposing factors for healthy behaviors. Also, health promotion education impacts the reinforcing factors for healthy breast behaviors by providing staff training and counseling from health professionals. Last, health education directly impacts local enabling factors such as community organizations and resources that facilitate adoption of healthy breast behaviors.

In the second component of Phase V, policy efforts are directed at encouraging community agency collaboration to implement the program for healthy breast behaviors. The policy component impacts the enabling or environmental factors effecting adoption of healthy behaviors. Completion of Phase V moves from the PRECEDE framework of the model. Phases VII-IX guide evaluation of the health promotion program (Green & Kreuter, 1991).

WOMEN'S HEALTH RESOURCE ROSTER

The third purpose of this research project was to compile a resources roster of available health services for women in the target area. The *Women's Health Resources Roster* (Landis & Cascio, 1992) will be useful to professionals providing healthcare and health-related services to women. It will also facilitate the communication and interaction process between providers and the women they serve, again promoting the goal of healing within this community. Further, it will be useful in future planning to identify and involve various service agencies in planning and intervention activities.

Various members of the local community provided assistance in identifying assets for inclusion in the *Women's Health Resources Roster*. Agencies identified included facilities concerned with obstetrical/gynecologic care, cancer treatment, rehabilitation, alcohol and drug treatment, and health and social services.

SUMMARY

The use of the PRECEDE-PROCEED Model in this community project is extremely valuable as a guide for presenting assessment and planning activities. It enables the Community Health Nurse to highlight the need for healing that targets a vital segment of the community: its women.

The current conceptualization of women's health is often bounded by the ages of 15 to 49 and by a sole focus on the reproductive system. The study reported here broadens this definition. Further, the establishment of a Community Advisory Board in the region provides a vehicle for strengthening community infrastructure and communications so vital to the achievement of mutuality and community cohesion, essential elements of healing. Women, as well as their healthcare providers, were immersed in the processes of appraisal and planning. Building a women's healthcare program that truly reflects women's healthcare concerns, not solely those of providers, is essential as a step toward healing within the community. Community assessment and planning approaches similar to those presented here empower our communities toward the ultimate goal of healing.

REFERENCES

Cascio, R. S., & Landis, B. J. (1992). *The woman's health resources roster: The women's health issues project*. Galveston, TX: Health Education Training Alliance of Texas.

Cascio, R. S., Landis, B. J., & Morris, D. (1992). *The household interview: The women's health issues project*. Galveston, TX: Health Education Training Alliance of Texas.

Green, L., & Kreuter, M. (1991). *Health promotion planning: An educational and environmental approach*. Mountainview, CA: Mayfield Publishing.

Horton, J. A. (Ed.). (1992). *The women's health data book: A profile of women's health in the United States*. Washington, DC: The Jacobs Institute of Women's Health.

Landis, B. J., & Cascio, R. S. (1992). *The interviewers's manual: The women's health issues project*. Galveston, TX: Health Education Training Alliance of Texas.

Morris, D., Hannigan, E., Dayal, H., Moore, R., Selwyn, B., McCandless, R., & Rosenthal, J. (1990). *South Texas needs assessment final report*. Austin, TX: Texas Cancer Council.

Public Health Service, Department of Health and Human Services. (1991). *Healthy people 2000: National health promotion and disease prevention objectives*. Washington, DC: U.S. Government Printing Office.

CHAPTER 44

Some Core Components of Healing: A Theory of Self-Reintegration: A Journey within Oneself

DORIS J. ROSENOW, PHD, RN, CCRN

Healing after an illness is a complex construct that entails a multidimensional personal experience with differing degrees of physiological, psychological, and social changes that reflect health promotion, health maintenance, and disease prevention actions for reintegrating holistic health. As a psychosocial phenomenon, healing has been studied as abandoning the sick role (Parsons, 1975), as a movement from a state of illness to a state of health or wellness (Naughton & Kolditz, 1975; Wilson-Barnett, 1981), and as a process of returning to normal as defined by pre-illness comparative standards of physical, social, and psychological well-being that progressed sequentially in three phases: passivity, activity resumption, and stabilization (Baker, 1989). Concomitantly, Dunn (1961) stated that high-level wellness is a direction that involves the whole being in a forward movement of reintegrating oneself within the social environment toward self-actualization.

Reintegration is bringing together parts of a whole. It becomes both the process and product of the self-healing journey whereby individuals find a motivational force, an interior activity, of bringing about a balance of harmony and wellness from a prior state of illness or disturbance. The healing process then becomes the energy that facilitates a person to mobilize resources for movement toward actualizing health potentials and well-being. This journey of growing toward health is based on the premise that resources are the building blocks in the healing process.

CONCEPT OF RESOURCES

Resources are internal and external substances that individuals draw upon for assistance in maintaining self-integrity in dynamic interactions with the environment. Hippocrates (400 BC) stated that human well-being is influenced by the totality of environmental factors, and health represents a generalized harmony among the factors of body, environment, and lifestyle (cited in Sahakian & Sahakian, 1966). Supporting these concepts, Knight (1974) defined health as a "harmonious integration of the person within himself and within his society, nature, and cosmos" (p. 274). Florence Nightingale (1859) noted that individuals possess inherent reparative powers to help them heal. These reparative healing powers are analogous to an individual's internal resources.

Powell (1989) eloquently posited a strong self-concept and self-esteem are analogous to healthy psychosocial residual resources as proposed by the theorist Erik Erikson (1963). These psychosocial residual resources serve as inner strengths that contribute to the individual's perception of well-being. Consistent with this view, Maslow (1970) claimed that all persons have a need for self-esteem (mastery, confidence, independence) and for esteem from others (attention, importance, status). As noted by Thoits (1983), the concept of perceived control of one's environment is often examined in association with feelings of self-esteem. As such, various writers have reaffirmed that gaining control and sustaining one's self-concept are significant factors in returning to a normal way of life after an illness (Ford, 1989; Frenn, Borgeson, Lee, & Simandl, 1989; Johnson & Morse, 1990). Because resources can be readily available to the individual or "they can exist as competencies for finding resources that are needed but not available" (Hilton, 1986, p. 12), they can supply the healing energy for a person to become whole on a higher level of harmony in the physical, psychological, cognitive, spiritual, and social domains (Eriksson, 1994; Erickson, Tomlin, & Swain, 1983; Newman, 1986; Scandrett-Hibdon, 1990).

In the health and wellness paradigm, individuals are encouraged to take a proactive approach to build adaptive strengths/resources as a way of preventing psychopathology and enhancing prospects for positive health outcomes. Therefore, individuals who can discover new ways of coping and relatedness with others are able to examine patterns of the healing process from a more adaptive and fluid perspective. According to Erickson et al. (1983), each individual possesses varied perspectives that result in a unique cognitive schema or model of experiences and these cognitive structures in turn regulate future person-environment interactions.

How individuals appraise their abilities and resources can affect their healing process for reintegrating holistic health (Erickson et al., 1983; Lazarus, 1966).

The theory of self-reintegration was based on an inductive–deductive scientific approach. To provide theoretical support for the theory of self-reintegration, an integrative theoretical and empirical review of literature on topics relevant to recovery, health, and resources was conducted.

PHILOSOPHIC AND CONCEPTUAL FOUNDATIONS OF SELF-REINTEGRATION THEORY

Gabriel Marcel

The French philosopher Gabriel Marcel (1962, 1967) developed a metaphysics of hope by describing the nature of man [sic] as Homo Viator, or man as a wayfarer. Marcel conceptualized life as a journey through which one develops or becomes; a condition of being-on-the way to one's relationship to oneself, others, and one's world. For Marcel, the main characteristics that shape man's journey are the search for meaning and for fulfillment. He described this search not in the sense of meaning and fulfillment of desires, but in the struggles with limits posed by reality, such as experiencing captivity (Aardema, 1984).

Marcel viewed captivity as the result of any stressor, such as illness, suffering, and loss that can lead man to despair. The process of despair "is one of the self turning against the self" (Aardema, 1984, p. 12); it is a state of hopelessness or "giving-up" (Engel, 1968) so that one cannot find meaning and fulfillment in life.

The resource of hope was perceived by Marcel as a perceptual adventure that becomes the motivation behind man as a wayfarer. Implied here is that hope is an important inner resource force "for survival in the face of captivity, trial, or entrapment" (Brown, 1994, p. 168). The hopeful man then is able to transcend the limits posed by the present situation and to recognize life as a journey, or process of finding meaning and fulfillment (Aardema, 1984; Brown, 1994).

Erik Erikson

Erik Erikson's (1982) theory of psychosocial development begins with infancy and continues through advanced age. He divides the entire life cycle into "the eight ages of man" which refer to the eight critical periods when certain lifelong ego concerns reach a climax. Two major principles underlying his theory are mutuality and epigenesis. Mutuality is defined as the coordination and exchange between individuals and their world. Epigenesis gives attention to the emergence of a particular aspect of development at a critical time. Erikson described the eight stages of psychosocial development through which we all progress. Each stage represents a developmental task that a person encounters and as one develops toward the positive poles of each developmental stage the resource of each stage becomes the residual strength that forms the core of a person's personality. Hope, self-control, purpose, competence, devotion, affiliation, production and renunciation are strengths that contribute to the health of the individual (Erickson et al., 1983). Because hope emerges from the very first crucial stage of infancy involving the poles of basic trust versus basic mistrust, Erikson viewed hope as the fundamental psychosocial strength affecting all stages of development from infancy onward. He stated, "hope bestows on the anticipated future a sense of leeway inviting expectant leaps, either in preparatory imagination or in small initiating actions" (pp. 59–60).

Theory of Modeling and Role-Modeling

The theory of Modeling and Role-Modeling (Erickson et al., 1983) represents a synthesis of concepts from theories of stress and coping (Engel, 1968; Selye, 1976), psychosocial development (Erikson, 1963), cognitive development (Piaget & Inhelder, 1969), basic and growth needs/self-actualization (Maslow, 1968) and attachment and loss (Bowlby, 1969; Klein, 1963; Winnicott, 1965). The major focus of the theory is that the core of a person's personality reflects the quality of basic needs satisfaction during growth and development that simultaneously affects the process of psychosocial and cognitive development, and ultimately, affects the organization of the cognitive schemata. These schemata are believed to reflect the "quality of the resolution of the Eriksonian psychosocial developmental tasks and the level of Piagetian cognitive development achieved" (Stein, 1988, p. 13).

Within this perspective, healthy psychosocial resources and a sense of basic need satisfaction can enable individuals to avoid or minimize the harmful and discomforting effects of the physiological and psychological expressions of stress. Therefore, individuals will predominantly experience a growth motivation characterized by an attitude of challenge and a desire for self-actualization (Kline, 1988). Concomitantly, individuals have an innate need to be close to and separate from significant others. This has been identified by Erickson et al. (1983) as the construct of affiliated-individuation. That is, there is a need for attachment to other humans "while simultaneously maintaining independence from one's support system" (p. 7). This relates to the feeling of both the "I" and "we" states of being and "to perceive freedom and acceptance in both states" (p. 47). Therefore, persons can act independently but at the same time rely on others and maintain a feeling of attachment to others.

Underlying the theory is the philosophical belief that the tripartite construct of self-care (knowledge, resources, actions) and coping have a reciprocal relationship in promoting growth-toward-health. Self-care knowledge is an individual's perceptions of the world in which he or she lives. Because self-care knowledge is knowing what one needs in life, each person has the key to what he or she personally needs. Self-care resources are both internal and external. Internal resources are the biophysical and psychosocial strengths that have been developed throughout an individual's psychosocial developmental process. External resources are aspects of the external environment, such as the support systems and social networks. Because self-care resources "have both enduring characteristics and are fluid, they respond to the continual changes individuals are faced with in life" (Kelly-Walsh, VandenBosch, & Boehm, 1989, p. 758). When individuals choose a course of action, self-care action is mobilizing self-care resources and utilizing self-care knowledge to act on one's own behalf. This conceptualization of self-care then implies that individuals freely choose to mobilize and acquire resources based on their personal needs.

COMPONENTS OF THE SELF-REINTEGRATION THEORY

Self-reintegration is defined as a self-creation process whereby individuals develop new capabilities by reorganizing the self and the environment so that there is a meaning and purpose in living that transcends the stressful experience. It is the inner journey toward wholeness and fulfillment. Some defining characteristics within this process are: (1) adjustment (Frenn et al., 1989); (2) self-responsibility (Blattner, 1981); (3) returning to normal life (Keller M. J., 1991); (4) affirmation of attitudes (Medich, Stuart, Deckro, & Freidman, 1991), and (5) obtaining a higher quality of life/well-being (Dunn, 1961).

Adjustment is the process where individuals must relinquish some activities that may have precipitated the illness or are too strenuous after the illness, and integrate new behaviors into one's lifestyle (Frenn et al., 1989). Within this integration process, individuals appraise their current behaviors with the recommended health value standards in order to reintegrate holistic health. This process allows a person to have a feeling of being capable of making decisions about one's life experiences (Erickson, 1984) as one attempts to repattern his or her personal and social behaviors (Frenn et al.,1989). It also allows the person to interact with others for supportive assistance to arrive at specific outcomes.

Self-responsibility is a state where an individual develops a desire and tendency for self-direction and determinism (Blattner, 1981). It is the belief that one is reliable, trustworthy, and accountable. Because self-responsibility begins with a prerequisite process of self-awareness, actions can be initiated by one-self to alter one's lifestyle patterning toward health.

Returning to a normal lifestyle (Keller C., 1991) arises when an individual develops self-care actions that represent the selected health promotion, health maintenance, and disease prevention activities. Because individuals recovering from an illness need to take a comprehensive risk management approach to improve their health, the activities of health promotion, health maintenance, and disease prevention are not mutually exclusive. The hallmark of healing is a moving forward journey process. Therefore, individuals after an illness must come to terms with coming back to the perceived self before the illness; yet, adjusting their lifestyle to integrate these self-care activities in an effort to improve their health and to reduce the risk of another illness.

Affirmation is developing an attitude in order to replace negative ideas with positive ideas that can assist in maximizing one's potential after the illness. This process allows individuals to: (1) reframe the illness to a health challenge; (2) reorder their values or standards; and (3) reclaim life satisfaction (Medich et al., 1991).

High level of wellness or obtaining a state of higher quality of life and well-being can become a direction and forward movement toward self-actualization that integrates and maximizes a person's physiological, psychological, spiritual, cognitive, and social well-being (Dunn, 1961). According to Dunn, "a person must have a concept of oneself in relation to both his (sic) inner self and outer world, and when a person can maintain his personal dignity within the social matrix he finds it easier to reintegrate himself and to solve his problems" (p. 230). Thus, high-level wellness is not an end or static goal, but an ongoing journey of self-creation toward a higher potential of functioning.

Some individuals may not emerge from the illness' stressful experience; consequently, these individuals are unable to move through the healing

process. Empirical studies dealing with the negative psychosocial responses indicate that individuals who develop a reactive depression are
less likely to adhere to the recommended medical regimen necessary for
the healing process than individuals who are able to move beyond the illness toward holistic health (Gentry, Foster, & Haney, 1972; Mayou, 1984).
These individuals can become powerless, live a life of fear, dependency,
and isolation or develop a state of hopelessness. Hopelessness means to be
ruled by a sense of the impossible, that life is too much to handle, and that
there are no resources to call upon (Lynch, 1965; Schneider, 1980). Rycroft
(1979) stated that if the sources of hope dry up or become exhausted, hope
ceases to be and is replaced by a negative condition of hopelessness. Hopelessness has been shown to be a factor in sudden death (Engel, 1968) as
well as in the development of physical illness (Engel, 1968; Schmale & Iker,
1966, 1971) and in vegetative signs of depression, apathy, and lack of motivation (Roberts, 1986).

CORE OF THE SELF-REINTEGRATION THEORY: RESOURCES

As a result of this theoretic and empirical review of literature and the resources that were identified from research studies (Hertz, 1991; Rosenow,
1992; 1993) that supported the conceptual linkages of self-care resources,
self-care knowledge, and self-care action as described in the theory of
Modeling and Role-Modeling (Erickson et al., 1983), the core of the self-
reintegration theory was based on the following integrated resource
concepts: (1) hope/inner strength; (2) growth-toward-health/sense of direction; (3) personal control/competence; and (4) social support and net-
works/affiliation. This core provides the individual the healing energy for
holistic well-being. Because these resources are consistent with the
strengths and virtues of a person's developmental stages of development as
described by (Erikson, 1963), the self-reintegration theory can be used as a
template for a variety of illnesses in assisting individuals to maximize their
potentials during the healing process.

Hope/Inner Strength

When individuals are able to grasp the wholeness of the illness event, the
phenomenon of inner strength (Rose, 1988) portrays expansion of energy
towards wellness. Inner strength closely aligns with Dossey's (1984) description of health as a way of being that allows a person to move "beyond

illness" to higher levels of self-awareness that facilitate one's own psychological process and self. Concomitantly, Brown (1994) stated that "the processes of hope are a bridge by which the individual is able to transform suffering and experience healing" (p. 170). According to Erikson (1982) "hope connotes the most basic quality of 'I-ness,' without which life could not begin or meaningfully end" (p. 62). Thus, the innate resource of hope underlies a person's inner strength.

The concept of hope has long been recognized as an intrinsic element of life for healthy coping (Engel, 1968; Erickson et al., 1983; Herth, 1990; Rines & Montag, 1976), a power resource for action (Miller, 1989), as a life force (DuFault & Martocchio, 1985; Lynch, 1965; Stoner, 1988), and is present in all stages of life, including dying (DuFault, 1985; Herth, 1990). Although Lynch (1965) theorized that the nature of hope is a function of the imagination an individual possesses, he also believed that hope needs a response from the environment and it has meaning only as an act of collaboration or mutuality with others. Without hope we do nothing, we have no energy, no wishing (Lynch, 1965).

Stotland (1969) defined hope in terms of expectation of goal attainment; a probability of success; a belief that the desired goal is obtainable. Rycroft (1979) described hope as fundamental to human life; a key to living. He believed that hope exists only contingently; that is, hope must have a source. If the sources of hope dry up or become exhausted, hope ceases to be and is replaced by negative condition of hopelessness. In support of these tenets, Korner (1970) stated that hope is a method of coping. Lazarus (1966) claimed that hope facilitates action and taking action during stressful situations is an efficacious coping tool.

McGee (1984) asserted that the "presence of hope fortifies the physiological and psychological defenses, and its absence has been correlated with an early demise" (p. 34). Similarly, Illich (1976) conceptualized hope as part of health and health as a process of adaptation. Based on the empirical studies, hope has been theorized as a multidimensional resource phenomenon that is linked with a person's adaptive powers and health outcome. Therefore, some of the dimensions of hope include optimism, courage, meaning in life, attainable goals, personal attributes, peace, and energy.

Growth-toward-Health/Sense of Direction

Growth-toward-health is a self-renewal pathway that represents a quantum leap of transformational development that is characterized by an understanding of the self and the environment. Because healing is the reintegration of self in the presence of suffering (Brown, 1994), the constructs of inner strength and hope closely align with Moch's (1989) conceptualization of a health-within-illness paradigm. Moch noted that this perspective posits illness as an event that can expand human potential by finding meaning in the illness through increased awareness and transformational change. Similarly, Moll (1982) noted that illness can be viewed as a positive opportunity for personal growth and health. Taylor (1983) reported a growth through crises with women who had experienced breast cancer. She noted that the cancer experience became the catalytic agent for restructuring some women's lives by forming a new meaningful attitude toward life. Cowie (1976) found that individuals who were able to understand why they had a heart attack were able to identify causal antecedents and were able to cope adaptively. He considered the reconstructive process to be an important part in the healing recovery process for an individual after an Myocardial Infarction (MI). Maslow (1970) identified this movement as growth motivation; an expansion of one's tendency to move toward further development.

Personal Control/Competence

Personal control can be defined as consisting of a person's beliefs of being capable of making decisions about one's own life experiences (Erickson, 1984). Jaffe (1985) noted that the self-renewal process after a stressful event is the rediscovery of some sense of meaningful psychological control over one's life. Taylor (1983) found that the force that facilitated people's recovery after they became ill was cognitive control. That is, individuals had control over the way they saw events and structure of their reality; it is the core of self-renewal because what changes is the person's sense of who they are and what is going on (Jaffe, 1985). Control research has suggested that personal control may underlie all forms of behavioral change (Cohen, 1990; Cousins, 1983; Erickson, 1984; Johnson & Morse, 1990; McSweeney, 1990).

Deci and Ryan (1985) claimed that control and feelings of self-determination are central to intrinsic motivation to achieve. Carver and Scheier's (1982) control theory is based on a hierarchical feedback loop process that consists of: (1) directing attention to the self; (2) comparing oneself with relevant and salient values; and (3) attempting to reduce the discrepancy between the perceived state and the reference value.

Therefore, the discrepancy between the present and desired valued behavior will motivate the individual to try to achieve the desired behavior. As such, the individual perceives some degree of control in achieving the desired goal. These patterns of control are also congruent with Brehm's (1966) reactance theory wherein the threat to freedom from uncontrollable circumstances creates its own motivation for control.

Social Support and Networks/Affiliation

The construct of social support and its relationship to other variables has been thoroughly investigated. Because people have needs that can be satisfied with social interactions with others (Thoits, 1982), social support and social networks have been identified as variables having either a primary effect or a buffering effect affecting a person's stress outcomes. That is, the functional aspect of social support and social networks may help individuals with more positive affective states, such as emotional sustenance (Bramwell, 1986), increased feelings of belonging, self-worth, self-esteem, and perceived control (Cassel, 1976; Cobb, 1976; Cohen & Willis, 1985), recovery from an illness (Christman et al., 1988; Mayou, Foster, & Williamson, 1978), positive health practices (Gottlieb & Green, 1984; Hubbard, Muhlenkamp, & Brown, 1984; Muhlenkamp & Sayles, 1986), and coping resources (Bruhn & Phillips, 1984; Thoits, 1982).

Although social support has been identified as an important external resource, both theory and research suggest that individuals vary in their need for support and networks because of individual differences (Erickson et al., 1983; Sarason & Sarason, 1985). This perspective is further explained within the theory of Modeling and Role-Modeling. Because people have needs to be "simultaneously close to and separate from significant others" self-care actions based on self-care knowledge and self-care resources may result in behaviors that can meet these needs (Erickson et al., 1983). Therefore, individuals can act independent in their self-care activities during the healing process after an illness; yet, at the same time rely on others for support and maintain a sense of attachment with them (Erickson et al., 1983). As noted by Vauz and Athanassopulou (1987), social networks have interactional dimensions that become resources for people. By providing this dimension, social networks then provide a link that joins people by becoming an external resource that facilitates support during the recovery process after an illness.

APPLICATION TO NURSING PRACTICE

Case

Tom is a young man in his early fifties who has had a three-vessel coronary artery bypass graft (CABG). The major behaviors he engaged in during the healing postoperative phase stemmed from the process of seeking normalcy (Keller, C., 1991). This phase is characterized by the restoration of himself to optimal functioning performance and the reintegration of himself into the affairs of daily living and society, commensurate with the limitation imposed by the disease process (Madden, 1977). For example, in spite of incisional pain and discomfort, Tom was eager to cooperate with the healthcare providers, and often expressed that "he wanted to do the right behaviors," such as early ambulation and faithful use of the incentive spirometer so that he could try to regain his health. He also expressed how much he valued the support from his family, friends, and staff. He stated that "all these people helped me to adjust and understand the importance of quitting smoking and making other lifestyle changes for the gains of longevity and functional ability." For Tom, the hallmark of the healing-recovery process following his CABG surgery is one of moving forward and enduring lifestyle changes in an effort to return to cardiovascular health.

The theory of Modeling and Role-Modeling (Erickson et al., 1983) states that human beings are holistic people who have multiple interacting subsystems. The theory also emphasizes the importance of human development and adds links to the theories of Maslow (1968, 1970) and Erikson (1963). By integrating these conceptual frameworks, the theory of Modeling and Role-Modeling facilitates our understanding of how people grow to be both alike and different. For example, Eric Erikson identified the first conflict state that every infant faces when born as trust versus mistrust. Like other infants, Tom was fed when hungry and nurtured, thus learning that his mother could be trusted to provide for his basic needs. Resolving this conflict allowed Tom to develop his inner strength of trust and the resource of hope. Tom was having his basic physical needs met which helped him feel safe, secure, loved and gave him a sense of belonging. By building these strengths and resources, this provided Tom with the energy to heal and recover after his surgery. In contrast, if Tom was not able to resolve some of the developmental conflict stages as described by Erik Erikson, he would have had very little internal strengths and resources to be mobilized to help him through his process.

Another component in the theory of Modeling and Role-Modeling (Erickson et al., 1983) is the adaptive potential assessment model (APAM). This model is a "useful investigative and clinical tool for describing and classifying an individual's potential to adapt to current and future stressors through the mobilization of internal and external resources" (Kline Leidy, 1989, p. 873). The APAM model integrates Selye's (1974) general adaptation syndrome, Engel's (1968) psychosocial indicators to stressors, and Lazarus' (1966) appraisal theory to stress. According to the APAM model, stressors exist in the environment at all times and exert their positive and negative effects on the person based on how a person appraises (Lazarus, 1966) the stressor and the available resources to cope with the stressor.

Empirical evidence suggests that personal and social resources mediate the relationship between stress and illness (Kobasa & Purcetti, 1983), and can reduce feelings of threat (Kline Leidy, 1989) because they represent the enabling factors that individuals draw upon to help them with their healing and growth toward health and wellness. Tom often expressed how he wanted to "do the right behaviors" (Kelly-Walsh et al., 1989) in order to help him get well, and how he valued the support he received from his family, friends, and the staff. Because of his innate ability and desire to be the best he could possibly be (Maslow, 1970), and a health within illness attitude (Moch, 1989), Tom was able to mobilize the internal resources of hope, growth toward health, and perceived personal control and the external resource of support to aid him in his healing-recovery period. Consequently, Tom was a hopeful person who had a self-directed, optimistic direction for cardiovascular health.

Major foci of health and social psychological theories are the understanding, explanation, and prediction of human interpersonal behavior and one's interaction with the environment. Based on the philosophical belief that a person is holistic (the mind and body are interrelated), the theory of self-reintegration provides a framework relevant to nursing practice in many diverse situations and settings. One important implication of this theory is focusing on the person's perception in order to understand the person's unique internal model. Since each person has a unique model (a specific way of getting basis needs met), each person also has the key to what he/she personally needs (Erickson et al., 1983). Thus, the self-reintegration theory incorporates the five aims of nursing interventions which reflect the theoretical bases and the linkages in the metaparadigm of Modeling and Role-Modeling (Erickson et al., 1983). The five aims and their principles are presented in Table 44.1.

TABLE 44.1. Relationships among intervention goals, principles, and aims.

Intervention goal	Principle	Aim
1. Develop a trusting and functional relationship between yourself and your client	The nursing process requires that a trusting and functional relationship exists between nurse and client	Build trust
2. Facilitate a self-projection that is futuristic and positive	Affiliated-individuation is contingent on the individual's perceiving that he or she is an acceptable, respectable, and worthwhile human being	Promote client's positive orientation
3. Promote affiliated-individuation with the minimum degree of ambivalence possible	Human development is dependent on the individual's perceiving that he or she has some control over life (while concurrently sensing a state of affiliation)	Promote client control
4. Promote a dynamic, adaptive state of health	There is an innate drive toward holistic health that is facilitated by consistent and systematic nurturance	Affirm and promote client's strengths
5. (a) Promote and nurture coping mechanisms that satisfy basic needs and permit growth-need satisfaction (b) Facilitate congruent actual chronological developmental stages	Human growth is dependent on satisfaction of basic needs and is facilitated by growth-need satisfaction	Set mutual goals that are health directed

Source: Reprinted with permission from Erickson, Tomlin and Swain (1983), *Modeling and Role-Modeling: A Theory and Paradigm for Nursing,* Englewood Cliffs, NJ: Prentice-Hall.

CONCLUSION

The art and science of nursing is to provide interventions that help individuals mobilize their resources, with hope being viewed as essential to life, and the cornerstone of one's self-concept and self-esteem (Lynch, 1965; Maslow, 1970). In addition, external resources such as perceived social support (Cobb, 1976), spiritual support (O'Brien, 1985), and social networks (Kobasa & Puccetti, 1983) enhance the healing process of individuals by buffering stress or directly enhancing behaviors that lead to a healthy lifestyle. By building on individuals' perception of resources needed after an illness, nurses can promote these strengths as enabling empowering factors that can help maximize their healing process.

Health promotion, health maintenance, and disease prevention are nursing goals for promoting holistic health. Understanding the factors that motivate people to take action to promote their own health is an important part of nursing. Therefore, nurses can facilitate individuals who have sustained an illness to integrate into their existing lifestyle the health behaviors that will promote the healing process. Although theory building begins with finding theoretical concepts to describe the phenomenon of concern, it is also important that empirical investigations be increased for the understanding and support of the resources as proposed in the theory of self-reintegration.

REFERENCES

Aardema, B. L. T. (1984). *The therapeutic use of hope.* An unpublished doctoral dissertation, Western Michigan University, Kalamazoo, MI.

Baker, C. A. (1989). Recovery: A phenomenon extending beyond discharge. *Scholarly Inquiry for Nursing Practice: An International Journal, 3*(3), 181-194.

Blattner, B. (1981). *Holistic nursing.* Englewood Cliffs, NJ: Prentice-Hall.

Bowlby, J. (1969). *Attachment.* New York: Basic Books.

Bramwell, L. (1986). Wives' experiences in the support role after husbands' first myocardial infarction. *Heart & Lung, 5*(6), 574-584.

Brehm, J. W. (1966). *Response to the loss of freedom: A theory of psychological reactance.* New York: Academic Press.

Brown, L., (1994). Hope as healing: Patient voices. In D. A. Gaut & A. Boykin (Eds.), *Caring as healing: Renewal through hope.* New York: NLN Press.

Bruhn, J. G., & Phillips, B. U. (1984). Measuring social support: A synthesis of current approaches. *Journal of Behavioral Medicine, 7,* 151-169.

Carver, C. S., & Scheier, M. F. (1982). Control theory: A useful conceptual framework for personality, social, clinical, and health psychology. *Psychological Bulletin, 92*(1), 111-135.

Cassel, J. (1976). The contribution of the social environment to host resistance. *American Journal of Epidemiology, 104*(2), 107-122.

Cay, E. L., Vetter, N., Philip, A., & Dugard, P. (1972). Psychological status during recovery from an acute heart attack. *Journal of Psychosomatic Research, 16,* 425-435.

Christman, N., McConnell, E., Pfeiffer, C., Webster, K., Schmitt, M., & Reis, J. (1988). Uncertainty, coping, and distress following myocardial infarction: Transition from hospital to home. *Research in Nursing and Health, 11,* 71-82.

Cobb, S. (1976). Social support as a moderator of stress. *Psychosomatic Medicine, 38,* 300-314.

Cohen, S. (1990). Control and the epidemiology of physical health: Where do we go from here. In J. Rodin, S. Schooler, & K. Warner Schaie (Eds.), *Self-directness: Cause and effects throughout the life course.* Hillsdale, NJ: Lawrence Erlbaum.

Cohen, S., & Willis, T. A. (1985). Stress, social support, and the buffering hypothesis. *Psychological Bulletin, 98*(2), 310-357.

Cousins, N. (1983). *The healing heart.* New York: Avon.

Cowie, B. (1976). The cardiac patient's perception of his heart attack. *Social Science and Medicine, 10,* 87-96.

Deci, E. L., & Ryan, R. M. (1985). The general causality orientations scale: Self-determination in personality. *Journal of Research in Personality, 19,* 109-134.

Dossey, L. (1984). *Beyond illness: Discovering the experience of health.* Boston: Shambhala.

DuFault, K., & Martocchio, B. C. (1985). Hope: Its spheres and dimensions. *Nursing Clinics of North America, 20*(2), 379-391.

Dunn, D. B. (1961). *High level wellness.* Arlington, VA: R.W. Beatty.

Engel, G. L. (1968). A life setting conducive to illness—a psychological setting of somatic disease: The giving-up-given-up complex. *Bulletin of the Menniger Clinic, 32,* 355-366.

Erickson, H. C. (1984). Self-care knowledge: Relations among the concepts support, hope, control, satisfaction with daily life and physical health status. *Dissertation Abstracts International, 46,* 06B, (University Microfilms No. 84-12, 136).

Erickson, H., Tomlin, E., & Swain, M. (1983). *Modeling and role-modeling: A theory and paradigm for nursing.* Englewood Cliffs, NJ: Prentice-Hall.

Erikson, E. H. (1963). *Childhood and society (2nd ed.).* New York: Norton.

Erikson, E. H. (1982). *The life cycle completed.* New York: Norton.

Eriksson, K. (1994). Theories of caring as health. In D. A. Gaut & A. Boykin (Eds.), *Caring as healing: Renewal through hope.* New York: NLN Press.

Ford, J. (1989). Living with a history of a heart attack: A human science investigation. *Journal of Advanced Nursing, 14,* 173-178.

Frenn, M., Borgeson, D., Lee, H., & Simandl, G. (1989). Life-style changes in a cardiac rehabilitation program: The client perspective. *Journal of Cardiovascular Nursing, 3*(2), 43-55.

Gentry, W. D., Foster, S., & Haney, T. (1972). Denial as a determinant of anxiety and perceived health status in the coronary care unit. *Psychosomatic Medicine, 34,* 39-44.

Gottlieb, N., & Green, L. (1984). Life events, social networks, life-style, and health: An analysis of the 1979 National Survey of Personal Health Practices and Consequences. *Health Education Quarterly, 11*(1), 91-105.

Herth, K. (1990). Relationship of hope, coping styles, concurrent losses, and setting to grief resolution in the elderly widow(er). *Research in Nursing & Health, 13,* 109-117.

Hertz, J. (1991). *The perceived enactment of autonomy scale: Measuring the potential for self-care action in the elderly.* Unpublished doctoral dissertation. The University of Texas at Austin, TX.

Hilton, A. (1986). *Coping with the uncertainties of breast cancer: Appraisal and coping strategies.* Unpublished doctoral dissertation. The University of Texas at Austin., TX.

Hubbard, P., Muhlenkamp, A. F., & Brown, N. (1984). The relationship between social support and self-care practices. *Nursing Research, 33,* 266-270.

Illich, I. (1976). *Medical nemeses: The expropriation of health.* New York: Bantam.

Jaffe, D. T. (1985). Self-renewal: Personal transformation following extreme trauma. *Journal of Humanistic Psychology, 25*(4), 99-124.

Johnson, J., & Morse, J. (1990). Regaining control: The process of adjustment after myocardial infarction. *Heart & Lung, 19*(2), 126-135.

Keller, C. (1991). Seeking normalcy: The experience of coronary artery bypass surgery. *Research in Nursing & Health, 14,* 173-178.

Keller, M. J. (1991). Toward a definition of health. *Advances in Nursing Science,* October, 43-52.

Kelly-Walsh, K., VandenBosch, T. M., & Boehm, S. (1989). Modeling and role-modeling: Integrating nursing theory into practice. *Journal of Advanced Nursing, 14,* 755-761.

Klein, M. (1963). *Our adult society and its roots in infancy.* London: Tavistock.

Kline, N. W. (1988). *Psychophysiological processes of stress in people with a chronic physical illness.* Unpublished doctoral dissertation. University of Michigan.

Kline Leidy, N. (1989). A physiologic analysis of stress and chronic illness. *Journal of Advanced Nursing, 14,* 868-876.

Knight, J. A. (1974). Spiritual psychology and self regulation, In G. M. Goldway (Ed.), *Inner balance: The power of inner healing.* Englewood Cliffs, NJ: Prentice-Hall.

Kobasa, S., & Puccetti, M. (1983). Personality and social resources in stress resistance. *Journal of Personality and Social Psychology, 45,* 839-850.

Korner, I. (1970). Hope as a method of coping. *Journal of Consulting and Clinical Psychology, 34,* 134-139.

Lazarus, R. S. (1966). *Psychological stress and coping process.* New York: McGraw-Hill.

Lynch, W. (1965). *Images of hope.* Baltimore and Dublin: Helicon Press.

Madden, B. (1977). Rehabilitation: Principles, philosophy, practice. *Nurs Digest, 5,* 35-40.

Marcel, G. (1962). *Homo Viator: Introduction to a metaphysics of hope.* New York: Harper & Row.

Marcel, G. (1967). Desire and hope. In N. Lawrence & D. O'Conner (Eds.), *Readings in existential phenomenology.* Englewood Cliffs, NJ: Prentice-Hall.

Maslow, A. H. (1968). *Toward a psychology of being* (2nd ed.). Princeton, NJ: Van Nostrand.

Maslow, A. H. (1970). *Motivation and personality* (2nd. ed.). New York: Harper & Row.

Mayou, R. (1984). Prediction of emotional and social outcome after a heart attack. *Journal of Psychosomatic Research, 28,* 17-25.

Mayou, R., Foster, A., & Williamson, B. (1978). Psychosocial adjustments in patients one year after myocardial infarction. *Journal of Psychosomatic Research, 22,* 447-453.

McGee, R. R. (1984). Hope: A factor influencing crisis resolution. *Advances Nursing Science, 6*(4), 34-44.

McSweeney, J. C. (1990). *Making behavior changes after a myocardial infarction: A naturalistic study.* Unpublished doctoral dissertation. The University of Texas at Austin, Austin, TX.

Medich, C., Stuart, E., Deckro, J., & Friedman, R. (1991). Psychophysiologic control mechanisms in ischemic heart disease: The mind-heart connection. *Journal of Cardiovascular Nursing, 5*(4), 10-26.

Miller, J. F. (1989). Hope-inspiring strategies of the critically ill. *Applied Nursing Research, 2*(1), 23-29.

Moch, S. D. (1989). Health within illness: Conceptual evolution and practice possibilities. *Advances in Nursing Science, 11*(4), 23-31.

Moll, J. A. (1982). High-level wellness and the nurse. *Topics in Clinical Nursing, 1,* 61-67.

Muhlenkamp, A. F., & Sayles, J. A. (1986). Self-esteem, social support, and positive health practices. *Nursing Research, 35,* 334-338.

Naughton, R. A., & Kolditz, D. (1975). *Patients' definitions of recovery from an acute illness.* Unpublished doctoral dissertation, Columbia University, New York.

Newman, M. A. (1986). *Health as expanding consciousness.* St. Louis: C.V. Mosby.

Nightingale, F. *Notes on nursing.* Philadelphia: Lippincott. (Original work published 1859)

O'Brien, M. E. (1985). Pragmatic survivalism. *Advances in Nursing Science, 4,* 13-26.

Parsons, T. (1975). The sick role and the role of the physician reconsidered. *The Milbank Memorial Fund Quarterly, 53,* 257-278.

Piaget, J., & Inhelder, B. (1969). *The psychology of the child.* New York: Basic Books.

Powell, P. (1989). Personal communications. *Class in Individual through the life cycle.* Educational Psychology Department. The University of Texas at Austin, TX.

Rines, A., & Montag, M. (1976). *Nursing concerns and nursing care.* New York: John Wiley.

Roberts, S. L. (1986). *Behavioral concepts and the critically ill patient* (2nd ed.). Norwalk, CT: Appleton-Century-Crofts.

Rose, J. F. (1988). *The voice of inner strength in women: A phenomenological study*. Unpublished doctoral dissertation. The University of Texas at Austin, TX.

Rosenow, D. J. (1992). *Multidimensional scaling analysis of self-care actions for reintegrating holistic health after a myocardial infarction: Implications for nursing*. Unpublished dissertation. The University of Texas at Austin, TX.

Rosenow, D. J. (1993). *Resources for cardiovascular health, using multidimensional scaling analysis*. Unpublished paper. The University of Texas at Galveston, TX.

Rycroft, C. (1979). Steps to an ecology of hope. In R. Fitzgerald (Ed.), *The Sources of Hope*. New York: Pergamon.

Sahakian, W. S., & Sahakian, M. L. (1966). *Ideas of great philosophers*. New York: Harper & Row.

Sarason, I. G., & Sarason, B. R. (1985). *Social support: Theory, research and applications*. Boston: Martinus Nijhoff.

Scandrett-Hibdon, S. L. (1990). The endogenous healing process in black women. *Journal of Holistic Nursing, 4,* 47-62.

Schmale, A. H., & Iker, H. (1966). The effect of hopelessness and the development of cancer. *Psychosomatic Medicine, 28,* 714-721.

Schmale, A. H., & Iker, H. (1971). Hopelessness as a predictor of cervical cancer. *Social Science & Medicine, 5,* 95-100.

Schneider, J. S. (1980). Hopelessness and helplessness. *Journal of Psychiatric Nursing and Mental Health Services, 18*(3), 12-21.

Selye, H. (1976). *The stress of life* (2nd ed.). New York: McGraw-Hill.

Stein, K. (1988). *Structure of the self and stability of self-esteem*. Unpublished doctoral dissertation. University of Michigan.

Stoner, M. H. (1988). Measuring hope. In M. Frank-Stromborg (Ed.), *Instruments for clinical nursing research*. Norwalk, CT: Appleton & Lange.

Stotland, E. (1969). *The psychology of hope*. San Francisco: Jossey-Bass.

Taylor, S. (1983). Adjustment to threatening events: A theory of cognitive adaptation. *American Psychologist, 38,* 1161-1173.

Thoits, P. A. (1982). Conceptual, methodological, and theoretical problems in studying social support as a buffer against life stress. *Journal of Health and Social Behavior, 23,* 145-159.

Thoits, P. A. (1983). Dimensions of life events that influence psychological distress: An evaluation and synthesis of the literature. In H. B. Kaplan (Ed.), *Psychosocial stress: Trends in theory and research*. New York: Academic Press.

Vauz, A., & Athanassopulou, M. (1987). Social support appraisals and network resources. *Journal of Community Psychology, 15,* 537-556.

Wilson-Barnett, J. (1981). Assessment of recovery: With special reference to a study with postoperative cardiac patients. *Journal of Advanced Nursing, 6,* 435-445.

Winnicott, D. W. (1965). *The maturational processes and the facilitating environment*. New York: International Universities Press.

CHAPTER 45

Interpretive Research Exploring the Healing Practices of Nurse Practitioners

KAREN A. BRYKCZYNSKI, RN, RNCS, FNP, DNSC
PHYLICIA H. LEWIS, RN, MS, MSN

Discovery of the theoretical and practical knowledge of healing in nursing practice is in its infancy with only a paucity of related literature available. Interpretive phenomenological research allows for an understanding of the healing practices of nurses as they go about their daily clinical lives. Benner (1984), Brykczynski (1985), and Lewis (1992) have conducted interpretive research studies related to the practical knowledge of nurses and nurse practitioners which highlight the phenomenon of healing and healing practices. This chapter illustrates the potential for discovery offered by such studies, and builds especially on Benner's (1984) contributions to understanding practical knowledge.

Practical knowledge is a perceptual kind of knowledge that develops through the practice of skills. It resists formalization because of several characteristics, including: (1) discretionary judgment is a central aspect, (2) background knowledge is necessary for skill development, and (3) the nature of these skills is experience-based. It is useful to discuss aspects of practical knowledge to enhance understanding of qualitative distinctions among them and to recognize these previously unidentified aspects of clinical knowledge. Exemplars of practical knowledge serve to illustrate selected competencies in the domains of nursing practice. *Competency* is used here as defined by Benner (1984): "an interpretively defined area of skilled performance identified and described by its intent, function, and meanings" (p. 292).

The authors would like to gratefully acknowledge the comments on an earlier draft of this chapter by Diane Heliker, RN, PhD.

The aspects of practical knowledge and the domains and competencies of nursing practice are not mutually exclusive, but closely interrelated. Illustrations of particular aspects of practical knowledge may also constitute exemplars of competencies in the domains of nursing practice and vice versa. Because aspects of practical knowledge, domains, and competencies are situational, their meanings are embedded in the context of whole situations. They are not to be abstracted and listed as context-free elements. A fully described clinical situation may constitute an exemplar of more than one aspect of practical knowledge and more than one competency.

Assessment Expertise

The theme, assessment expertise (Brykczynski, 1985), can be used to illustrate this interplay between aspects of practical knowledge and competencies of nursing practice. In terms of the identification and description of practical knowledge, assessment expertise conveys two aspects of practical knowledge, specifically qualitative distinctions and maxims (Benner, 1984). Exemplifying situations here illustrate both the clinical ability to recognize qualitative distinctions and the maxim "real disease declares itself." At the same time, exemplars of assessment expertise can be depicted as illustrations of the competency, "detecting acute and chronic disease while attending to the experience of illness," in the domain of managing Patient Health/Illness Status Over Time (Brykczynski, 1985). Domains are clusters of competencies that have similar intents, functions, and meanings (Benner, 1984).

In Brykczynski's (1985) study of the clinical judgment of nurse practitioners, assessment expertise appears as a recurring theme with spending time, recognition of subtle cues, and listening identified as three central aspects. Illustrative here is the following excerpt, where a nurse practitioner saw a 32-year-old man who was complaining of excessive sleepiness:

> *In my first hour with him, I never even examined him. He was just so anxious, so upset, and had so much to tell me that all I ever got out of him was his history that first entire hour. I just (you know how you get that overwhelming sense when someone is really anxious), they finish and you feel anxious. I just felt claustrophobic in the room with this man.*

The nurse practitioner described her ability to discriminate among ambiguous cues as having that "sixth sense." She explained how she used herself as a kind of personal barometer by attending to personal cues, such as feeling very anxious, and sorting out whether these feelings were generated from herself or were communicated by the patient. Feelings of lack of closure, of uneasiness, incompleteness, or discomfort (which she described as a sense that something was going to come up) were other personal cues to which she attended that aided her in her assessments. After spending two entire hours with this man, the nurse practitioner related:

> *All I could think of was that it was my sixth sense that he was more than neurotic. He had a kind of whiny, neurotic personality, which I knew was probably the reason that other providers hadn't listened to him and looked any further. I just had this sense that something was going to come up.*

This excerpt describes experience-based recognition of subtle cues in a patient's presentation and getting an overall initial impression or gestalt about the patient situation in the first few moments which are later confirmed by events. In this case, the man was found to have an inoperable glioma thus validating the nurse practitioner's sense that something was going to come up.

In addition to providing a rich exemplar of the ability to recognize qualitative distinctions (an aspect of practical knowledge), this case illustrates that the nurse practitioner not only diagnoses diseases, but also attends to the meaning of the disease in the patient's life (a nurse practitioner competency). The nurse practitioner learned that even though the patient's disease was terminal, he found "knowing" preferable to the stress of the unknown he suffered as he searched for a definitive diagnosis. At this point in his care, the nurse practitioner then attended to anticipatory guidance as he identified and accomplished what was most important to him before his death, such as arranging an agreement with his ex-wife to grant him visiting privileges to see his son, applying for disability benefits, and planning for his mother to come from out of town to spend his last months with him.

HEALING RELATIONSHIP

Benner (1984) describes "establishing a healing relationship" as a competency within the domain of: The Helping Role of the Nurse. A nurse practitioner in Brykczynski's (1985) study described her ideas about the healing relationship as follows:

If I could say what I want to be when I grow up—I would say I'd be a healer. I guess there is something magical about being a healer. I think there are two levels: the level of what you know, and then there is the level of a relationship you have with patients that makes them feel that you will heal them. There is that element of the healer that goes throughout healthcare and part of it is belief.

This excerpt refers to commitment to healing and the importance of belief. The suggestion that something magical takes place makes one contemplate the power of human connectedness. The magical aspect of the healing relationship that involves belief, hope, commitment, and involvement is unsettling to many because it is not completely understood. Yet, this nurse practitioner felt quite comfortable about this even though she could not explain this phenomenon. She realized it existed and tried to make it work for her in patient care situations. She did not apologize for it, but simply accepted it and benefited from it when possible.

The competency "establishing a healing relationship" involves mobilizing hope for the nurse as well as the patient. The aspect of practical knowledge called *common meanings* helps clarify how nurses mobilize hope. Benner described "situated possibility," an example of a common meaning, which signifies that nurses recognize and enable possibilities in the self and the situation. This aspect of practical knowledge gives the nurse the vision for the proposed trajectory of mutually constructed outcomes and sets up the situation for a healing transaction to occur.

Several illustrations of this phenomenon of mobilizing hope for the nurse as well as the patient were described in Brykczynski's (1985) research. The ability to interpret "stability" or "maintaining the status quo" as indicative of a positive achievement or outcome in a long-term complex multiproblem situation is one way a nurse practitioner remains hopeful and committed to a patient's care. This is illustrated by the following situation where a nurse practitioner explains that she has learned to accept that there are certain things that are not going to change about people's lives and sometimes behavior may change to the point of being less destructive even if it's not optimal; maybe that's the best that a person can do at that time. She looks for positive achievements in a persons' lives that help her connect with them and allow for a healing relationship to develop, as she describes in the following excerpt referring to a patient who was the mother of one of the clinic staff:

I've always liked her and despite the fact that she's been real destructive in her life, she's done some very positive things in her life, too. I mean she's raised a family; she still takes care of her grandchildren. Her kids are really crazy about her. She has a husband who's an alcoholic, as she is, and she constantly talks about leaving him, but they've been together for many years and I suspect that she'll continue to talk about him and how she is going to leave him and maybe she won't. So, I don't know, I mean maybe I don't have any expectations as such, except to just sort of be there—you know to provide a service. Maybe if I set low expectations then I can't be disappointed . . . But also, I guess her behavior at this point is less destructive than it has been in the past. I mean the alcohol is not good, but it's better than IV heroin and she seems to have a certain stability in her life that makes her functional.

In mentioning "being there" as a nurse to "provide a service," this nurse practitioner brings up a very significant component of the healing relationship: she is being there for the patient, sensing her needs and tailoring the expectations for the patient's situated possibility while at the same time mobilizing and maintaining her own energy and belief in continuing to work with this woman by seeing stability as positive and alcohol as less destructive than IV heroin. This nurse practitioner has been the primary care provider for this woman for many years. She can point to several successes, such as the fact that she no longer takes IV drugs, she successfully recovered from a life-threatening episode of pneumonia following the nurse practitioner's prompt, accurate assessment and intervention, and she now has a certain stability in her life.

Several of the nurse practitioners in Brykczynski's (1985) study mentioned that one of the ways they maintain and mobilize hope in themselves as well as in their patients is by recognizing that the phenomenon of "readiness to change, grow, or learn" varies over time. They have learned to bring up the topic of smoking or drinking alcohol every time they see a patient where it is an important factor. Patients may interpret a provider not mentioning these habits as evidence of condoning them. These nurse practitioners maintain their hope because they believe that when they bring up these habits some patients will be open to listening and changing and they don't really know when this will occur, so they always mention it when it is pertinent to the situation. They remain committed to this practice because if even once it helps, they feel it is worth it.

One nurse practitioner reported that one of her patients expressed his gratitude by presenting her with his 5-year sobriety medal from AA. He credited the nurse practitioner with motivating him to stop drinking. Even though the nurse practitioner tried to negate her part in the patient's successful behavior change and explained that the patient deserved the credit for being able to break that cycle of dependence, the patient insisted that if it were not for the nurse practitioner's belief in him and his ability to change he would not have tried to stop. This is a powerful example of the potential impact of mobilizing hope.

Another example of mobilizing hope that creates a climate for healing was evidenced by a situation where a nurse practitioner (who normally worked in the GI clinic, but was helping out in the General Episodic Medical Clinic one afternoon) helped a twenty-two-year-old single woman who felt immobilized by the crisis of an unintended pregnancy. The young woman was paralyzed with anxiety and the only thing she was sure about was that she did not want her parents to know she was pregnant. The nurse practitioner actively listened to the young woman's predicament, explored possible options with her, with attention to the specific details of her unique situation and careful consideration of the personal ramifications of the options available to her, obtained information about available resources for her, and encouraged and supported her to actively make her own decision. In the following excerpt, the nurse practitioner describes how she helped the woman sort out her feelings and thoughts. The nurse practitioner's attention to the lived experience of this crisis is apparent in her account of the situation as follows:

Investigator: You said she was really very upset. Did you see any kind of cues or did you pick up anything that gave you the impression that this sorting out of her feelings was of assistance to her?

Nurse Practitioner: Well, I think she was calmer when she left and she said, "That's what I need to do. I need to sit down and think about this." And I explained to her that she is the one who is ultimately responsible—that she has to make this decision for herself regardless of what the sister, the ex-boyfriend, or her parents think or anyone else. I think she felt a little—to me she looked like her mind was really clicking whereas when she came in she just looked really frazzled.

Investigator: I wonder being only 22, how many times she's ever had to really make an important decision like that.

Nurse Practitioner: Oh, we talked about that, too—that she was young and it was a very difficult decision for her to make. But it wasn't something that she could just trust to her whim. She couldn't just get involved in anxiety and allow the pregnancy to go beyond a point when abortion wouldn't be available to her. She had the opportunity and the resources to do something about it. So she had to think about it—NOW. And she had a place in deciding what was going to happen and she had to be active in that process.

The nurse practitioner personalized the situation to this particular young woman by recognizing that she had little experience in making significant decisions in her life. The nurse practitioner did not try to "take over" and solve the problem for the young woman nor did she thrust the problem back to her to deal with alone, instead she spent time with her exploring possibilities and supporting her ability to make the best decision for herself. The nurse practitioner's ability to counsel this young woman was enhanced by her nursing knowledge, as well as her personal experience with pregnancy (the nurse practitioner was pregnant at the time and this was a factor in triaging this patient to her). She was aware of the significant changes that having a baby can make in someone's life. This encounter transformed the patient's situation from a woman immobilized and in crisis to a woman who, now fully understanding the available options, can reach her own decision that she will be able to live with.

Transition from Helping to Healing

Brykczynski's interpretive research of skilled nursing practices important to healing began with further delineation of aspects of practical knowledge and expansion of competencies in Benner's domain of The Helping Role of the Nurse. The education committee of the National Organization of Nurse Practitioner Faculties (NONPF) used Brykczynski's nurse practitioner adaptation of Benner's domains and competencies of nursing practice to develop national guidelines for nurse practitioner curricula (Zimmer et al., 1990). A draft of the guidelines was presented for discussion at the annual meeting of the organization in 1989 and feedback was received from nurse practitioners and nurse practitioner educators across the country. At the NONPF annual meeting in April 1989, the suggestion to change the name of the Domain: "The Helping Role of the Nurse" to "The Healing Role of the Nurse" was made and adopted. It was felt that the term "healing" was more robust and descriptive than the term "helping."

In Brykczynski's research, nurse practitioners described their approach to patients as personal, egalitarian, collaborative, and involving mutuality. The personal approach to care is not just simply friendly, rather it has implications in terms of the accuracy of diagnoses and the success of outcomes. The careful history of the present illness is variously touted as eliciting the correct diagnosis in 70 percent to 98 percent of clinical situations. The more comfortable patients feel the more likely they will be to disclose concerns about what is really bothering them. A nurse practitioner describes her approach to patients as follows:

> I try to spend a lot of time with patients; treat them very individually; do a lot of patient education; and help them calm down and make them more comfortable when they're here. I make a real effort to let them know who I am and give them my phone number and tell them to call me if they have questions or problems.

Research examples such as these help decipher the process behind the outcome in clinical care. Further study to understand and document these practices that nurses employ which make patients feel more comfortable is needed.

EXEMPLARS OF HEALING PRACTICES

Lewis (1992) was interested in healing and conducted a study to further expand understanding of the healing role of the nurse practitioner for her master's thesis. Her research question was: What healing practices do nurses engage in and how do they create a climate for healing? She used the Domain: "The Healing Role of the Nurse" as adapted by NONPF (Zimmer et al., 1990) for a portion of the interpretation of the narrative data collected in her study. An aspect of practical knowledge that Lewis identified in her study was the maxim "Healing begins with listening." Healing was described as listening, attending, and presencing—being with the patient. An exemplar illustrating this maxim involved a 27-year-old man who had been experiencing episodes of severe chest pain for several months. The nurse practitioner relates:

> Here's an example of how important listening is. This guy had been in and out of emergency rooms and spent thousands of dollars on tests and EKGs and various other things . . . He ended up here out of frustration and exhaustion. I saw him in the ambulatory clinic after the ER triaged him over. He presented with his mother. I remember walking into the room and seeing that they were frustrated, scared, and upset about the fact that he was having all this severe pain. With all the money spent and all the tests having been done, nobody knew what was wrong with him, and no one was able to fix it at this point. I did the same thing with him as far as listening as I do for all my

patients. I put the chart down and didn't look at it. I had him start at the very beginning. He had six or eight months of these periodic bouts of severe squeezing chest pain. His mother was sitting over there almost in tears thinking he's going to die.

After listening, I tried to summarize what he had told me to validate the story. Finally, I looked at him and said, "What are you concerned about?" His mother answered, "We're concerned about his heart. We think he's having a heart attack." My first statement was, "If it was a heart attack, he'd be dead by now, and they could have found that out on all these EKGs they were doing. Obviously, it's not that because they've been stone cold normal." Just then you could see the relief in her face—like nobody had ever said that or brought it down to that level. They were like, "Whew! I feel better already."

We then started working through the possibilities, and I introduced the idea of esophageal spasms being in his chest with squeezing tight pain. He looked at me and said, "That sounds exactly like what's going on!" Taking time to listen to his story made the whole thing come together. I remember the tension that they came in the room with and the relief they went out with, which was a significant difference. It was just like healing had occurred, and they felt better immediately.

As this narrative excerpt illustrates, it was not some special test or secret strategy the nurse practitioner used to understand this patient's situation, but rather taking the time to really listen and comprehend the lived experience of this patient's symptoms. This excerpt also depicts "the straight talk" often evidenced in dialogue between nurse practitioners and their patients. She "tells it like it is" by stating that he would be dead already if it had been his heart all this time. This honest, direct communication on the patient's level was immediately effective in relieving both his and his mother's anxiety. Instead of simply stating that all the tests were negative and nothing could be found to account for his symptoms and sending him on his way, the nurse practitioner acknowledges the patient's experience thereby validating him as a person, but explains that it could not be his heart given the history of the situation. She then goes on to explore with the patient what could possibly be going on to account for his symptoms. This encounter was transformative for the patient and his mother in that they were no longer fearful of his imminent death. The nurse practitioner recalled that she prescribed an antispasmodic medication for him and referred him to a primary care physician for follow-up, but she did not receive any further feedback.

"Responsible risk taking" was a new competency that Lewis identified in the domain of the Healing Role of the Nurse. Of particular interest here is that the skilled healing practice of "personal persuasion" described by Brykczynski (1985) was further delineated and extended by Lewis.

"Personal persuasion" was initially described as an especially complex healing practice which must not be confused with officious, impersonal paternalistic persuasion. In relating situations involving personal persuasion, nurse practitioners in both studies used the metaphor of the heart saying that they were convinced in their hearts of their interpretation of the situation and this in turn provided the moral courage to pursue the appropriate course of action in the situation. Personal persuasion involves commitment and involvement along with mutual trust and vulnerability. In such situations, the nurse practitioner responds more as if the patient were one of her own family members. The close, intimate nature of the relationship is central to the effectiveness of this practice. The nurse's personal, contextual, and holistic understanding of the particular situation is what makes it *constructive* instead of *controlling* because the intervention is developed in active mutuality with the patient (Kritek, 1994).

Responsible risk taking as described by Lewis, requires moral courage to pursue a course of treatment or intervention in the face of uncertainty or doubt. It incorporates responsibility and accountability for the decision-making process as well as the ultimate choices made on behalf of the patient. It is a conscious decision by a nurse to take a calculated risk in order to effect changes in health outcomes.

An example of a situation that illustrates responsible risk taking from Lewis' study is evidenced in the following excerpt where a nurse practitioner speaks plainly and directly to a young girl with a brain tumor who was denying her poor prognosis:

> *I was trying to get one little girl to go to summer camp. She was reluctant, and I said "Go. You will have the time of your life. It's not overly regimented." She answered "But I don't want to be around all those other kids." I told her "You are one of those other children. It's like you're here and they're there, but that's not so."*
>
> *She didn't say anything right away. I think she needed to know that this is something she will be dealing with for the remainder of her life.*

The nurse practitioner felt the need to be forthright and honest about the young girl's need to face her situation so she could take advantage of opportunities such as summer camp for children with cancer. The nurse practitioner was committed and concerned about promoting the best possible experience for this girl. It took courage for her to risk the young girl's anger as she confronted her denial and used her close personal relationship with the girl to try to convince her to attend the camp. The nurse practitioner reported that the girl decided to go to camp and had a very positive experience.

Several situations involving "personal persuasion" from Brykczynski's research constitute powerful exemplars of this more fully delineated competency "responsible risk taking." When reinterpreted in this way they help us understand the mutuality of decision making more clearly. In the following excerpt the nurse practitioner describes her interaction with a woman (the mother of one of the clinic employees) who was very ill with pneumonia and needed to be hospitalized, but was adamant about refusing to be hospitalized. The nurse practitioner relates:

> *After sitting there and thinking about it for a while, I finally went back into the room and told her, "Listen, I know you want to go home, but if you were my mother, I'd make you stay." And I said, "You know you could die from pneumonia. Not only that—there's no one at home to take care of you." And I told her that I couldn't force her to stay, but that I absolutely thought she should stay and be admitted. So she said, "Well, all right."*

Here is another example of the nurse practitioner using direct, honest communication on the patient's level. The intimate, personal nature of their long-term relationship, characterized by mutual trust, is evident in the nurse practitioner's personalization of this situation.

There is a complex balancing involved in promoting autonomy while at the same time upholding the principle of beneficence without being overly paternalistic or maternalistic. Because care providers are skilled at recognizing significant illness in patients, they sometimes find themselves in situations where they must use their influence to provide appropriate care for patients whose limits of knowledge and understanding at the time may result in autonomous wishes that are harmful to them. Anxiety, for example, often impedes understanding in illness situations. The context of the specific situation provides the key to understanding the situation and dictates the appropriate action as it did in this instance. The nurse practitioner continues her description of how the situation unfolded:

> *So we got her ready for admission and actually she was getting worse and we started IVs and sent her over to the hospital with oxygen. At*

that point she was feeling so bad that she didn't much care about not wanting to be hospitalized. Well, the lab reports showed that her blood cultures were positive for bacteremia, her potassium was very low, and she was dehydrated. And not only was she admitted, but the next day she was transferred to the ICU. On the third day she had delirium tremens even though she claimed she hadn't been drinking at all. So I realized afterwards that if she'd gone home she might have died. I thought about that when I got home at night and just sort of started trembling because there was a point when I wasn't going to hospitalize her against her wishes. My consulting physician had agreed that she could go home on oral antibiotics and the only thing that really convinced me was that I knew that she wasn't very healthy.

The nurse practitioner commented that this situation showed the significance of having some kind of continuity with patients. She had a sense of this woman's overall condition, her living situation, she knew her and her family well, she could see that she was very sick, and she had established a relationship with her over time so that her recommendation for hospitalization was accepted by the patient who in turn knew the nurse practitioner well and realized that she cared about her and was concerned for her overall well-being as a person. This situation was transformative for both the patient and the nurse practitioner. The nurse practitioner related that on a follow-up visit after discharge from the hospital, they shared the meaning of that situation where the woman had said "Hello" to death.

Another example follows where a nurse practitioner recognized that a patient's wishes were incompatible with safe care. The nurse practitioner states:

A woman with diabetes refused to have anything to do with insulin. I pointed out that she now had hemorrhages in her eyes and that her blood sugar was out of control. I told her that I just couldn't do it any other way. I just had to recommend insulin. She insisted that she didn't want insulin. I said, "I'm going to write it down here in the chart and I want you to sign it that you don't want insulin." Then she said, "Well, let me think about it and ask you some questions... What if I want to sleep late on Saturday morning? What if ...? What if ...?" So I just asked her to wait until she was ready and she took the insulin and called me a week later and said, "I feel so good."

This is another example where a concerned and committed approach to the patient results in the nurse practitioner risking making the patient angry by going against her expressed wishes. In both situations, the quality of the nurse patient relationship was very personal and not officious or authoritarian. There was a lack of professional distancing and a real commitment to helping the patient understand the reality of the ramifications of her chosen actions.

The nurse practitioner used the concrete measure of requesting that the patient sign a note in her chart that she would not take insulin in order to convince the patient of the danger of her preferred course of action and how seriously concerned the nurse practitioner was about it. This strategy was effective in requiring that the patient actively commit herself to refusing insulin and not allowing her to continue to sit back and simply passively refuse to take insulin. In this situation the nurse practitioner skillfully coached the patient to experience the difference between passive inaction and active commitment to a choice thereby enabling the patient to choose the necessary treatment.

The nurse practitioner's strategy proved to be successful in this instance and the patient responded well to the treatment that they both came to accept as necessary in this situation. The nurse practitioner assessed that failure to use insulin would very likely be life threatening and at the very least would contribute to further secondary complications. It is important to point out that this strategy was appropriate and effective in this situation, but it should not be taken out of context and applied as a routine measure in the care of diabetics. A discrete sense of timing involving the ability to notice patient readiness to change and the presence of a trusting relationship are essential for implementing such an intervention.

A final exemplar that illustrates a different aspect of the competency of responsible risk taking is described by a nurse practitioner who was so sure that there was something seriously wrong with a patient who complained of back pain that she argued with a prestigious physician about the necessity of sending an ambulance to bring him to the hospital to be examined. When asked about how she could be so confident in her assessment, she replied:

Nurse Practitioner: I've always had confidence in knowing when there's something wrong with somebody, but what nurse practitioning has done is give me the history and physical skills so that I can figure it out myself.

Investigator: So your confidence in your ability to sense that something is wrong really developed a long time ago.

Nurse Practitioner: Yes. And learning to argue with doctors . . . I really do believe that you learn from confrontation and negative experiences as well as positive ones. It broke the rules around here because nobody ever argued with an attending physician before. It wasn't easy to do that.

In this situation, the nurse practitioner had examined the patient at an earlier date and felt that further evaluation of his condition was beyond her expertise. The patient was transported to the outpatient clinic by ambulance and was seen by a physician as the nurse practitioner had requested. However, the patient was sent home by the physician after the examination. The man's wife called the nurse practitioner back the next day and asked what they should do now. The nurse practitioner and the wife both sensed that there was something really wrong with the patient. Fortunately, he had an appointment that day at another facility and the nurse practitioner advised them to go there.

They went to the other facility where the man was admitted and cancer was subsequently diagnosed. This situation illustrates that the nurse practitioner's concern and advocacy for the patient takes precedence over her allegiance to her institution. After this incident, the nurse practitioner arranged a meeting with the attending physician and they discussed the situation. She reported that they both learned from it and have developed mutual respect for one another.

This situation shows a real collaborative relationship between the nurse practitioner and this couple. The nurse practitioner and the wife were united in their assessment of the gravity of the man's situation. The wife felt comfortable enough to call the nurse practitioner back to try to determine what to do. They were both sure something serious was wrong. The wife had faith in the nurse practitioner and the nurse practitioner risked ridicule, social chastisement, and possible dismissal from her position by advocating for this man and his wife. This example serves to extend the competency of responsible risk taking to include situations of conflict over possible courses of action. In this situation the nurse practitioner and the couple were united, and instead of risking anger on the patient's part as in previous examples, the nurse practitioner risked the anger of her peers, other healthcare providers, and hospital administrators.

There is overlap between and among the aspects of practical knowledge and the domains and competencies of nursing practice. Exemplars of aspects of practical knowledge often relate to a variety of competencies just as exemplars of competencies often contain various illustrations of aspects of practical knowledge. The three exemplars of the competency responsible risk taking from Brykczynski (1985) also constitute exemplars of the maxim "real disease declares itself." The interpretations are interrelated in a holistic fashion, yet they can be differentiated for heuristic purposes. They are not intended to be decontextualized and abstracted out into rigid classifications to form lists divorced from the situational context. Understanding of interpretive accounts is enhanced by the accompanying presentation of narrative excerpts of the situational context. This is so because their meanings are embedded in whole situations and decontexualization may produce distortion.

DISCUSSION

Gadow's (1980a) concept of existential advocacy provides a useful perspective for interpreting the exemplars described here. Existential advocacy is defined by Gadow (1980a) as the nurse's participation with the patient in discerning the personal meaning which the particular situation is to have for that individual. The nurse and the patient become engaged in a joint endeavor to reach a shared understanding of the situation and the available options. Gadow (1980b) describes the nurse as the "mediator between the abstract, objective medical assessment of the benefit and the personal understanding of benefit which the patient possesses" (p. 47). She explains that "the nurse assists patients to develop as fully as possible that unique existential knowledge of their situation that medicine cannot provide" (p. 47).

Gadow (1983) further characterizes existential advocacy as a partnership model. The advocacy partnership involves helping patients "become clear about what they want in relation to a clinical situation; assistance in discerning and clarifying patients' own beliefs, values, and goals; then help in examining available courses of action" (p. 65). This model involves trying out "how best to participate with patients in defining their situation, that is, in constituting their personal truth" (p. 67). The nurse *enables* patients to see possibilities in the situation rather than merely *allowing* patients to constitute their personal meaning of the situation. Thus, the nurse's role as partner is directed toward overcoming the initial inequality inherent in the professional nurse-patient relationship "by assisting patients to be self-determining rather than to conform because of habit, deference, or inexperience" (p. 67).

The exemplars of healing practices presented here constitute clinical situations from actual nursing practice that illustrate Gadow's (1980a) concept of existential advocacy and validate and extend understanding of Benner's (1984) aspects of practical knowledge, domains, and competencies of nursing practice. These examples open a window of understanding on the processes of "being with"—of presencing oneself in the lived experience of the patient's world and trying out ways to participate with patients in making decisions and learning to live with their particular health and illness situations.

CONCLUSION

Enhanced understanding of healing practices of nurses will bring to open discourse aspects of nursing care that have been largely covered over and not acknowledged explicitly. Once identified, such healing practices can be studied to contribute to knowledge development. The exemplars presented here extend our knowledge of some of the complex processes of nursing practice. By identifying and describing exemplars of healing practices, we can learn from our nursing practice and develop creative ways to manage problematic clinical situations where there is provider-patient incongruence regarding treatment options. The skill of successfully resolving interdisciplinary conflict between providers is perhaps even more complex and in need of continued study and development. Interpretive phenomenological research can be valuable in further developing understanding of a broad range of clinical practices.

REFERENCES

Benner, P. E. (1984). *From novice to expert. Excellence and power in clinical nursing practice.* Menlo Park: Addison-Wesley.

Brykczynski, K. A. (1985). Exploring the clinical practice of nurse practitioners. (Doctoral dissertation, University of California San Francisco, School of Nursing). *Dissertation Abstracts International, 46,* 3789B. (University Microfilms No. DA8600592).

Gadow, S. (1980a). Existential advocacy: Philosophical foundation of nursing. In S. F. Spicker & S. Gadow (Eds.), *Nursing. Images and ideals* (pp. 79-101). New York: Springer.

Gadow, S. (1980b). A model for ethical decision making. *Oncology Nursing Forum, 7*(4), 44-47.

Gadow, S. (1983). Basis for nursing ethics: Paternalism, consumerism, or advocacy? *Hospital Progress*, 62–67, 78.

Lewis, P. H. (1992). *Exploring the healing role of the nurse practitioner.* (Master's thesis. The University of Texas Medical Branch at Galveston, School of Nursing). (University Microfilms No. 1350919).

Kritek, P. (1994). *Healing, a central nursing construct.* Unpublished Doctoral Program White Paper. The University of Texas Medical Branch School of Nursing, Galveston, TX.

Zimmer, P., Brykczynski, K. A., Martin, A., Newberry, Y., Price, M., & Warren, B. (1990). *Advanced nursing practice: Nurse practitioner curriculum guidelines.* Seattle, WA: National Organization of Nurse Practitioner Faculties.

CHAPTER 46

A New Paradigm for Promoting Healing in Communities

DONNA L. MORRIS, RN, CNM, DRPH

I have spent the better part of my career in nursing either practicing in the community, teaching students about the community, or testing health service delivery models in the community. My doctoral preparation was in public health. Until in preparing this chapter I attempted to identify my convictions about the promotion of healing in communities, I thought, rather smugly, that I knew a lot about working in communities. I, the dedicated, well-intentioned, middle-class, educated Anglo woman, had the "answers." It was only after I struggled with a definition of what a healthy community was that I realized that I had accumulated many experiences; that I had learned much about the varying characteristics, organizations, politics, and people of communities; that I had even learned reasons why some interventions "succeeded" while others "failed"; but I was no longer clear about how to define a healthy community. I could repeat others' descriptions of what contributes to health, but those definitions focused on only a small segment of health, much like a few pieces in a much larger and more complex puzzle.

We commonly describe the "health" of a community by quoting morbidity and mortality statistics; the change in the infant mortality rate and other leading causes of death have been used to represent how well the community is combating disease. Immunization rates and time of entry into prenatal care are used to demonstrate progress in the prevention of disease. These data are important criteria and they are measurable. However, can we say that the people in a community are healthy simply because fewer of them become ill from infectious diseases or that they die less frequently from chronic diseases or violent causes? Lelonde (in Norris & Lampe, 1994) reported that "human health status depends 50 percent on lifestyle and behavior, 20 percent on environment and socioeconomic class, 20 percent on heredity, and 10 percent on medical care and access"

(p. 5). Norris and Lampe, in their discussion entitled "Healthy Communities, Healthy People," argued that in order "to address health in a meaningful way, we must redefine what health is and consider the relationship between wellness and key components of our living and working environments" (p. 5). I would take that one step further and suggest that we must also consider the individual's perspective of his or her state of health, wellness, or illness, the "quality of life," and the degree to which that individual is experiencing an "expanding consciousness and awareness" (Newman, 1993).

As a society we are beginning to realize that health is much more than the absence of illness; that health is a resource used to enhance our lives (Ottawa Charter, 1986). Miller (cited in Labonte, 1993) defines health as "the increased becoming of what we are most deeply." Weil (1995) describes healing as " 'making whole'—that is, restoring integrity and balance" (p. 6). Labonte (1993) conducted a series of workshops with health professionals, during which he asked them to construct "phrases describing a recent time they felt 'healthy' and a recent time they experienced 'community' " (p. 19). Participant descriptions of health included: "(1) feeling vital, full of energy, (2) having good social relationships, (3) experiencing a sense of control over one's life and one's living conditions, (4) being able to do things one enjoys, (5) having a sense of purpose in life, and (6) experiencing a connectedness to 'community.' " Their experiences of community included: "commitment, connectedness, shared values, discipline, action, sharing/caring, openness, belonging, loved/loving, respectful, working hard, having a purpose, predictability, equitable, fair, [and] fun." These phrases do not state that one must be free from illness or disease in order to experience "health" and "community." It seems to me that they refer more to the "quality of life." As I wrote, I began to realize that our approach to promoting community health has been heavily influenced by the medical perspective. Weil (1995) stated that "a major focus of scientific medicine has been the identification of external agents of disease and the development of weapons against them. An outstanding success in the middle of this century was the discovery of antibiotics and, with that, great victories against infectious diseases caused by bacteria. This success was a major factor in . . . convincing most people that medical intervention with the products of technology was worth it, no matter the cost" (p. 4). Our vision of health of the individual and the community has been influenced by the dominant scientific paradigm, a paradigm that more and more contemporary citizens, healthcare providers, and scientists are beginning to challenge.

To measure "quality of life," "expanding consciousness," or "the restoring of integrity and balance" presents additional challenges for those working in and with communities. If we are indeed aware of a higher order of existence, it may be difficult to articulate, let alone to measure or quantify. How, for example, do we measure the degree to which people feel happy, fulfilled, purposeful, or in control of their environment? We will need to explore modified and perhaps, new, ways of describing health or healing in a community.

EXTERNAL FORCES AFFECTING COMMUNITY PARTNERSHIPS

As professionals, we may be thwarted in our work with communities by the very organizing frameworks to which we subscribe. As nurses, we have been socialized to use the nursing process as a basis for practice. Although that process implies patient involvement, it does not necessarily incorporate the patient as a "partner," an active and equal participant in the process. In addition, Western medicine encourages health professionals to start with the assumption that a problem exists, and to "fix" it at whatever cost and with whatever means are available. This mentality can easily be interpreted by a community as paternalism. We may be seen as the self-appointed authorities, the "outsiders" who presume to know the solutions or answers to *their* problems (as we have identified them). Labonte (1989) suggests that "our role as health professionals in community health promotion is to remove what obstacles we can that impede the process of community empowerment. The first obstacle we can remove is our own need to define health problems for the community. The power of defining health must belong to those experiencing it" (pp. 24–25).

As health service researchers in the community, we may face funding requirements that place additional impediments in the way of promoting a partnership with the community. Funding is generally granted to the project that most successfully convinces reviewers of the severity of the problem or problems faced by a community and the efficacy of the interventions to be employed in ameliorating and/or resolving those problems. This approach assumes that: (1) funding is attainable only by demonstrating weaknesses and deficiencies in a community; (2) funding is more likely to be granted if interventions are aimed at specific problems, for example, increasing the proportion of women who receive cervical cancer screening; and (3) extensive preliminary work has been accomplished with the community in establishing priorities and intervention plans prior to submission of a proposal for funding.

Several problems are inherent with these assumptions. As Labonte (1989) so aptly wrote, the concept "'community' has become essential to all our actions. Unfortunately, we tend to define 'community' in the static vocabulary of data: the poor community, the unemployed community, the black community, the native community, the women's community. We define it by geography. . . . Although community has elements of both affinity and geography, it is much more. . . . Community embodies the quality of sharing; . . . the dynamic act existing in the reality of people being together" (p. 24). Labonte went on to state that "we consistently presume [that] our major task is to motivate individuals and groups to take greater responsibility for their health. We define their deficiencies, and calculate how we might manipulate them into acting in ways we think best. We deny people choice and, intentionally or by accident, subtly or blatantly, rob them of their own capacity for power" (p. 24). McKnight (1995) and Kretzman and McKnight (1993) argue that this approach that emphasizes the community's problems and ignores its assets perpetuates a community identity of deficiency, powerlessness, and dependency upon health or other professionals to modify the condition or conditions. They, instead, recommend that we approach communities from an assets-based approach, where the strengths of the individuals, families, organizations and various sectors of the community are identified and these community members (however community is defined by them) become actively involved in the process of planning for the future.

Second, to aim interventions at a specific problem identified by the funding agency (for example, increasing mammography screening in an attempt to reduce mortality from breast cancer) is to ignore the priorities within the community, and the complexity and interaction of issues and conditions between all sectors of the community. Wainwright (in Anderson & McFarlane, 1995) describes her work with a rural Arkansas community made up of middle class, somewhat conservative, white residents. According to the traditional data used to assess health issues within a community, she noted an unusually high teen pregnancy rate. In her work with community leaders, she recognized that a program focus on the prevention of teen pregnancy was neither recognized as a priority nor considered socially acceptable by community residents. Providing accessible and safe prenatal care for teens once they were pregnant was, however, seen as an important objective. Thus, a successful plan was initiated by the community to assist pregnant teens. Several

years later, community participants identified the prevention of pregnancy as a priority and moved to develop a strategy to address the issue.
Had Wainwright pushed for an intervention program to promote family
planning or other prevention programs among teenagers to address the
priorities she assumed to be most important or those of a funding
agency, she potentially would have jeopardized the whole program with
subsequent loss of community support and participation.

Finally, it is certainly desirable and, in almost all cases, critical to the
long-term success of community interventions, that we as investigators
have worked with individuals and groups to identify priorities and plans of
action prior to submitting funding proposals. However, in reality, requests
for proposals frequently are submitted to potential grantees with very little
notice of the intent of proposals sought and a brief turn around time for receipt of proposals. Rather than work closely with communities to develop
proposals, we as investigators sometimes write and submit proposals with
limited input from the community in order to meet funding agency dead-
lines and our own needs to "conduct" community projects.

INTERNAL FORCES AFFECTING COMMUNITY PARTNERSHIPS

As specialists in community health practice, we naturally bring our own
biases with us as we approach communities. Our motives may be sincere
and usually have something to do with bringing additional resources into
the community and working with the community so that its members will
become more empowered. Inherent in our role as specialists and consultants is the built-in prejudice that we have something important to offer
to the community, that we may even have the "answers" or "solutions" to
their problems. We, and they, may be seduced into believing that we can
tell them, in fact, how to "fix" their problems.

Not only does this approach undermine the development of independence, leadership, creativity, initiative, and empowerment among community residents, but it also perpetuates the myth that we as experts have all
the answers, that all communities are alike, that the same solutions will
work in every community, and that change can occur without the commitment and participation of community members. This leads to an exploration of the concept of community participation versus community
involvement. Involvement has been described (Labonte, 1993) as a process in which the agent (for example, the researcher or community health
consultant) or those representing an agency maintain control over the

planning and implementation of the project, with little input from or formal decision-making authority by community representatives. Community participation, on the other hand, is seen as a more active process, with a shared decision-making authority among community and other "outside" participants. In other words, those who will be affected by the project or program are key to the process and share in the power and control.

The problems and subsequent interventions identified through this process are more likely to be "owned" by community residents, and integrated into their ongoing activities. Ultimately, the chance of successfully resolving the problems, or in the proposed new vernacular, of maximizing and expanding the strengths and assets of the community, is increased. The process itself, in addition to the desired outcomes, may be central to promoting healing in a community. How, then do we move from an agency-sponsored and controlled effort to one that is more collaborative, one in which all partners are recognized to possess and/or are allowed to develop skills at effective negotiations, and to develop their own destinies; a process in which partners, both community and agency, have equal power to influence the process and the outcome?

Negotiating Successful Alliances

Negotiating successful alliances, then, becomes essential to the promotion of healing in communities. Kanter (1994) studied business partnerships all over the world in an attempt to understand the critical elements involved in producing a successful alliance. She wrote that "Intercompany relationships . . . seem to work best when they are more familylike and less rational. Obligations are more diffuse, the scope for collaboration is more open, understanding grows between specific individuals, communication is frequent and intensive, and the interpersonal context is rich" (p. 100). Although Kanter's discussion was focused on business partnerships, many of the elements which her research identified seem to apply equally well in community settings. For example, she emphasized the importance of each partner's clear understanding of how their organization would benefit from the partnership, the fact that the partners have complementary assets and skills, and that no one partner can accomplish the long-term objectives alone. The partners make a commitment to the relationship through financial or other resource investment, formal recognition of the partnership, with clear responsibilities and decision processes; and open and honest communication among the various partners (Kanter, 1994).

Key to the success of the alliance is the shared definition of collaboration reached by the partners. Gray (cited in Labonte, 1993) defined successful intergroup collaboration as "a mutual search for information and solutions." Fielding (1995), in his discussion about the formation of public-private partnerships, indicated that "Even the strongest agencies recognized that they alone are unable to solve the multifactorial refractory health problems that account for a disproportionate share of our premature deaths, disability, and illness." The key may be in understanding that a successful collaborative effort involves a process, one in which each partner's contribution is valued (Kanter, 1994; Labonte, 1993); one which must be "nurtured" regularly through frequent, active exchange (Kanter, 1994); and one in which change is the major constant (Flynn, 1994).

Case Study Experiences

Between 1990 and the present time, my university colleagues and I, with the encouragement and financial support from state and federal agencies, have tested a variety of health service delivery models related to early detection and treatment of cervical cancer among women in communities along the Texas-Mexico border. Our approach has been community-based, with involvement of community leaders from the health, social, and business sectors. The program interventions included the identification and elimination of barriers to cervical cancer screening (Morris et al., 1990), continuing education for nurses to provide breast and cervical cancer screening (Morris et al., 1991), a collaborative agency model to provide evaluation and treatment for women with cervical dysplasia (Morris et al., 1991), and a model using nurse practitioner colposcopists to evaluate and treat cervical dysplasia (Morris et al., 1991). A variety of factors have contributed to the sustainability or lack of sustainability of the projects. In one community in which we worked with a community coalition to establish a cervical dysplasia clinic for indigent women, the coalition conducted a feasibility study to assess the need, collaborated to obtain funding, and jointly established a dysplasia clinic (Morris et al., 1991). After a couple of years, the majority of the key agency players changed, as a result of seeking other jobs and the sudden death of one agency head. Although the original clinic did not survive, the university has re-established the clinic in collaboration with a community agency and services are being offered in the community currently. In a second project (Morris et al., 1991), a program designed to remove reported barriers to Pap screening reported by Mexican-American women, another community coalition provided one-time Pap screening in settings located throughout the county and "vouchers" for no-cost Pap smears at participating agencies. Just over 300 women received Pap screening through the project, demonstrating their willingness to seek this form of preventive healthcare when adequately informed and provided access to the service. One year later and with no additional program intervention, 25 percent of these "hard to reach" women had obtained repeat Pap screening (Morris, Hannigan, Dayal, & McLean, 1992).

Our various projects have continued in some fashion, albeit to a limited extent in some cases. We have consistently worked with community coalitions (which we called community *advisory* boards), believing that the community was determining the course of action. In retrospect, we probably did not follow the guidelines for establishing effective alliances as described. Our conscious intentions allowed for active participation of the community partners. However, it is clear that our "vote" held more power than theirs in most cases, creating an unequal partnership. In some cases, the community agencies' priorities and agendas were different from ours. Our academically oriented goals (to explore a new way of offering services and to document and evaluate the outcomes of those programs) were not in conflict with the goals embraced by community participant agencies (to provide additional services to those in need of healthcare). However, the priorities we each assigned to accomplishing the project's goals were sometimes not in synchrony and had to be negotiated repeatedly; for example, our need to collect data and their need to provide service. Issues occasionally arose within the communities which affected the project. In more than one case, territoriality, or the need by one local agency to control aspects of the project without regard for the other agencies, resulted in disharmony among the community participants and had to be addressed. It is now clear to me that we (our academic group *and* the community groups) have been on a pathway of learning—primarily of how to create community-based, public-private-academic alliances that "work."

LESSONS FROM A SPECIAL CASE

One community, which I will call LaFrontera, stands out in my mind from the others, not only in its approach and its degree of commitment, but also in its inherent "culture." It is a community of around 130,000 individuals who are culturally and ethnically homogeneous, with the majority having a Mexican-American heritage. LaFrontera is located in a semi-arid area along the Rio Grande River and is geographically separated from other communities of any size except for its sister city in Mexico. LaFrontera has three international bridges connecting it with Mexico, and experiences significant flow of foot, auto, truck, and train traffic between Mexico and the United States. It is seen as a gateway between the two countries. Because of its geographic and social "isolation" from other Texas cities and its clearly defined boundaries, LaFrontera has a true sense of community, of being "close knit." In many respects, it functions much like a rural town, where everyone knows or is related to everyone else.

In our original work, my colleagues and I approached healthcare leaders from several communities, with information that an excessive proportion of women in their communities were dying unnecessarily from cervical cancer, and that moneys were available to address the problem. All of the communities, except LaFrontera, accepted the information and agreed with moderate enthusiasm to participate in the project. Unlike the other communities, health professionals in LaFrontera questioned the statistics, looked up the cases of women who had died and, in general, became concerned that women in *their* community were dying unnecessarily. They immediately recommended the formation of an Advisory Board to investigate the situation, with involvement of colleagues in the public and private sectors, the business community, and the schools. After their investigation, community participants agreed that the problem should be addressed.

One of the local hospitals, a religious institution, established a cervical dysplasia clinic, with medical input from the private sector, and assigned support staff from the hospital. A nurse practitioner was hired and sent to a colposcopy course so that she could assist the physician in providing the necessary follow-up evaluation and care for women. A referral network was developed and implemented. In addition, the Advisory Board agreed that an insufficient number of providers was prepared to provide breast and cervical cancer screening for indigent women. Thus, they requested that the university offer a continuing education course for local nurses. Not only did they participate in the planning and implementation of the course, but they also arranged for clinical experiences for course participants. A commitment to deal with the problem was evident from the beginning. Although the health agencies in the community did not always get along politically and, in fact, were feuding publicly over the division of services and who should receive health dollars, representatives from the agencies were able to leave their differences outside the door and sit down at the table to negotiate programs that were best for the community. Sometimes the agency heads didn't participate in the meetings, but they gave approval and support for the participation of their department directors.

Administrative hostilities were recognized but, surprisingly, were not a part of the discussions and negotiations involved in planning and implementing a project that would benefit members of the larger community. It is unclear to me how they were (and are) able to orchestrate this sense of cooperation.

The continuing education program planned by the Advisory Board was implemented through a collaborative effort between community participants and us as university representatives and was considered to be a success by the community. The Advisory Board members even requested additional continuing education, which we were unable to provide due to the lack of external funding.

Several years later, I was contacted by a LaFrontera funding agency and invited to develop a program proposal to submit to a larger private foundation. The LaFrontera agency was willing to provide matching funds for the project. Again, my colleagues and I convened an Advisory Board, with many of the same members as the original Advisory Board. After discussing the options, the Advisory Board members agreed that a mobile van was needed in order to provide healthcare to residents living in *colonias* outside of the city limits. The intent of the proposal was agreed upon, the methods were developed, the budget negotiated, and the proposal was submitted and subsequently funded. The Advisory Board has developed into a strong collaborative alliance which has realized that it can accomplish much more and has a better chance of sustaining the program as a partnership than as individual agencies. The coalition has readily pulled in additional community resources, such as the county judge and commissioners, the local department of transportation, the EMS (emergency medical service) members, the environmental health agency and, most importantly of all, the *colonias* residents. The religious hospital originally involved has continued its commitment to the dysplasia clinic and has expanded its support to include a variety of outreach activities in the community at large and in the *colonias,* in particular. It also provides laboratory and x-ray services for *colonias* residents. The community health center accepts outpatient referrals from the project, and the hospital negotiates with local physicians for specialist and inpatient care as needed.

I do not want to portray this project as a utopia, for it is not. It has experienced the normal start-up delays, difficulties in hiring and retaining staff, and territorial disputes typical of any community-based project. However, there are indications that this community is moving along a pathway of healing. Disputes are being resolved in a mature, caring manner, with respect for the ultimate goal. *Colonias* residents are actively participating in the project. They have planned fund raising, consciousness raising and health screening events for their communities. Their advisory board selected the additional sites to locate the mobile health clinic and they determine whether the mobile van may be used for other activities. Residents are beginning to take responsibility for promoting their own health; for example, several women in one of the *colonias* have initiated a walking program. Both *colonias* residents and other participants in the coalition are beginning to look toward their own inner resources, to evidence an expansion of their own consciousness, a sign of healing.

If we look back, then, and try to determine what is different about the community of LaFrontera, and what has moved them further along this continuum of healing, the indicators are "soft" and difficult to measure. There is a commitment to a higher goal, a sincere effort to promote open and honest communication and equalized power among the participants, a recognized value to each partner's contributions, and a sense of "nurturing" of the partnerships and the project. We, as academicians/researchers/community health "specialists," have worked to support the process unfolding within the community at large. It has truly been an experience of growth and, to a large extent, healing on our part. We are still learning how to be good partners; how to support community efforts without expecting to control them; how to step back and "allow" (and accept) the development of community leadership and ownership; and how to recognize, accept and support their growing sense of empowerment within the community.

It is too soon to know whether more children are getting immunized or more individuals are receiving screening for cancer or diabetes or hypertension. It is too soon to know whether fewer babies will die during the first year of life. But it is not too soon to know that a process has been initiated in this community. Perhaps it was already in motion prior to this program, and we happened along at an appropriate moment to help nurture its continuation and to become a part of its momentum. We as individuals and as a group have moved a little further toward "health" in a true qualitative sense.

REFERENCES

Anderson, E. T., & McFarlane, J. M. (Eds.). (1995). *Community as partner: Theory and practice in nursing.* Philadelphia, PA: Lippincott-Raven Publishers.

Fielding, J. E. (1995). *Community health improvement and public-private part-nerships.* Background paper prepared for the Leadership Action Forum: Building bridges between public and private sectors for community health improvement, Atlanta.

Flynn, B. C. (1994, May/June). Partnerships for health. *Healthcare Forum Journal, 55-56,* 73.

Kanter, R. M. (1994, July/August). Collaborative advantage: The art of alliances. *Harvard Business Review,* 96-108.

Kretzman, J. P., & McKnight, J. L. (1993). *Building communities from the inside out. A path toward finding and mobilizing a community's assets.* Evanston, IL: Center for Urban Affairs and Policy Research Neighborhood Innovations Network, Northwestern University.

Labonte, R. (1989, March). Community and professional empowerment. *Canadian Nurse, 85,* 3, 22-28.

Labonte, R. (1993). *Practice frameworks.* Centre for Health Promotion, University of Toronto ParticipACTION, 1-2, 8-80.

McKnight, J. (1995). *The careless society. Community and its counterfeits.* New York: Basic Books.

Morris, D., Hannigan, E., Dayal, H., Moore, F., Selwyn, B., McCandless, R., & Rosenthal, J. (1990). *South Texas needs assessment final report.* Texas Cancer Council, Austin, TX.

Morris, D., Hannigan E. V., Dayal, H., & McLean, C. (1991). *Screening and treatment of cervical cancer in South Texas final report.* Texas Cancer Council, Austin, TX.

Morris, D. L., Hannigan, E. V., Dayal, H., & McLean, C. H. (1992). *Evaluation of screening and treatment of cervical cancer in South Texas.* The University of Texas Medical Branch, Galveston, TX.

Newman, M. (1993). Health as expanding consciousness. In J. Marchione (Ed.), *Notes on nursing theories.* Newbury Park, CA: Sage.

Norris, T., & Lampe, D. (1994, Summer-Fall). Healthy communities, healthy people. *National Civic Review,* 2-11.

Ottawa Charter for Health Promotion. (1986, November). An International Conference on Health Promotion: The Move towards a New Public Health, Ottawa, Ontario, Canada.

Styles, M. M. (1984). Reflections on collaboration and unification. *Image: The Journal of Nursing Scholarship, XVI,* Winter (1), 21-23.

Weil, A. (1995). *Spontaneous healing.* New York: Knopf.

CHAPTER 47

Adolescents and Young Adults and Violence

ROBERTA K. LEE, RN, DRPH, FAAN

Some years ago, a disease accounted for substantial morbidity and mortality in the United States and elsewhere. At the time of the Industrial Revolution, it became rampant in urban areas, especially among poor people who lived in substandard, crowded conditions and in ethnic and racial minority groups. Healthcare providers had little to offer in response. It was considered a social problem that was not amenable to prevention. Sanitariums were available for people with financial resources, quarantine was suggested for those without. That disease is tuberculosis. Prior to the 1940s, Chowder (1992) notes that America was gripped with the fear of acquiring this infection much as we fear becoming victims of violence today.

In this chapter, I will describe aspects of my work in the area of the epidemiology of violence and violent injury, and current thinking about strategies to reduce violence. I have used one model of healing (Figure 47.1) to consider a variety of issues and problems in the field of violence research and prevention (Labonte, 1992). I will focus specifically on research regarding victims and theoretical approaches to violence research, and will conclude with several recommendations I wish to propose.

Sources of Data

In public health, the current definition of violence or intentional injury includes deliberate self-harm (attempted suicide and suicide) and deliberate interpersonal injuries such as homicide, rape, and deaths associated

---

Based on a presentation given at Violence: Nursing Debates the Issues, American Academy of Nursing, Nov. 15-16, 1993, Washington, DC.

Personal	Small Group	Community Organization	Coalition Advocacy	Political Action
developmental casework	improving social support	developing local actions on community defined health issues	lobbying for healthier public policies	support for broad-based social movements
enhancing personal perceptions of control & power	promoting personal behavior change	critical community/ professional dialogue	achieving strategic consensus	creating vision of sustainable, preferred future
conflict resolution	conflict management	raising conflict to conscious level	collaboration and conflict resolution	enhancing participatory democracy
	empowerment			

FIGURE 47.1.   Healing.

with domestic altercations. In this chapter, *violence* includes all "behaviors by individuals that intentionally threaten, attempt, or inflict physical harm on others" (National Academy of Science, 1993), excluding deliberate self-harm. Violence includes all manner of assaults, regardless of whether injury occurs and regardless of the relationship between the assailant and the other person. This definition includes rape, family and intimate assault, assault and homicide, child abuse (including child sexual abuse), elder abuse, and firearm injuries. At a national level, there are two major sources of information regarding violent injuries. These are the National Centers for Disease Control (CDC) and the National Institutes of Justice (NIJ).

The CDC collects information regarding fatal injuries from our death registration system which provides information such as these:

- In 1991, 38,317 people died nationwide as a result of firearm injuries, including 17,986 homicides and 18,526 suicides (U.S. National Center for Health Statistics, 1993).
- Over the past thirty years, while suicide rates in the United States have decreased for those aged 45 and older, the rate for youth between the ages of 15 and 24 has nearly tripled (Alcohol, Drug Abuse, and Mental Health Administration, 1989).
- In 1990, firearms surpassed motor vehicle crashes to become the leading cause of injury mortality in Texas (Zane, Preece, Patterson,

& Svenkerud, 1991) and are projected to do so in the nation by the year 2004 (CDC, 1994).

Thus, at local state and national levels, we can characterize these deaths according to variables on which we have relatively complete data—age, race, sex, and place of residence. But, what about violent injuries that do not result in death?

At the national level, we have little information. The National Hospital Discharge Survey data is usually not coded in a manner that permits identifying the underlying cause of hospitalization, although some states are beginning to use the external cause codes (E-codes) in the *International Classification of Disease, 9th Edition.* While universal use of external cause codes would improve our ability to characterize violent injuries, this still excludes injuries that are serious enough to warrant medical attention but not serious enough to require hospitalization. And, as acuity levels mandating hospitalization have changed over time, it is impossible to make comparisons over time.

National surveys are another way to estimate the impact of violent injuries. However, between 1972 and 1990, the National Health Interview Survey did not include questions that would allow estimates of injuries according to external cause. The 1990 youth supplement to the Health Promotion and Disease Prevention Survey included this question: Have you carried a weapon to school in the past 30 days? The response surprised many people in the United States as one in five adolescents answered yes (CDC, 1990). Because of these limitations in our public health data, we look to other sources in order to gain a better understanding of violence. These sources include criminal justice and law enforcement agencies.

The NIJ implements a crime registration system (Uniform Crime Reports) based on reports to local police, similar in logic to our death registration system. The NIJ also conducts a survey of people's experiences as victims of crime. From those reports, we learn the following:

- Only 16 percent of adolescent rapes are committed by strangers (Massachusetts Department of Public Health, 1990).
- Only about half of criminal victimizations are reported to police (National Institutes for Justice, 1993).
- Victimization rates peak in the adolescent and young adult years for both males and females (National Institutes for Justice, 1993).

From these two major sources of national data, it is clear that violence, especially homicide, disproportionately affects minority youth who live in urban environments.

From other sources, we can make the following observations:

- 1.2 million households in the United States combine the risk factors of firearms and an unsupervised child in the home (Lee & Sacks, 1990).

- Studies of firearm injuries in Galveston County, Texas, have yielded the following findings: 12 percent to 14 percent of people who died as a result of firearm suicide attempts bought the weapon the same day they committed suicide; the overall incidence rate of handgun injuries exceeded the incidence rate for lung cancer; the incidence rate of firearm injuries among African-Americans approached their incidence rate for all cancers; and 45 percent of nonfatal firearm assaults were perpetrated by a person or persons the victim knew (Lee, Waxweiler, Dobbins, & Paschetag, 1991).

- Estimates concerning the prevalence of spouse abuse suggest that approximately 12 percent to 20 percent of adult women in the United States have been physically abused at least once by a male intimate (Strauss, Gelles, & Steinmetz, 1980).

- In 1986 alone, according to the annual 50-state survey of the National Committee for Prevention of Child Abuse, an estimated 1.6 million reports of child abuse and neglect were filed, which represented a 6 percent increase over the number of reports in 1985 (US-DHHS, 1988).

NATIONAL RESEARCH COUNCIL'S REVIEW OF VIOLENCE

In the late 1980s, the National Academy of Science convened several select, multidisciplinary panels to summarize our knowledge regarding violence and to present recommendations for research and action. This effort resulted in a series of publications including *Understanding and Preventing Violence* (National Research Council, 1993), *Losing Generations* (National Research Council, 1993), and *Understanding Child Abuse and Neglect* (National Research Council, 1993). And, the CDC published the position papers from the Third National Injury Control Conference (USDHHS/PHS/CDC, 1993), and Prevention of Youth Violence (USDHHS/PHS/CDC, 1993).

Understanding and Preventing Violence includes a model which is useful in thinking about violence research, risk factors, and prevention. The model jointly considers units of analysis and temporal sequence of predisposing, situational, and activating factors. This is useful in characterizing the complex web of risk factors associated with violent events. In both public health and criminal justice data, the determination of who is the victim and who is the perpetrator occurs after the violent event and is often determined by factors such as age, race, and sex. The available data on violence strongly suggest that public policy strategies aimed at preventing and controlling violence must recognize and account for diverse factors including factors affecting young males, particularly young males from indigent backgrounds and minority groups. However, these data are *extremely* limited and we have much to learn if we are going to reduce the toll of social violence. These available data do not include income or other socioeconomic factors nor combinations with characteristics such as who is drunk, who is better armed, who is a better shot, or who has been socialized in a manner which increases risk of victimization.

THEORETICAL FOUNDATIONS OF VICTIMIZATION

The National Research Council explored a variety of research studies regarding risk factors for violence, including those which pertain at the level of individual people. These include psychosocial as well as biologic models for analysis.

Psychosocial Perspectives

From a psychosocial viewpoint, aggressive childhood behaviors correlate with a higher potential for violent adult behavior. However, of the young children who exhibit aggressive behavior patterns, little data exist regarding why a few become violent adults while most do not. One of the determining factors may be socioeconomic status. Adult violent behavior is concentrated in low income neighborhoods.

Social learning theories suggest that aggressive and violent behaviors are learned responses to frustration, that these behaviors can be learned as a means for achieving goals, and that learning occurs through observing models of such behavior. Modeling of aggressive behavior may be observed by children through the mass media, in the family, among peers, or in their neighborhoods.

Biological Perspectives

Some studies have yielded evidence pointing to genetic influences on the development of antisocial personality disorder in adults, a diagnostic category which includes persistent assaultive behavior. However, the relationship has not been studied in U.S. samples and evidence of a genetic influence specific to violent behavior is mixed. Future research may find that genetic processes account for individual or family level deviations from overall patterns within societies.

Neurological processes refer to the complex electrical and chemical activities which occur in specific brain regions and underlie externally observable human behavior. Neurobiological research on violent behavior should be expanded and integrated with research on the macrosocial and psychosocial causes of violence. However, to date, no known neurobiological patterns are precise enough to be considered reliable markers for violent behavior.

Community Perspectives

The effects of social interaction are vital in understanding the origins of violent behavior. For example, socioeconomic status and ethnicity interact. At low socioeconomic levels, African-Americans are more likely to be homicide victims than whites. Research points to several structural factors which account for this variation in risk of victimization:

- Concentrations of poor families in geographic areas and greater income differences between poor and nonpoor (income inequality);
- Measures associated with differential social organization such as population turnover, community transition, family disruption, and housing/population density, all of which affect a community's capacity to supervise young males; and
- Markets and opportunities associated with violence, such as illegal markets in drugs and firearms.

Some individual level risk factors for violent behavior point to possible community level causes. Drug use, ineffective parenting, school failure, and a poor employment history are all likely to occur in communities in which illegal markets are more available than prenatal and pediatric care, good schools, and legitimate job opportunities. Communities that differ in occasions for learning violent behavior can be expected to exhibit different distributions of developmental sequences.

A critical need exists to understand the ways in which these risk factors interact. For example, there are poor communities with low levels of violence. Interactions between ethnicity and community characteristics are difficult to disentangle because poor minorities are much more likely than poor whites to be concentrated in communities with a large percentage of impoverished residents.

These indicators of community disorganization appear to mirror the breakdown of social capital, including the ability to transmit positive values to younger generations. This breakdown manifests itself in such intangibles as parents' inability to distinguish neighborhood youth from outsiders, to join with other parents in solving common problems, to participate in friendship networks, and to monitor neighborhood common areas. Working single parents have less time for such activities, and continuous family turnover in large multidwelling housing complexes makes it difficult to maintain these activities. Many neighborhood elders who once took responsibility for local youth have emigrated from inner city communities, and the status of those who remain is diminished by the rise of successful entrepreneurs in illegal markets.

The economic, organizational, and social niches in which poor people live are disadvantaged in ways that defy easy measurement. For example, many poor neighborhoods and people are isolated from legitimate economic opportunities and from personal contacts with those who control resources in the larger society. Structural economic transformations over the last decade have reduced employment opportunities for low-income urban minorities, and increased the number of such families living below the poverty line. Economically stable and secure families have moved away from poor inner city neighborhoods, contributing to the decline of institutions of socialization and informal control.

To make progress in the understanding, prevention, and control of violent behavior, the panel recommended a balanced program of initiatives with both short- and long-term benefits in carefully evaluated prevention and research programs.

Recommendations for Prevention

Promising interventions need to occur not only with individuals and families, but with community-based programs and multidisciplinary interventions such as the following:

- Community health nursing or similar home visitor programs to prevent child abuse and reduce the intergenerational nature of family abuse,
- Comprehensive neighborhood and community programs characterized by "one-stop shopping" for services,
- Measures to ensure safe schools and safe havens in public housing projects,
- Measures designed to reduce access to guns,
- Measures designed to increase individual, neighborhood, and community empowerment,
- A consumer orientation by helping professionals, and
- Evaluation research focusing on program outcomes.

Recommendations for Research

The National Research Council's analysis also included recommendations for further research. The panel specifically recommended that sustained problem-solving initiatives be undertaken in six areas for which systematic intervention design, evaluation, and replication could contribute to the understanding and control of violence. In addition to further research, I noted three specific areas of particular interest to nursing:

1. Intervening in the biological and psychosocial development of individuals' potential for violent behavior with special attention to preventing brain damage associated with low birth weight;
2. Modifying places, routine activities, and situations that promote violence, including schools; and
3. Implementing a comprehensive initiative to reduce partner violence.

In 1993, I was invited to a conference sponsored by the National Academy of Science, CDC, and the Kennedy School of Government at Harvard to review the major conclusions in the recently published monographs and to discuss implementation of the recommendations. Multidisciplinary teams representing researchers in several fields, mayors of urban cities and police chiefs were presented with a case study and asked to make recommendations for immediate, short- and long-range responses to the problem of violence in urban communities (National Research Council, 1994). I was struck by how easily we, the work groups, responded to crisis intervention and how difficult it was to develop strategies which have potential for prevention, especially long-range prevention. When the small work group presentations were made at the end of the conference, I observed several themes.

First, the social construction of violence which has occurred cannot be resolved by individuals and families alone; it is necessary to also address the consequences associated with the public policies of a generation ago which have had the result of placing high-risk people and families in high-risk environments while also fragmenting social services. We need to confront our racism, classism, and elitism.

In this country, we describe events according to characteristics we can easily count. But who defines these characteristics and who defines the problems? Whose worldview is represented in the definition? Who is at the table when the problem if framed? It is striking to me that we spend much more time defining and redefining the description of the problem and much less time securing new data which has potential to explain why the problem exists. If we understood more about why the problem exists, we might come closer to defining the problems multidimensionally. Violence needs to be defined within the context of community. We need to deconstruct this issue rather than aggregating it based on race, class, and sex. We need to look at the institutional and systemic barriers that contribute to these stereotypes and the problems that come with them—unemployment, lack of meaningful work, educational discrimination, the distribution of tangible resources, and power.

Armed with new data that is based on the experiences and views of those at the table (I refer to those who experience the problem and who should be at the table) we might do something. So far, we have done little beyond counting the recounts and wondering why, despite our increasing capacity to partition the variance and covariance, we demonstrate our racism and classism when we imagine violence to be a social rather than a nursing problem. We should think about the context of violence—its market context, its community context as well as its individual context. Violence should be a major focus in nursing's agenda and in our efforts in healthcare reform.

So, what does this mean for us; what does this mean for nursing? Nursing is about healing—healing ourselves and healing our communities. Healing implies a process that leads to structural integrity (Figure 47.1). There are many possibilities ranging from improving our willingness to identify victims of violence in our emergency rooms to supporting development of the capacity of our local health departments to provide home-based nursing care to mothers and babies, to evaluate impacts of comprehensive programs in which nurses participate in terms of outcomes for people, families, and neighborhoods. The concept of healing should be expanded and applied to the study of violence. This would require that nurses develop and promote an ethic of health that emphasizes prevention of violence rather than its medicalization as currently expressed in our toll in mopping up our nation's emergency rooms.

RECOMMENDATIONS FOR THE NURSING PROFESSION'S CONSIDERATION

While we await research results and evaluations of community programs and randomized intervention trials, we can begin to interrupt this multicausal mechanism now. Specific recommendations that nursing might consider include the following:

- Support measures such as the Brady bill to restrict access to firearms.
- Improve our proactive political capacity in order to promote policies consistent with individual beliefs as well as with professional nursing's organizational policies.
- Utilize our capacity to conduct qualitative research because much remains unknown about the contributors to violent behavior.
- Improve our knowledge about the quantitative effects of racism, based on new variables and concepts.
- Implement methodologically sound interventions such as visiting nurse programs initiated prenatally to improve pregnancy outcomes, programs designed to detect and treat child abuse/neglect, and other programs emphasizing prevention of violence.
- Increase our linkages with the various communities engaged in interdisciplinary research on violence.
- Support multicultural qualitative research with those affected by violence so that we better understand what we ought to be quantifying. Research that deals with contextual relationships may give more explanatory power to our quantitative outcomes.

Unless we make a commitment to participate in solving these problems, we will continue to demonstrate a paradox in which we are simultaneously victims and perpetrators, individually and collectively.

CONCLUSION

While we ponder this issue today, 32,000 people in the United States will experience criminal victimization and 210 people will die due to discharge of firearms. Nationally, in 1990, we spent about $20 million on violence research. Is it any wonder that we do not have a "magic bullet" or antibiotic available to give our "target" population? Rather, I hope we choose to be pro-biotic.

REFERENCES

Alcohol, Drug Abuse, and Mental Health Administration (1989). *Report of the Secretary's Task Force on Youth Suicide, Vol. 1: Overview and Recommendations.* DHHS Pub. No. (ADM) 89-1621. Washington DC: U.S. Government Printing Office.

CDC (1990). Weapon-carrying among high school students—United States. *MMWR, 40,* 681–4.

CDC (1994). Deaths resulting from firearm—and motor-vehicle-related injuries—United States, 1968-1991. *MMWR, 43,* 37–42.

Chowder, K. (1992). How TB survived its own death to confront us again. *Smithsonian, 23,* 180–194.

Labonte, R. (1992). Heart health inequalities in Canada: Model, theory and planning. *Health Promotion International, 7,* 119–28.

Lee, R. K., & Sacks, J. J. (1990). Latchkey kids and guns in the home. *Journal of the American Medical Association, 264,* 2210.

Lee, R. K., Waxweiler, R. J., Dobbins, J. G., & Paschetag, T. (1991). Incidence rates of firearm injuries in Galveston, Texas, 1979–1981. *American Journal of Epidemiology, 134,* 511–21.

Massachusetts Department of Public Health (1990, Feb.). *Shattering the myths: Sexual assault in Massachusetts 1985-1987.* (Pub. No. 16, 367-62-1000-6-90-CR). Boston: Bureau of Community Health Services.

National Institutes of Justice (1993, Dec.). *Criminal victimization in the United States, 1991: National crime survey report.* Washington, DC: Bureau of Justice Statistics.

National Research Council (1993). *Understanding and preventing violence.* Washington, DC: National Academy Press.

National Research Council (1993). *Losing generations: Adolescents in high risk settings.* Washington, DC: National Academy Press.

National Research Council (1993). *Understanding child abuse and neglect.* Washington, DC: National Academy Press.

National Research Council (1994). *Violence in America: Mobilizing a response.* Washington, DC: National Academy Press.

Reiss, A. J., Jr., & Roth, J. A. (Eds.). (1993). *Understanding and preventing violence: Panel on the understanding and control of violent behavior.* Washington, DC: National Academy Press.

Strauss, M., Gelles, R., & Steinmetz, S. K. (1980). *Behind closed doors: A survey of family violence in America.* New York: Doubleday.

USDHHS (1988). *Study findings: Study of national incidence and prevalence of child abuse and neglect.* Report of contract 105-85-1072. Washington, DC: DHHS.

USDHHS/PHS/CDC (1993). *Position Papers from the Third National Injury Control Conference: Setting the National Agenda for Injury Control in the 1990s.* Atlanta: CDC.

USDHHS/PHS/CDC (1993). *Prevention of Youth Violence: A Framework for Community Action.* Atlanta: CDC.

U.S. National Center for Health Statistics (1993). *1991 United States detailed mortality data* (public use data tape).

Zane, D. F., Preece, M. J., Patterson, P. J., & Svenkerud, E. K. (1991). Firearm-related mortality in Texas (1985-1990). *Texas Medicine, 87,* 78-83.

CHAPTER 48

Healing: The Underground Experience

MARY V. FENTON, RN, DRPH

Nursing as a discipline is at a crossroads. We are facing the future and challenge of healthcare reform knowing that we will be asked to carry out many functions that ten to twenty years ago would never have been considered part of the scope of nursing practice. With changes in health profession regulation, the boundaries of our scope of practice are beginning to blur even more with that of other health professionals. Therefore, we are asking ourselves again, "What is unique or different about the practice of nursing?"

This discourse is not new. Professional nursing was first defined by Florence Nightingale's classic *Notes on Nursing* published in 1860 which is still in print today (Nightingale, 1860). It was an auspicious beginning that lasted through the early 1900s when the developing discipline of medicine laid claim to most of healthcare through the regulation process, forcing the nursing profession in the process to define a future scope of practice outside of medicine. This led to a search for a definition of nursing that was broad enough to encompass the scope of nursing practice but did not infringe on medicine's claim to healthcare. It was an almost impossible task that has led to endless discourse about defining health and defining nursing. In the last century, the question has been asked over and over in nursing schools and professional meetings. All nurses can recall discussions when someone said, "Define nursing for me." Older nurses are probably dying with this question on their lips: "What is nursing? If only I had figured out what exactly, nursing is!"

Nursing's knowledge base is beginning to be defined in a scientific manner, and we have produced researchers and scholars who are developing skills to answer this question. Nursing theories derived inductively have provided some guidance to struggling nursing scholars, but often the practicality of the theory and its application to nursing practice is not clear. Both students and faculty often find the utility of the concepts difficult to grasp and apply in practice. Consequently, there has been a move away from the use of nursing grand theories to guide curriculum and research, but the dilemma about the scope of nursing practice has remained. We already know our scope of practice, but it is not well documented nor always obvious to the public or to other professions and, in many cases, not even to practicing nurses.

OUT OF THE MAINSTREAM NURSING CARE

At the University of Texas Medical Branch (UTMB), I have watched faculty and other nurses provide care to friends, family, and colleagues that could be considered "out of the mainstream." It is not the care they necessarily espoused in class nor taught on the clinical units. It was often carried out at home and, if in the hospital or in a clinical setting, was still outside the traditional care system. Modern medicine was woven into the plan of care as necessary, including initial diagnosis, lab tests, treatments and use of medications, especially for pain control and relief of symptoms; it was, however, only a component of the care rather than the main focus. Nursing took over quietly, seemingly unseen or somehow overlooked by other involved healthcare professionals. The focus became one of guiding and assisting the person, the family, and friends to cope, adapt, accept, and come to terms with the illness, problems, and prognosis. Nurses have used all types of interventions including physical, psychological, social, spiritual, and cultural. Concurrently, they serve as patient and family advocates to force the healthcare system and other agencies to respond. Alternative and complementary therapies are also utilized as adjuncts to care when indicated and especially when nothing else is available. It has become apparent to me that the focus of this behind-the-scenes process was healing at the physiological, psychological, social, spiritual, and cultural levels.

UNDERGROUND NURSING

To describe these phenomena, I coined the term *underground nursing*. It was not the first time in my career that I had observed this process. In the 1980s, I carried out an ethnographic study of the expert practice of Clinical Nurse Specialists in a hospital setting that included both interviews and participant observations (Fenton, 1985). I discovered that much of the expert practice of Clinical Nurse Specialists was hidden from the general knowledge of the hospital bureaucracy and other care givers. The Clinical Nurse Specialists quietly went about getting patients' needs met through personal contacts throughout the system when the bureaucracy failed to respond to patients' and/or families' needs. Behind closed doors, and sometimes in full view, they used their listening, presencing, comforting, and touching skills in ways that were not always apparent to other professions.

Weaving Healing into Clinical Situations

In one episode, I observed a Clinical Nurse Specialist assist an older man through a radiation therapy treatment. She quietly assessed the knowledge level and fears of the man and his wife as they moved through the clinic procedures. No one else paid attention or was aware of what was occurring in the interaction in the busy clinic atmosphere as the assessment and intervention were expertly woven into the clinical routine. The Clinical Nurse Specialist discovered that neither the man nor his wife understood the prognosis and both were convinced he was dying, when in fact the prognosis was very good and he was responding well to treatment. When the man became nauseated at one point, I saw the Clinical Nurse Specialist quietly use therapeutic touch without any other technician or staff in the room even realizing what she was doing. The effect was dramatic relief without medication. I asked her afterwards how she decided when to try therapeutic touch and I have never forgotten her answer, "When I know nothing else will work." My last picture of this episode was as they left. The man's wife stopped and hugged the CNS with tears in her eyes. She was laughing and crying with relief about her husband's prognosis and for having experienced a truly healing encounter.

Learning to Heal and Live

Since that time I have continued to observe such encounters. I watched faculty members contribute to the care of a nurse colleague who had been diagnosed with untreatable cancer. She had been given six months to live with no real options for life. She went home from the hospital with no defined plan of care or follow-up, not even for pain control. I watched a frightened woman with the help of her colleagues take back control of her life and live over two years of productivity outside the hospital. I watched and was told how she learned to cope with her situation through prayer, meditation, imagery, therapeutic touch, and by learning to focus on her body's response to her fear and pain. In addition, arrangements were made to take her to another city to see a cancer pain specialist, so she had the benefit of expert pain relief. The result of this process was remarkable, as I would see her in the grocery store and realize that if I did not know the diagnosis, I would never have identified her as ill. Her eventual peaceful death at home was a tribute to all the nurses who cared for her during this time.

Behind-the-Scenes Plan of Care for Healing

In another example, the son of a colleague was injured in an accident in which the immediate prognosis was potentially very serious. Immediately, faculty and other nurses not directly involved in caring for her son organized a plan for support of the family. As problems were revealed, they were analyzed and solved. Again, the plan of care was developed out of the mainstream of the hospital care and integrated when necessary. The most striking example was the suggestion that a local Reiki healer be asked to treat the son. The results were very positive; the healer taught the parents to continue the treatments, and the physician wrote on the chart "massage three times a day," to make it "legal." In these and other cases, the faculty and nurses literally mobilized a plan of care outside the medical or nursing plan even if the person was in the hospital. Certain aspects were shared with other involved health professionals but only if necessary, and only if they seemed to be open to it. Those nurse administrators who were part of these "underground" plans constantly monitored what was happening and were often instrumental in making sure that certain select physicians and nursing staff were involved in the case. Otherwise, the plan was carried out almost behind the scenes.

Testing Alternative Healing Therapies

Most nurses can probably relay similar stories concerning the care of their family members and friends where they greatly influenced the outcome without officially being a caregiver assigned to the case. I once unofficially specialed my mother following complicated surgery for a suspected abdominal tumor that turned out to be a ruptured spleen and an abscess that involved an incidental cholecystectomy. My agreement with the nurses on the floor was that I would focus on my mother's comfort but would monitor her vital signs, IVs, drains, catheter, and need for medication and would notify them of any problems. They, in turn, would check on us periodically. This arrangement worked very well as I was able to control all the timing of her care. She was able to continue sleeping when she was asleep, and got immediate attention when she became restless.

This was in the 1970s and I was in the process of learning about the use of alternative healing therapies, so I decided to try my new skills out on my mother. Since the nature of her surgery limited my access to her, I concentrated the use of massage, reflexology, and accupressure on her feet, hands, head, neck, and shoulders. I also used therapeutic touch on these areas as well as other areas of her body and constantly gave her feedback as to how she was doing. Her progress was so remarkable that when her surgeon came in that afternoon to examine her and look at her chart, he turned to me and asked, "What are you doing? She is progressing too fast." At that time, I was not confident enough in what I was learning to tell him. However, in retrospect, I should have as he was truly open to the sharing of information. He had a standing order on all his patients that the patient and family could have access to the medical chart any time they wanted to look at it.

My mother went home two days early with no complications or setbacks. Perhaps most remarkable was that she required very little pain medication. Her vital signs never fluctuated. She did not have an elevated temperature even through she had had an abscess and a fever before the surgery. Her pulse rate was slow and regular, and her blood pressure remained at her normal value throughout her recovery. I later asked her what she remembered about what I did. She said she did not really remember all the things I did except that she knew I was there. What she did remember was that she would have reocurring thoughts of panic and every time that would happen, whatever I said or did enabled her to calm herself. I am including this story in this chapter in hopes that other nurses who have had similar experiences that they were not comfortable sharing because they seemed out of the mainstream will begin to acknowledge that these experiences reflect the level of nursing care that we should be and are capable of providing.

WHY HEALING IS UNDERGROUND

The term "underground" implies that it goes against the status quo of the current authorities. It implies that if those in charge knew about it they would at one extreme end the practice and punish the practitioners or, to a lesser extreme, be very nervous and wary and attempt to undermine or discredit the practice. These are normal responses to threats or changes in the status quo. I believe nurses have been so socialized to follow the rules that they fear the consequences of having those in authority such as nursing administrators, hospital administrators, and medical staff know how adept and powerful they have become in providing healing therapies. By hiding these practices, nurses are able to practice a much broader and higher level of practice without fear of consequences—only the patients, their families, and trusted colleagues know about it.

The downside to hiding these practices is that the majority of patients do not have access to this level of care. Although based on empirical evidence and reviews of many nurse-patient interaction studies, it appears that patients given this level of care may have fewer complications and heal faster. However, these practices are not acknowledged or deemed relevant when costs of care are examined. Therefore, many of the nursing practices that we deem to be most essential to promote healing are not named, described, studied, documented, acknowledged, or owned. They are kept "underground."

We are not always teaching students to provide the type of care that faculty and other nurses I have described prefer to give to their own family, friends, and colleagues. We are not studying the impact and outcomes of such care and integrating the results into our educational programs and serving as role models for students. Healing describes what nursing accomplishes at the highest level of practice. Healing is often a missing link in our education of nurses at both the generic and advanced level. It is a major component of the expert case manager, advocate, and comforter role and all advanced practice roles. We keep creating new roles trying to make things better, but if we move to the concept of healing as a central component of the nursing role, all of those roles become clearer and legitimate.

It has become clear to many of the UTMB nursing faculty that the development of a conceptual model of healing as a nursing construct is essential to the scope of practice of nursing. The response to this concept by faculty has been phenomenal. It has given direction to teaching, to scholarship, to research, and to practice. It appears to literally free up known nursing knowledge to be utilized in more practical and logical ways and is broad enough to provide direction to most research carried out by nurses today, including physiological, psychological, social, and spiritual healing. It is easily applied to individuals, families, groups, and whole communities. Once adopted, it gives nurses a reason for seeking to turn the healthcare bureaucracy into a healing environment. For example, if the concept of healing is adopted, it demands that the fears, concerns, and wishes of patients and families must be considered priorities. It places the healthcare provider in a more comfortable role as all practices and policies of institutions and providers can be measured against the criterion of healing. If an action or policy does not promote healing in the broadest sense, it can be considered inappropriate. It is time that the healing provided by "underground nursing" becomes the standard of professional nursing care and part of the mainstream of healthcare.

REFERENCES

Fenton, M. (1985). Identifying competencies of clinical nurse specialists. *Journal of Nursing Administration, 15*, 31-37.

Nightingale, F. (1860). *Notes on nursing: What it is, and what it is not.* London: Harrison.

Afterword: Beginning a Dialog on Healing

PHYLLIS BECK KRITEK, RN, PHD, FAAN

When the project that became this book was initiated, it was my hope that some members of the UTMB faculty would decide to share some of the wisdom, knowledge, skills, attitudes, abilities, competencies, and scholarship that had characterized our collective journey toward a commitment to healing as a central construct in our school's mission and work. That hope was met and exceeded. The rich array of perspectives and insights afforded in this book are valuable precisely because of their diversity and multiplicity. As such, we have prepared not a seamless garment, the illusional image of many who seek truth, but instead a patchwork quilt of images, ideas, ideals, and destinies.

You may find you do not agree with everything in this book. I know I don't. Agreement is not the goal. Rather, to begin to explore the concept of healing from a myriad of perspectives, to begin to tease apart its complexity and its promise, to see what new paths it reveals and what new problems it presents. Certainly the richness and robustness of healing as a central idea becomes apparent. And in the very diversity and differences lurks the opportunity. It is our hope, collectively, that the many perspectives in this book will serve to stimulate you, the reader, to your own clarity of thinking about your views about healing and healing processes in nursing practice. It is our hope that this book will start a more deliberate, focused, open and articulate dialog about healing, and encourage all nurses to make this central construct a guide for discovery and quality patient care.

We conclude with an invitation to that dialog. What are your views on healing? How does it shape your teaching or practice or scholarship? Is it within the scope of your practice, and if not, why not? If we are not committed to healing, can we then practice nursing? These are important questions for every nurse. It is our hope that this book heightens the consciousness and the urgency that surrounds the questions.

In order to honestly ask and answer these questions for oneself requires that we take leave of what was and move toward what can be. This is difficult for all of us at some point. We are ultimately change aversive humans. We cling to our past patterns even when we know that they are dysfunctional or inadequate. As the rate of change continues to escalate, our facility in moving beyond the past and into the future is sorely tested. Skillful evolution becomes a priority. To conclude this book, we have one last contribution, a parable about healing from loss and change. It emerges from an alternative therapy, appropriately, and points to the path we can elect as we take leave of a past that no longer is and move into a future that we might choose to create, one committed to the promotion of healing.

Dream as Healing Parable

PHYLLIS BECK KRITEK, RN, PHD, FAAN

PHYLLIS WATERS, RN, MS

"Look to love and you may dream,
and if it should leave then give it wings."

Enya, "Hope Has a Place": The Memory of Trees Album

I sighted the woman at the bottom of the path, shortly after I had gone over the gentle rise. It was a sunny clear day, but on seeing her, the day seemed to turn cloudy and cool. I stopped to study her. People born in mountain country always called the plains flatland. Accustomed to extremes in terrain, they miss these gentle rolls and valleys, and the opportunity to be startled coming over a slight hill.

She was of indeterminate age, her head bowed and her hair, long and dark, covered her entire face. She walked slowly, a yoke resting heavy on the back of her neck and on her shoulders. The yoke was a wooden pole about five feet long, I estimated, about the thickness of my forearm, dark and smooth. On each end of the pole hung a large bucket of the same wood. Judging by her struggle to carry the yoke, I sensed that the buckets were very heavy, full of something I could neither see nor imagine. She wore a simple, loosely fitting cream gown. She seemed to fit no time or space I knew, yet I was drawn to her instinctively. I knew she was there for me.

A voice asked "Why do you continue to carry these burdens?" She did not look up but she responded, quietly, resigned, "I am weary, unable to go on, but I do not believe that I can put these burdens down." The voice

---

The authors have for several years shared a process of energy work focused on healing, incorporating dimensions of Reiki, Therapeutic Touch, and Acupressure. In this work, they have found that they share awarenesses experienced as dreamwork. Phyllis Waters tends to experience these as images; Phyllis Beck Kritek tends to experience these as words and ideas. Combined, they generate parables such as this.

then gently shifted to advisor. "Turn them to doves and set them free." I was incredulous. "How can she do that?" I asked sullenly. I understood the burdens, and reacted to this simplistic advice.

Quietly, she shifted the pole so it rested on her right shoulder, then reached out to the bucket before her. She took it in her large hands and began to knead and shape it, as if it were clay. She worked silently, slowly turning the bucket into a malleable mass that faded gradually to white. She began to shape a dove from the mass, carefully and reflectively. When she had completed this, she placed the dove she had shaped on her right shoulder. It perched there briefly, still and stoney. Then abruptly it was full of life, and flew away.

She seemed to move in slow motion. She turned the pole so it rested on her left shoulder, and once more took the bucket on this end of the pole and began shaping it. Completing the second dove, she placed it on her left shoulder. It too sat in stoney silence, then abruptly found life and flight. She stood silently with the pole, then layed it down on the edge of the path. the voice returned. "If these burdens are yours to carry, they will return to you. If not, you have set them free."

A year later, I met her again, this time in a shallow gully cut through a small patch of forest. Once more it was a sunny clear day, and bands of sunlight filtered down through the trees creating a warm glow around us. This time it was I who had the burdens, carried on my back in a wicker backpack of sorts. She approached me, concerned and attentive. "Why do you continue to carry these burdens?" she asked. "It is behind you." Her concern heightened my sense of soft frustration.

"These are people I love; I couldn't just leave them behind." She nodded quietly, and I realized that she understood what I had said and meant. I sensed her compassion for me, her awareness that while the burden was troublesome, I also wished to keep faith with these loves. She stepped forward, stood beside me and gently removed the strap from my left shoulder, then from my right, and took the bundle on my back and solemnly handed it to me. I took it in my arms like an infant, and held it gently close to myself. She began to slowly walk out of the gully, up the hill. She did not speak.

I did not know where we were going, but I knew I was to follow her, carrying my bundle in my arms. I watched her feet as she moved forward stepping as she had stepped. We are moving to higher ground, I thought to myself. We walked slowly and deliberately for some time on an upward incline until she stopped walking. I looked up and saw about 20 feet away from me a funeral bier like those I had seen constructed by tribes in early

America, a platform of tree branches among the living trees on the uppermost ridge of this small valley. She stopped by the platform, turned to me as she pointed to the funeral bier.

"You can lay them down here and you can still honor them." she stated quietly.

The Last Word

"Sisters Are Doin' It For Themselves . . ."

Annie Lennox and Dave Stewart
Eurythmics

Index